Reproductive Surgery

Reproductive Surgery

The Society of Reproductive Surgeons' Manual

Edited by

Jeffrey M. Goldberg
Cleveland Clinic, Cleveland, OH

Ceana H. Nezhat
Nezhat Medical Center, Atlanta, GA

Jay I. Sandlow
Medical College of Wisconsin, Milwaukee, WI

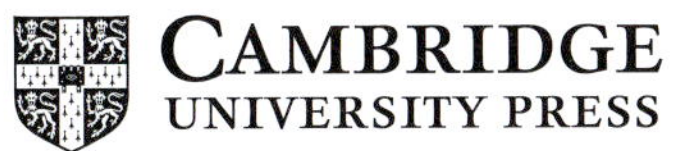

CAMBRIDGE
UNIVERSITY PRESS

CAMBRIDGE
UNIVERSITY PRESS

University Printing House, Cambridge CB2 8BS, United Kingdom

One Liberty Plaza, 20th Floor, New York, NY 10006, USA

477 Williamstown Road, Port Melbourne, VIC 3207, Australia

314–321, 3rd Floor, Plot 3, Splendor Forum, Jasola District Centre, New Delhi – 110025, India

79 Anson Road, #06-04/06, Singapore 079906

Cambridge University Press is part of the University of Cambridge.

It furthers the University's mission by disseminating knowledge in the pursuit of
education, learning, and research at the highest international levels of excellence.

www.cambridge.org
Information on this title: www.cambridge.org/9781107193963
DOI: 10.1017/9781108150064

First published 2018

Printed and bound in Great Britain by Clays Ltd, Elcograf S.p.A.

A catalogue record for this publication is available from the British Library.

Library of Congress Cataloging-in-Publication Data
Names: Goldberg, Jeffrey M., editor. | Nezhat, Ceana, editor. | Sandlow, Jay I., editor.
Title: Reproductive surgery : the Society of Reproductive Surgeons' manual /
edited by Jeffrey Goldberg, Ceana Nezhat, Jay Sandlow.
Other titles: Reproductive surgery (Goldberg)
Description: Cambridge, United Kingdom; New York, NY: Cambridge University Press, 2018. |
Includes bibliographical references and index.
Identifiers: LCCN 2018031527 | ISBN 9781107193963 (hardback)
Subjects: | MESH: Urogenital Surgical Procedures | Reproductive Techniques | Genital Diseases,
Female – surgery | Genital Diseases, Male – surgery | Endoscopy.| Practice Guideline
Classification: LCC RD571 | NLM WJ 168 | DDC 617.4/6–dc23
LC record available at https://lccn.loc.gov/2018031527

ISBN 978-1-107-19396-3 Hardback

....

Contents

Videos

The video content listed below can be accessed directly from the Society of Reproductive Surgeons at www.reprodsurgery.org. Please refer to corresponding chapters for discussion of the video content.

Contributors

Sara Arian MD
Department of Obstetrics and Gynecology
Cleveland Clinic
Cleveland, OH

Phil V. Bach MD
Department of Urology
Weill Cornell Medicine
New York, NY

Bala Bhagavath MD
Division of Reproductive Endocrinology and Infertility
University of Rochester Medical Center
Rochester, NY

Peter T. K. Chan MD, CM, MSc, FRCS(C), FACS
Director of Male Reproductive Medicine
Department of Urology
McGill University Health Center
and
Professor
Department of Surgery
McGill University
Montreal, Quebec, Canada

Kathryn D. Coyne MS
Department of Obstetrics and Gynecology
Boonshoft School of Medicine
Wright State University
Dayton, OH

Christopher M. Deibert MD, MPH
Assistant Professor
Division of Urologic Surgery
Department of Surgery
University of Nebraska Medical Center
Omaha, NE

Tommaso Falcone MD
Department of Obstetrics and Gynecology
Cleveland Clinic
Cleveland, OH

Rebecca Flyckt MD
Department of Obstetrics and Gynecology
Cleveland Clinic
Cleveland, OH

Antonio R. Gargiulo MD
Assistant Professor
Harvard Medical School
Boston, MA

Julian A. Gingold MD, PhD
Department of Gynecology and Obstetrics
Cleveland Clinic
Cleveland, OH

Jeffrey M. Goldberg MD
Professor and Head of Reproductive Endocrinology
and Infertility
Department of Gynecology and Obstetrics
Cleveland Clinic
Cleveland, OH

Linnea R. Goodman MD
Department of Gynecology and Obstetrics
Cleveland Clinic
Cleveland, OH

Daniel Greene MD
Resident Physician
Glickman Urologic and Kidney Institute
Cleveland, OH

Brooke A. Harnisch MD
Assistant Professor
Department of Urology
University of Connecticut
Farmington, CT

Keith B. Isaacson MD
Newton Wellesley Hospital
Harvard Medical School
Boston, MA

Nisha A. Lakhi MD, FACOG
Assistant Professor Department of Obstetrics and Gynecology
New York Medical College
Valhalla, New York
and
Director of Research
Co-Director of Minimally Invasive Surgery
Richmond University Medical Center
Staten Island, New York

Vadim V. Morozov, MD, FACOG FACS
Minimally Invasive Gynecology
MedStar Washington Hospital Center
Washington, DC

Ceana H. Nezhat MD, FACS, FACOG
President, Society of Reproductive Surgeons
Fellowship Director
Nezhat Medical Center
and
Medical Director of Training and Education
Northside Hospital
and
Adjunct Professor of Gynecology
and Obstetrics
Emory University
Atlanta, GA

Nigel Pereira MD
Center for Reproductive Medicine
Weill Cornell Medical Center
New York, NY

John C. Petrozza MD
Massachusetts General Hospital
Boston, MA

Samantha M. Pfeifer MD
Associate Professor Clinical Obstetrics and Gynecology
Associate Professor Clinical Reproductive Medicine
The Ronald O. Perelman and Claudia Cohen Center for Reproductive Medicine
Weill Cornell Medical Center
New York, NY

Katherine Rotker MD
Division of Urology
Brown University
Providence, RI

Edmund Sabanegh, Jr. MD
Department Chair of Urology
Glickman Urologic and Kidney Institute
Cleveland, OH

Jay I. Sandlow MD
Professor and Vice Chair
Department of Urology
Medical College of Wisconsin
Milwaukee, WI

Christina Salazar MD
Newton Wellesley Hospital
Harvard Medical School
Boston, MA

Peter N. Schlegel MD
Department of Urology
Weill Cornell Medicine
New York, NY

Mark Sigman MD
Professor and Chairman
Division of Urology
Brown University
Providence, RI

Foreword

It's about time. In the age of artificial reproductive technology (ART) when all attention is assisted on the latest advances in in vitro fertilization (IVF), leaders of the Society of Reproductive Surgeons present us here with a definitive manual for surgeons operating on females and males with the hopes of preserving or enhancing their reproductive capacity. You will find everything you need to know when contemplating your next case. From simple hysteroscopy, caring for or preventing adhesions, various approaches to myomectomy, ovarian surgery for routine cystectomy, and routine tubal anastomosis to the more difficult müllerian anomaly surgery, endometriosis cases, and female fertility preservation surgery – it is all here. For the male, you will find a complete coverage of the contemporary surgical challenges also provided by the experts: from vasectomy reversal and varicocele repair to surgical sperm retrieval methods, management of ejaculatory duct obstruction, and other scrotal surgeries.

The SRS Manual is filled with the best photos and figures collected over time by the experts that will allow the reader to easily understand the surgical techniques used. The minimally invasive approach to topics is highlighted here and, when necessary, the authors turn to laparotomy. In short, this manual will be an excellent resource for novices and experts providing reproductive care globally.

Drs. Goldberg, Nezhat, and Sandlow are to be congratulated on assembling this treatise that covers contemporary reproductive surgery. Once again, the Society of Reproductive Surgeons has stepped forward with a very timely initiative that has filled a much-needed gap.

Richard H. Reindollar, MD
CEO, ASRM

Preface

The Society of Reproductive Surgeons (SRS) is one of the few societies in the world dedicated solely to female and male reproductive surgery. It is therefore fitting that SRS write the comprehensive manual for modern surgical procedures for treating female and male infertility. All contributing authors are SRS members and are highly recognized authorities in their respective areas of expertise. It is our intention that this book illustrates the benefits of reproductive surgery, as well as how to perform these procedures using the latest advances, so practitioners can offer their patients all of the current treatment options in this competitive field.

Historically, reproductive endocrinology and infertility specialists (REIs) were the pioneers and early adopters of minimally invasive gynecologic surgery. Over the last three decades, the focus of reproductive health has shifted away from reproductive surgery in favor of in vitro fertilization (IVF). Currently, most REI fellowship programs are not preparing their trainees to perform reproductive surgery. Strong evidence-based studies have shown that in many cases, surgery is the more cost-effective choice for achieving a pregnancy and should be the primary treatment option. Many patients also prefer surgical correction as it is more "natural" than IVF. Reproductive surgeons abide by conservative microsurgical principles and possess a tactical eye for preventing postoperative adhesions aimed at both fertility enhancement and preservation. Reproductive surgery should be viewed as complementary to IVF, as operative management of pelvic pathology may enhance IVF success rates in select cases. The ability to perform reproductive surgery makes REI physicians more "complete" as they can offer patients all available modalities.

This text is aimed at reproductive medicine specialists (both for male and female infertility) as well as general gynecologists and urologists in practice or in training. The procedures are described in a logical step-wise sequence and supplemented with intraoperative color photos and videos. The implementation and teaching of these procedures will assure that current and future infertility patients will continue to derive the benefit of having access to the full array of treatment options. We trust that our readers will find this to be a useful, well-rounded, and educative resource.

Hysteroscopy: Office and Operative – Myomectomy, Polypectomy, and Adhesiolysis

Christina Salazar and Keith B. Isaacson

1.1 Introduction

Hysteroscopy has become a mainstay within a gynecologic surgeon's practice for endoscopic examination of the uterine cavity due to the benefits of its relatively low-risk methods and accurate diagnostic capabilities. The hysteroscopic approach provides excellent visualization and is minimally invasive in that no incisions are required for therapeutic procedures. New tools are constantly being developed for the office as well as for the operating room, broadening the options available to address a wide variety of intrauterine pathologies.

1.2 Hysteroscopes

The first hysteroscopes that were developed in the late nineteenth century were rigid-rod lens systems. This is still the most commonly used design, but flexible fiber-optic hysteroscopes and digital hysteroscopes are currently available. The flexible hysteroscopes are 3.2–3.5 mm in diameter with a tip that deflects over a range from 90° to 120°, and have the advantage of not requiring preliminary dilation of the cervix or use of anesthesia. They are most commonly used for office hysteroscopy. The disadvantage is that because they are single-channel scopes with 1 mm working channels having a noncontinuous flow, they can only be used for diagnostic purposes and they are more costly, less durable, and cannot be sterilized within an autoclave as is the standard for most rigid hysteroscopes. Digital hysteroscopes such as the Endosee© have recently become available for diagnostic use; they are cordless and utilize single-use cannulas.

Rigid hysteroscopes come with several options for viewing angles: 0°, 12°, 15°, 25°, or 30°. The 12° viewing angle is helpful for surgical procedures because it keeps the working instruments in the field of view at all times. On the other hand, the 30° viewing angle is advantageous because only small rotational movements are needed to visualize the entire cavity, thereby causing less discomfort to the patient. Typically, the single-flow sheath of the rigid hysteroscope has a 2.9 mm diameter and is used in combination with an outer sheath whose diameter ranges from 3.2 to 5.3 mm, creating a continuous flow system as well as permitting the passage of semi-rigid operating instruments such as scissors, graspers, or biopsy forceps. Small 5 French bipolar electrodes can be passed through the working channels of the continuous flow hysteroscopes and can be used for resection of small myomas, polyps, scar tissue, and septa.

For the purpose of definition, a resectoscope is a hysteroscope operating with radiofrequency or mechanical energy and ranging in diameter from 21 to 28 French. The working instruments employed with the resectoscope include loop electrodes, roller balls, and barrels as well as vaporizing electrodes. Resectoscopes may employ monopolar radiofrequency energy where the current flows from the active electrode (i.e., the loop) through the tissue via random diffusion to a remotely located large dispersive electrode. Electrodes in a ball or barrel have a larger surface area than cutting loops and serve well for tissue desiccation and are used to perform endometrial ablations. Monopolar electrodes necessitate the use of nonconductive fluid distention media such as glycine, sorbitol, or mannitol (see "Distending Media" section later in the chapter). Bipolar resectoscopes allow the current to arc only through the tissue, which comes into direct contact with the loop and its return electrode, and require a conductive electrolyte-containing distention medium to be used.

1.3 Morcellators

Hysteroscopic morcellators became available in the United States in 2005 as an option for mechanical resection of intracavitary lesions in which thermal energy is not utilized, and may be used with isotonic electrolyte-rich distention media such as normal saline. The reciprocating blades of the instrument cut while the suction element removes the tissue. Consequently, a morcellator cannot cauterize blood vessels. Due to their side-opening cutting design, the morcellators have limited utility in cases with myomas that have deep involvement into the myometrium. The clear advantage of morcellators is the ease in attaining visibility due to the continuous suction and collection of the resected tissue into a specimen bag [1]. Classic loop resectoscopic surgery can be challenging secondary to the aggregation of tissue chips, formation of gas bubbles, and blood clots obstructing visualization. The time involved in removing chips can be cumbersome when taking into account the multiple removals and reinsertions of the resectoscopic device into the cavity. When using a morcellating device, on the other hand, clearing the cavity can be achieved by activating the device and allowing the suction element to remove the visual field of the debris.

1.4 Distention Media

The options for distending medium include both fluid and gaseous media. Carbon dioxide (CO_2) is the only gaseous media used because it is highly soluble in blood, and currently is only an option for diagnostic procedures because the field of view is obscured when the gas encounters blood. CO_2 gas is readily soluble in the blood stream and can lead to serious risk of gas embolism, and if the volume of the gas embolism is large, it can result in catastrophic cardiovascular collapse and death.

Low-viscosity fluid is the distention media of choice for current hysteroscopic technologies. High-viscosity media such as Dextran-70 (Hyskon) has fallen out of favor secondary to the low maximum infusion volume of 300 mL, as higher volumes can be associated with adverse outcomes such as pulmonary edema and right-sided heart failure secondary to its impact on expanding the patient's plasma volume. Furthermore, there are concerns of anaphylaxis as well as strict regimens for cleaning instruments when used in high-viscosity fluids, which have further limited the practical use of this media.

The available low-viscosity media vary in electrolyte content as well as in osmolality. The common electrolyte-free media include 1.5% glycine, 5% mannitol, and 3% sorbitol. The electrolyte-free fluids have unique features that vary in their osmolality and have different pathways of metabolism with resultant breakdown by-products. Plasma absorption of electrolyte-free media can lead to hyponatremia and other electrolyte disturbances. The signs of their systemic absorption included nausea, vomiting, and cardiac arrhythmias as well as a range of neurological symptoms such as cerebral edema, seizures, tremors, and even coma or death. On the other hand, 5% mannitol is near isotonic to plasma. However, because it lacks electrolytes, excess absorption can still cause hyponatremia with all the risks noted earlier. As a general rule, the serum sodium will be reduced by 10 mEq/L for every 1 L of electrolyte-free media absorbed. Subsequently, the American Association of Gynecologic Laparoscopists (AAGL) guidelines recommend concluding the procedure that employs hypotonic solutions when the fluid deficit reaches 1,000 mL [2].

On the other hand, electrolyte-rich solutions such as normal saline are isotonic, and thus are safer when they are systemically absorbed as they do not cause an electrolyte imbalance or hyponatremia. AAGL guidelines for operative hysteroscopy using isotonic distention media such as normal saline recommend limiting the fluid deficit to 2,500 mL in order to restrict intravasation of significant volumes of fluid and thereby prevent the onset of dangerous sequelae associated with fluid overload such as right-sided heart failure, hypoxia, difficulty with ventilation, and pulmonary edema [2]. Electrolyte-rich fluids can be used with bipolar radiofrequency surgical instruments but are not an appropriate fluid of choice for monopolar radiofrequency surgical instruments due to the dispersion of current.

For patients with compromised cardiovascular systems or who are elderly, the AAGL recommendation is to limit the maximum fluid deficit to 750 mL, regardless of the composition of the distention medium.

1.5 Office Hysteroscopy

The most common use of diagnostic office hysteroscopy is to evaluate both pre- and postmenopausal patients who complain of abnormal uterine bleeding (AUB) for intracavitary pathology. Additionally, systematic evaluation of the uterine cavity can be helpful in diagnosing unsuspected abnormalities in infertility

patients [3,4]. The advantage for the physician is an expedited pathway to diagnosing and treating the etiology of the AUB and/or infertility via a safe procedure with few complications. For the patient, resumption of daily activities begins immediately and the risks of undergoing anesthesia are avoided.

Patients should be selected appropriately for office hysteroscopic procedures. Select those who are ASA Class I or II, whose procedures are not complicated, and can be completed successfully within a brief period of time. Avoid patients who have poor pain tolerance or unrealistic expectations of in-office procedures. Further considerations regarding cardiac and pulmonary medical history should be taken into account if moderate or deep sedation is involved.

1.5.1 Indications for Office Hysteroscopy

- Abnormal uterine bleeding (polypectomy, myomectomy)
- Infertility evaluation
- Intrauterine synechiae evaluation and treatment
- Retained products of conception evaluation and treatment
- Uterine malformation evaluation and treatment
- Retrieval of intrauterine device (IUD) or foreign bodies
- Evaluation of defects from hysterotomy at the time of cesarean section (isthmocele)
- Placement of permanent contraceptive implants

Scenarios of complications that can be encountered when performing office procedures include vasovagal reactions, local anesthetic toxicity, uterine perforation, hemorrhage, allergic reaction, and respiratory arrest secondary to excessive sedation.

Vaginoscopy is a technique employed in order to enter the vaginal, cervical, and uterine cavity without use of a speculum or a tenaculum. A common reason for failing to complete an office hysteroscopic procedure is pain. The stimulus of pain is generated from the cervix and the vagina often by use of the tenaculum, the speculum, as well as manipulation of the instrument within the endocervical canal. The pain sensation is conducted by autonomic fibers up to the S2 to S4 spinal ganglia via the pudendal and pelvic splanchnic nerves. Pain from intraperitoneal structures that occurs during the instillation of fluid into the uterine body is conducted by autonomic fibers via the hypogastric nerves to the T12 to L2 spinal ganglia. A 2010 meta-analysis of nine randomized controlled trials (RCTs) involving 1,296 patients compared the effectiveness and safety of different types of pharmacological interventions for pain relief and concluded that the use of local anesthesia during outpatient diagnostic hysteroscopy significantly reduces the mean pain score in comparison to placebo both during the procedure as well as 30 minutes after the procedure. On the other hand, no significant reduction of pain was found with the use of nonsteroidal anti-inflammatory drugs (NSAIDs) or opioids when compared to placebo at both those time points.

1.6 Choice of Analgesia

The choice of anesthesia is surgeon dependent. The options range from NSAIDs to combinations of intravenous (IV) or general anesthesia with or without adjunct administration of local anesthesia. Surgeons may choose to avoid a paracervical block secondary to the discomfort caused by performing the block itself, which is not insignificant. Moreover, potential complications from local anesthesia can occur when patients are given an overdose of the analgesia, have an allergic reaction, or when the analgesia is inadvertently injected intravascularly. Manifestations of systemic injection include dizziness, tremor, oral paresthesias, blurry vision, and seizure. More serious sequelae include bradycardia secondary to myocardial depression, as well as respiratory depression and apneic episodes. To reduce the risks associated with systemic injection, the addition of epinephrine (1:100,000) can be used to enhance local vasoconstriction and thereby minimize the absorption of the analgesic.

If vaginoscopy is not performed, a total infiltration of 20 mL of a local anesthetic (such as 1% lidocaine buffered with 2 mL sodium bicarbonate) can be used as a paracervical block. The block consists of the following technique: 2 mL injected superficially into the anterior lip of the cervix at the 12 o'clock position prior to placement of a tenaculum, and the remaining 18 mL injected at the 4 o'clock and 8 o'clock positions along the cervicovaginal junction (9 mL at each site). Maximum dosing should not exceed 4.5 mg/kg of 1% lidocaine without epinephrine, or 7 mg/kg of 1% lidocaine with epinephrine.

1.7 Cervical Ripening Agents

Cervical dilation is the first step at the commencement of an operative hysteroscopic procedure to gain access to the uterine cavity. Some surgeons may elect to pretreat with cervical ripening agents in an effort to gain easier passage through the endocervical canal. Nearly 50% of hysteroscopic complications are related to difficulty of entry into the cervix. Thus cervical ripening can reduce complications associated with difficult entry such as creation of a false passage, cervical lacerations, and uterine perforation.

A commonly used cervical ripening agent is synthetic E1 prostaglandin (PGE1) known as misoprostol. Its administration in 200–400 mcg tablets taken orally or vaginally 12–24 hours before surgery for cervical ripening is considered an off-label, investigational use in the United States despite the existence of high-quality evidence from RCTs that suggest it improves cervical dilation as well as decreases the risk of traumatic entry in premenopausal patients [5]. In postmenopausal women, there is evidence to suggest that pretreatment with 25 μg of vaginal estradiol for 2 weeks in combination with 400 μg of vaginal misoprostol 12 hours prior to the procedure can help facilitate cervical dilation in hysteroscopic procedures [6,7]. Side effects of misoprostol include fevers, chills, vomiting, diarrhea, vaginal bleeding, and uterine cramping. Other options include a natural prostaglandin E2 (PGE2) known as dinoprostone, or hygroscopic dilators that are placed within the endocervical canal. Hygroscopic dilators gradually dilate the endocervical canal radially via osmosis-induced expansion over a period of hours and may be a good option for women with contraindications to prostaglandin use; however, the

limited available evidence is mixed regarding the efficacy of this method [5]. Given that laminaria require time to hydrate and dilate, this method requires an office visit the day prior to surgery or at least 6 hours pre-operatively for intracervical placement.

Injection of a dilute solution of vasopressin (0.05–0.2 U/mL of normal saline) can also promote cervical dilation as well as improve hemostasis by inducing contraction of the myometrium, thereby decreasing the fluid absorption. Associated toxicity can include arrhythmias. This technique consists of a total of 8–10 mL of dilute vasopressin, with 4–5 mL injected intracervically at 3 o'clock and at 9 o'clock positions. See "Vasopressin Administration" section under Hysteroscopic Myomectomy for further details.

It is rarely necessary to soften the cervix for office hysteroscopy due to the narrow diameter of the hysteroscopic equipment. The surgeon must beware that oversoftening of the cervix will make it difficult to maintain uterine distention during the hysteroscopic procedure.

1.8 Hysteroscopic Lysis of Adhesions

Intrauterine adhesions, interchangeable with the term Asherman's syndrome, typically present secondary to trauma of the basalis layer of the endometrium. This most often occurs after a uterine curettage for management of postpartum hemorrhage or incomplete spontaneous abortion. However, they can also develop after common procedures such as hysteroscopic myomectomy. Granulation tissue forms secondary to the trauma and creates tissue bridges between the walls of the uterine cavity, resulting in occlusive adhesions.

1.8.1 Indications for Procedure

Patients may present with secondary amenorrhea and severe dysmenorrhea with hematometria if cervical adhesions are dense and cause menstrual outflow obstruction. Oligomenorrhea or diminished menstrual flow with irregular spotting is also a common presenting complaint. With adhesions of the cavity diminishing the viable endometrial surface, patients may also frequently present with infertility or recurrent miscarriages.

1.8.2 Diagnosis and Treatment Guidelines

Hysteroscopy is the gold standard for the diagnosis and treatment of adhesions as it is very effective in restoring normal menstruation and improving fertility and reproductive outcomes [8]. If hysteroscopy is not available for diagnosis, hysterosalpingography and hysterosonography are considered reasonable alternatives. There is no role for medical management alone or blind D&C for these patients.

It is important to obtain a transvaginal ultrasound in order to evaluate the endocervical canal and endometrial lining of the uterine cavity. If there is no lining visible, it is suggestive of obliteration of the cavity, and the surgeon should consider intraoperative transabdominal ultrasound guidance as this can be particularly useful to prevent inadvertent uterine perforation when attempting lysis of adhesions because there are no anatomic landmarks.

Box 1.1 ASRM Classification of Intrauterine Adhesions

Extent of cavity involved	<1/3	1/3 to 2/3	>2/3
	1	2	4
Type of adhesions	Filmy	Filmy and dense	Dense
	1	2	4
Menstrual pattern	Normal	Hypomenorrhea	Amenorrhea
	0	2	4
Stage I	(Mild)	1 to 4	
Stage II	(Moderate)	5 to 8	
Stage III	(Severe)	9 to 12	

There are a variety of classification systems proposed for intrauterine adhesions. A commonly used system in the United States is provided by the American Society for Reproductive Medicine (ASRM), which defines the severity of intrauterine adhesive disease based on the extent of cavity involvement (<1/3, 1/3 to 2/3, >2/3); the type of adhesion seen (filmy, filmy and dense, dense), as well as the menstrual pattern (normal, hypomenorrhea, amenorrhea). Points are assigned to each finding and the patient is staged from 1 to 3 corresponding to mild, moderate, or severe, based on the total score (Box 1.1) [9].

If the adhesions are minimal to moderate (occupying <2/3 of the cavity) and the patient does not have cervical stenosis, then office hysteroscopic adhesiolysis can be considered and this procedure offers the advantage of avoiding IV sedation for anesthesia.

1.8.3 Pain Management

In the outpatient setting, we do not routinely pre-medicate our patients with NSAIDs. However, patients can elect to take 600 mcg of ibuprofen before or after the procedure, however they prefer. We do not use local anesthetic blocks for this procedure as taking down scar tissue should not cause pain unless the adhesiolysis has extended into the wrong plane, such as into the myometrium. During outpatient office adhesiolysis, the patient's vocalization of discomfort can provide the surgeon with important clinical cues that otherwise are not available when the patient is under IV sedation.

1.8.4 Pre-Procedure Planning

Patients whose procedures you anticipate will take <15 minutes are candidates for outpatient adhesiolysis. For extensive adhesiolysis, we offer patients IV sedation under monitored anesthesia care in the operating room. We do not pre-treat our patients with prostaglandins, as the small 5 mm caliber rigid hysteroscope can be advanced into the uterus without the necessity of cervical dilation. No prophylactic antibiotics are indicated for this type of procedure. The optimum timing for hysteroscopic procedures is during the early proliferative stage (menstrual day 4–11), as this is when the endometrial lining is the thinnest.

1.8.5 Surgical Approach

Treatment consists of sharp hysteroscopic adhesiolysis using the 5 mm rigid hysteroscope with 12° viewing angle and blunt-tipped scissors, with the primary objective to restore the normal volume of the cavity as well as the communication between the cavity, cervical canal, and fallopian tubes. Blunt dissection can lyse filmy adhesions easily using only the tip of the hysteroscope or with blunt use of the scissors. Our practice avoids use of electrosurgical instruments for adhesiolysis as the approach itself further damages the endometrium and thereby predisposes the patient to recurrent adhesive disease. In addition, since the procedure has an inherently higher risk of perforation, using electrosurgery for the procedure has the potential to cause thermal injury to surrounding organs. The choice of distention medium for our practice is isotonic electrolyte-rich fluids such as normal saline.

1.8.6 Surgical Technique

See Video 1.1

1. Place patient in the dorsal lithotomy position.
2. Perform pelvic exam to determine the position and size of the uterus.
3. Sterile prep the patient.
4. Using the vaginoscopic technique, the hysteroscope is introduced into the vagina and distend the vaginal vault with normal saline. Slowly raise your hand to lower the tip of the scope into the posterior fornix, directly visualizing the upper third of the vagina as you pull back to locate and visualize the external os. Guide the scope into the endocervical canal and drop your hand toward the ground to keep the internal os centralized at the 12 o'clock position in order to avoid digging the scope into the posterior wall of the endocervical canal. Do not advance the scope with force if you are met with resistance as this can result in formation of a false passage. Successful entry into the cavity is achieved by placing one hand on the light cord and the other on the camera while rotating the entire scope back and forth between 4 o'clock and 8 o'clock positions and advancing gently along the axis of the cervical canal.
5. Once the uterine cavity is entered, obtain a panoramic view to assess the extent of adhesive disease and locate any lesions if present (Figure 1.1). Take a systematic

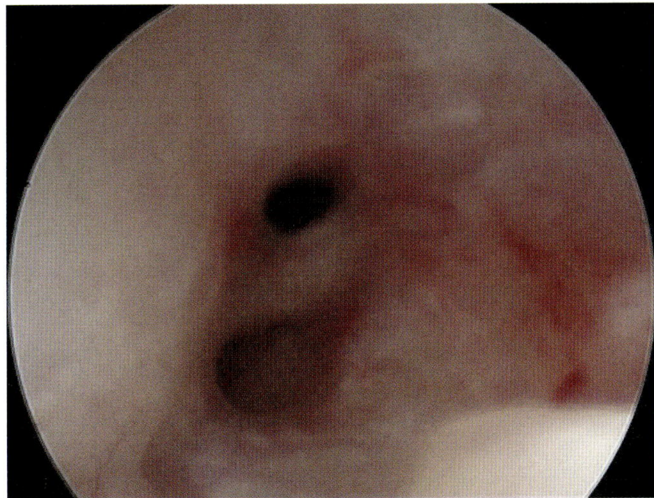

Figure 1.1 Hysteroscopic view of fundal adhesions.

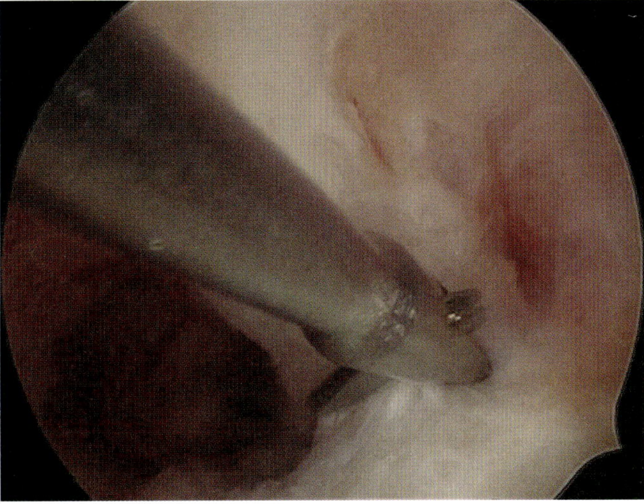

Figure 1.2 Lysis of intrauterine adhesions with scissors.

approach and note if either ostium is visible. Classify the severity of adhesive disease by the degree of uterine cavity involvement as described earlier. With more significant adhesive disease, anatomic landmarks are no longer recognizable and make spatial positioning difficult. In those cases, intraoperative transabdominal ultrasound guidance can be helpful.

6. Advance the blunt-tipped scissors, using both the sharp dissection to take down synechiae as well as blunt dissection by spreading the tips of the scissors (Figure 1.2). If you encounter bleeding, this is a cue that you are no longer dissecting scar tissue and have encountered the myometrium. Continue adhesiolysis until the normal cavity is restored (Figure 1.3). In cases with obliterated cornua, it may be difficult to visualize the tubal ostia after adhesiolysis secondary to the small size of the ostia.

7. While extracting the hysteroscope, evaluate the endocervical canal.

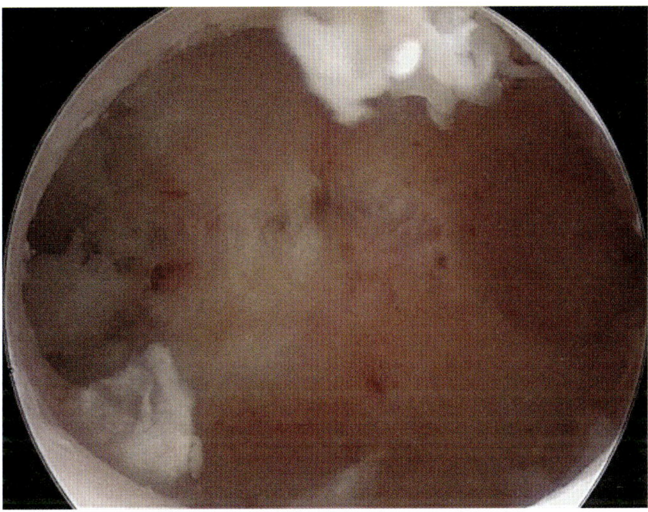

Figure 1.3 Restoration of the uterine cavity.

1.8.7 Postoperative Management

There is no consensus on postoperative management of patients with Asherman's syndrome. Estrogen supplementation is given postoperatively to stimulate endometrial growth; however, there is no standard dosing length or regimen [10]. Following the procedure, we recommend a 25-day course of 4 mg of oral estradiol (2 mg tablet by mouth twice daily) along with 5 days of medroxyprogesterone acetate (10 mg tablet by mouth once daily on days 21–25 of the cycle) for withdrawal. We perform a second-look office hysteroscopy within 2 weeks of the initial procedure in order to bluntly break the newly forming synechiae before they become dense [11]. The patients then return for another hysteroscopy 4 weeks later to assess the cavity, and additional sharp lysis of adhesions can be performed if needed.

Additional methods to reduce the recurrence of adhesions include intrauterine balloons or catheters and intrauterine devices. Options include insertion of a size 8 French pediatric Foley catheter with a 5 mL balloon placed into the uterine cavity for 3–10 days, or placement of a Malecot catheter for up to 10 days. Prophylactic antibiotics (Doxycycline 100 mg tablet by mouth twice daily × 10 days) should be considered when inserting a foreign body into the uterus. Insertion of an inert IUD for a period of several weeks is another option to keep the uterine walls apart following adhesiolysis. However, it should be noted that none of the above methods have been shown to be effective as the studies were few in number and underpowered [12,13].

1.8.8 Outcomes

Prognosis largely depends on the stage of adhesive disease. Recurrence rate of intrauterine adhesions can be as high as one in three women with minimal to moderate adhesions, whereas two in three women with severe adhesive disease may experience recurrence. Follow-up reassessment after two to three menstrual cycles is recommended if the patient has not achieved pregnancy or has not re-established a normal bleeding pattern.

1.9 Hysteroscopic Polypectomy

Endometrial polyps are exophytic overgrowths of hyperplastic endometrial glands and stroma that are soft in consistency and present in a multitude of shapes, sizes, and numbers. Increasing age, obesity, hypertension, and diabetes are all well-known risk factors for the development of endometrial polyps. Tamoxifen use is associated with malignant transformation as well as with large (>2 cm) and multiple polyps [14].

1.9.1 Indications for Procedure

Polyps represent one of the most common etiologies of abnormal uterine bleeding in both premenopausal and postmenopausal women, but it can also be asymptomatic. Focal malignancy can occur in 1–2% of the patients [15]. However, the vast majority of polyps are benign. Endometrial polyps are also thought to adversely impact fertility, as they are space-occupying lesions that could interfere with embryo implantation [16]. In patients with unexplained infertility, current evidence supports resection of endometrial polyps and has been shown to improve assisted reproduction conception rates [17]. The natural course of endometrial polyps is largely unknown and small polyps may resolve spontaneously in 25% of the cases. However, the definitive treatment is surgical resection and is widely practiced [18]. Data regarding the relationship between hormonal therapy and endometrial polyps are contradictory; thus medical management of polyps has a limited role and is not supported by evidence.

1.9.2 Diagnosis and Treatment Guidelines

Saline infusion sonogram can be very useful for diagnosis and determining the location and shape of the lesion in comparison to transvaginal ultrasound alone. Endometrial biopsy is a basic part of the workup for abnormal uterine bleeding; however, there is low sensitivity for diagnosis of polyps when compared with direct visualization and guided resection via the hysteroscopic approach.

Typically, hysteroscopic polypectomy can be performed in the office and offers the advantage of avoiding additional IV sedation for anesthesia.

1.9.3 Pain Management

In the outpatient setting, premedication is not universally necessary. However, patients can elect to take 600 mcg of oral ibuprofen 20 minutes before the procedure.

1.9.4 Pre-Procedure Planning

It is not necessary to pre-treat patients with prostaglandins, as the small 5 mm caliber rigid hysteroscope can be advanced into the uterus without necessity of cervical dilation. No antibiotics are indicated for this type of procedure. Optimum timing for hysteroscopic procedures is during the early proliferative stage (menstrual day 4–11), as the endometrial lining is the thinnest during this time.

1.9.5 Surgical Approach

Hysteroscopic visualization of the polyp using the 5 mm rigid hysteroscope with a 12° viewing angle is the preferred modality, as blind curettage may miss the polyp and provide inadequate treatment. The polyp(s) are excised with hysteroscopic scissors and removed from the cavity with hysteroscopic grasping forceps or tenaculums under direct vision.

If multiple polyps are present, an electrosurgical loop may be more effective to achieve resection of the lesions. For infertility patients, we recommend sparse use of electrosurgery so as not to damage the underlying endometrium. In our practice, we use the resectoscope loop to bluntly lift the base of the polyp away from the underlying myometrium and activate the loop only when directly on polyp tissue. The distention medium with use of the bipolar resectoscope is isotonic electrolyte-containing fluids such as normal saline.

1.9.6 Surgical Technique

See Video 1.2

1. Place patient in the dorsal lithotomy position.
2. Perform pelvic exam to determine the position and size of the uterus.
3. Sterile prep the patient.
4. Introduce the hysteroscope vaginoscopically as described earlier.
5. Once you have entered the uterine cavity, obtain a panoramic view as polyps can be located anywhere along the endometrial cavity and can be varied in dimension and shape.
6. Advance the blunt-tipped scissors to use sharp dissection to dissect 90% of the base of the polyp off of the underlying endometrium (Figure 1.4). Introduce the hysteroscopic graspers or 5 French tenaculum to then grab the polyp and twist in a circular motion to avulse the remaining connected fibers (Figure 1.5). Directly visualize the specimen in your graspers in front of your

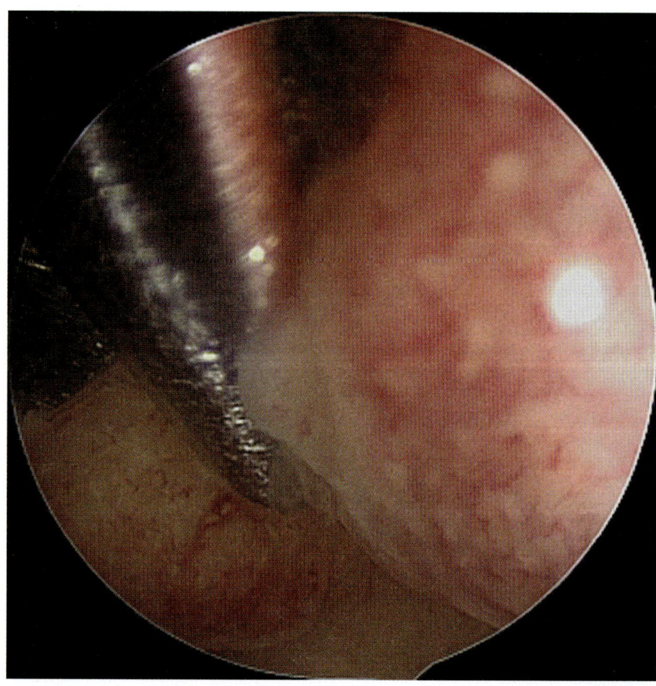

Figure 1.4 Polyp stalk is incised with scissors.

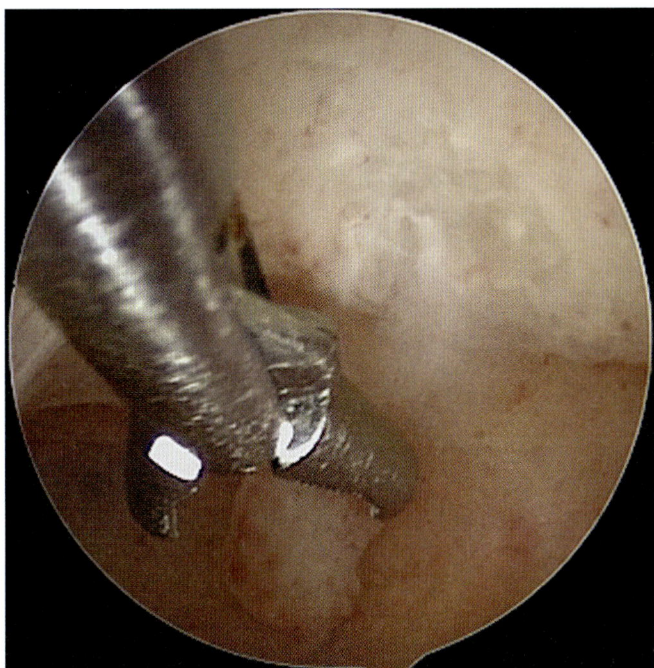

Figure 1.5 Remainder of the polyp stalk is grasped with polyp forceps and avulsed.

hysteroscopic lens as you extract the tissue. This method avoids losing the specimen in the cavity, as it is important to send it to pathology for review. Note that when utilizing a hysteroscopic morcellator device, polypectomy is then best approached from the distal end, advancing the tip of the device toward the endometrial wall as the polyp is being resected. However, unless the polyp is extremely large, this is not a cost-effective use of this device.

7. Reintroduce the hysteroscope to confirm complete removal of the polyp.

1.9.7 Outcomes

Recurrence rates vary between 2.5% and 13%, and widely depend on the length of follow-up and nature of polyp [19,20]. Among subfertile patients, the subsequent pregnancy rates can vary between 60% and 70% [21].

1.10 Hysteroscopic Myomectomy

Uterine fibroids are monoclonal tumors that derive from the myometrial layer of the uterus, and have a varied presentation depending largely on their size, number, and location. Submucous fibroids disrupt the vasculature of the endometrial lining and inhibit the uterine contractile capacity, and thus can present with heavy flow, irregular menstrual bleeding, and iron-deficiency anemia as well as issues related to recurrent pregnancy loss or infertility. Among women with abnormal uterine bleeding, a systematic review reported that 23% will have submucous leiomyomas identified as one of the contributing etiologies [22]. There are three main techniques for myomectomy: (i) monopolar and bipolar electrosurgical loops, (ii) mechanical morcellation, and (iii) vaporization, which is performed with a large surface area bipolar electrode.

1.10.1 Indications for Procedure

Fibroids are the most common benign pelvic tumors in women, and indications for transcervical resection of symptomatic submucous myomas present when they negatively impact quality of life secondary to abnormal uterine bleeding among women who desire to maintain their uterus. There is an extensive body of evidence for the deleterious effect on implantation that a submucous myoma exerts, leading to significantly decreased pregnancy rates [23]. Uterine leiomyoma are common and malignancy is very rare. For resectoscopic surgery, the incidence of malignancy has been reported to be as low as 0.13% [24].

1.10.2 Diagnosis and Treatment Guidelines

It is important to evaluate the location, size, and extent of depth into the myometrium for each fibroid either via saline infusion sonography (SIS), or a combination of diagnostic hysteroscopy with transvaginal ultrasound. SIS may not be effective when uterine distention is encumbered by enlarged fibroids (e.g., ≥14-week-sized uterus on pelvic examination). Magnetic resonance imaging (MRI) provides accurate location and size of the fibroids; however, it is expensive and not routinely indicated.

1.10.3 Pain Management

Local anesthetic blocks for this procedure such as 2% chloroprocaine without epinephrine can be utilized, but the anesthetic relief when combined with IV sedation or general anesthesia has not been well studied [25,26]. Either 15 or 30 mg of IV Ketorolac helps to mitigate postoperative cramping if the patient can tolerate NSAIDs.

1.10.4 Pre-Procedure Planning

Routine pre-operative evaluation should include pregnancy testing for reproductive-age women as well as a serum hematocrit as these patients are frequently anemic. Anticipated blood loss for these procedures does not typically exceed 100 mL. In our practice, we do not pre-treat our patients with prostaglandins or GnRH agonists. No antibiotics are indicated for this type of procedure. Optimum timing for hysteroscopic procedures is during the early proliferative stage (menstrual day 4–11), as this is when the endometrial lining is the thinnest.

1.10.5 Surgical Approach

When considering the options for transcervical approach, classification of the submucous leiomyoma into three subtypes can be useful for guidance and counseling of the patient [27]. Fédération Internationale de Gynécologie et d'Obstétrique (FIGO) put forth one of the most commonly used classification system for the extent of myometrial involvement, describing Type 0 lesions as completely within the endometrial cavity, Type I lesions as those that extend <50% into the myometrium, Type II lesions as those in which ≥50% are within the myometrium, and Type III lesions are 100% intramural and abut the endometrium but do not distort the endometrial cavity [28] (Figure 1.6). The goal of submucous myomectomy is to remove

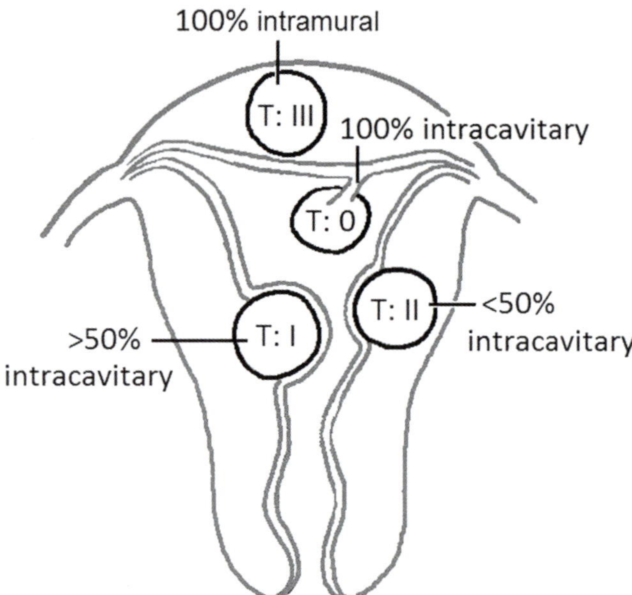

Figure 1.6 FIGO classification of myomas. (Modified from Munro MG, Critchley HO, Broder MS, Fraser IS. The FIGO Classification System ("PALM-COEIN") for causes of abnormal uterine bleeding in non-gravid women in the reproductive years, including guidelines for clinical investigation. *Int J Gynaecol Obstet.* 2011;113:3–13.)

100% of the fibroid. Complete hysteroscopic resection yields high patient satisfaction between 85% and 95%, and patients can avoid hysterectomy with few recurrences of symptoms [29]. Removal of 100% of a Type I or II myoma can be safely achieved as long as one stays within the pseudocapsule and does not cut myometrium because a fibroid (not adenomyoma) will displace myometrium and not invade it. Even myomas that extend close to the uterine serosa can be safely removed using this technique as the myometrium thickens as the myoma is resected [30].

Patients with Type III myomas should only have hysteroscopic resection by very experienced hysteroscopic surgeons. Similarly, transcervical resection of low lying is challenging in that the cervical canal often obstructs the outflow channels of the resectoscope, making visualization very difficult.

When fibroids are on opposing uterine cavity walls (either the anterior, posterior, or lateral walls of the uterus), consideration should be given to performing surgery in two stages, as intrauterine adhesions can form between the two surgical sites if opposing myomas are resected at the same surgery.

In our practice, we most often select a size 24 French bipolar resectoscope (7.5 mm diameter) with a 12° viewing angle for resection of leiomyomas. For patients who are postmenopausal and/or have a small myoma, we may select a size 22 French bipolar resectoscope (7.3 mm diameter). Patients should be counseled that a second procedure may be necessary to completely excise lesions for those with multiple fibroids, large fibroids (>3 cm), and/or those whose fibroids penetrate deeply into the myometrium. Multistage procedures are generally performed at least 6 weeks after the initial procedure.

Hysteroscopic myomectomy carries a greater risk of excess fluid absorption because breeches in the integrity of the myometrium allows fluid intravasation into the venous bed secondary to the higher hydrostatic pressures (>50 mmHg) compared to venous intravascular pressures (10–12 mmHg). It is important to follow the current fluid absorption guidelines published in 2013 by the AAGL. The key to minimizing fluid overload is to keep the intrauterine pressure at the lowest level that allows for adequate visualization. If it is feasible to keep the intracavitary pressure lower than the patient's mean arterial pressure (MAP), then the risk of significant fluid intravasation is drastically reduced. See the earlier section on "Distending Media" for further details regarding fluid management.

1.10.6 Additional Methods to Decrease Fluid Absorption

Active engagement with the anesthesiologist is important for resectoscopic cases. They should be notified that myomectomies are associated with risk of higher volumes of fluid intravasation, and that the IVF should be running at a slow infusion rate that only keeps the vein open.

1.10.7 Pre-treatment with GnRH Agonists

GnRH agonists may be administered for 2–3 months prior to hysteroscopic myomectomy to correct significant anemia as well as to reduce the size of very large myomas to facilitate surgery. In addition, GnRH agonists may decrease myometrial vascularity to help limit fluid intravasation. However, premenopausal women are more susceptible than postmenopausal women to hyponatremic hypotonic encephalopathy secondary to estrogen's inhibition of the Na^+/K^+-ATPase pump, and thus are more likely to die or have permanent brain damage [31].

1.10.8 Intracervical Vasopressin Administration

Intracervical injection of 8 mL of a dilute solution of vasopressin (0.05 U/mL of normal saline) has been shown to decrease fluid absorption during resectoscopic surgery via its primary mechanism of inducing vasoconstriction [32]. The dilute injection can be repeated at 20-minute intervals. Avoid intravascular injection, as systemic absorption can result in vagal-mediated bradycardia as well as coronary artery vasospasm provoking cardiac arrest. In situations of cardiac arrest, chest compressions should be initiated along with 1 mg epinephrine, 0.5 mg of atropine as well as 100% oxygen. Do not exceed the maximum dosage of approximately 5 U of Vasopressin.

1.10.9 Surgical Technique

See Video 1.3

1. Place the patient in the dorsal lithotomy position.
2. Perform pelvic exam to determine the position and size of the uterus.
3. Sterile prep the patient.
4. Insert an open-sided speculum into the vaginal vault. Grasp the anterior lip of the cervix with a single-toothed tenaculum and place tension on the tenaculum in order to straighten the axis of the uterus into a midline position.

5. Gently dilate the cervical canal up to the diameter that is equivalent to the hysteroscopic sheath in order to prevent inadvertent uterine perforation, cervical laceration, or creation of a false passage. Overdilating the cervix may make it difficult to maintain adequate distention.

6. Introduce the resectoscope into the endocervical canal with your dominant hand, and utilize the other hand to straighten the cervix with traction on the single-tooth tenaculum with your index finger placing countertension on the cervix as you advance into the cavity in order to prevent tearing of the cervix by the tenaculum. Drop your hand toward the ground to keep the internal os centered at the 12 o'clock position in order to avoid digging the scope into the posterior wall of the endocervical canal. Do not advance the scope with force if you are met with resistance as this can result in formation of a false passage. Successful entry into the cavity is achieved by placing one hand on the light cord and the other on the camera while rotating the entire scope back and forth between 4 o'clock and 8 o'clock positions and advancing gently along the axis of the cervical canal.

7. Once you have entered the uterine cavity, obtain a panoramic view and locate the lesions present. Take a systematic approach and note if bilateral ostia are visible.

8. Controlled variation of the intracavitary pressure is an important step throughout the procedure. Initially, briefly decreasing the pressure will allow for better identification of the lesions as higher pressure may obscure them by compressing them into the myometrium. Further along in the procedure, making special note of the intracavitary pressure in relationship to the patient's MAP will be important. The goal is to keep the distention of the cavity adequate enough for resection with as minimal pressure required so as to diminish the amount of fluid intravasation.

9. Readjust your hands so that you are now holding the camera head steady with your non-dominant hand, and with your dominant hand hold the working element of the resectoscope with your thumb and third finger in the handles of the scope.

10. Place your foot comfortably next to the pedal that actives the electrode of the loop. Begin by opening the handles to extend the loop of the resectoscope out into the uterine cavity, and place the loop squarely behind the fibroid. Be aware of the space behind the fibroid and the proximity of the surrounding uterine walls to avoid inadvertent injury to the normal endometrium. Slowly bring the loop slightly toward the lens by closing the handles without applying current. This enables you to have countertension placed on the lesion and ensures you are in the correct position prior to initiating energy for resection. Next, activate the cutting current and continue closing the handles to bring the loop towards the lens in a linear motion until you have reached the edge of the fibroid (Figure 1.7). You should visualize the fibroid as dense, white fibers that are distinct from the appearance of the surrounding pink myometrium. Shave evenly and systematically along the fibroid in a

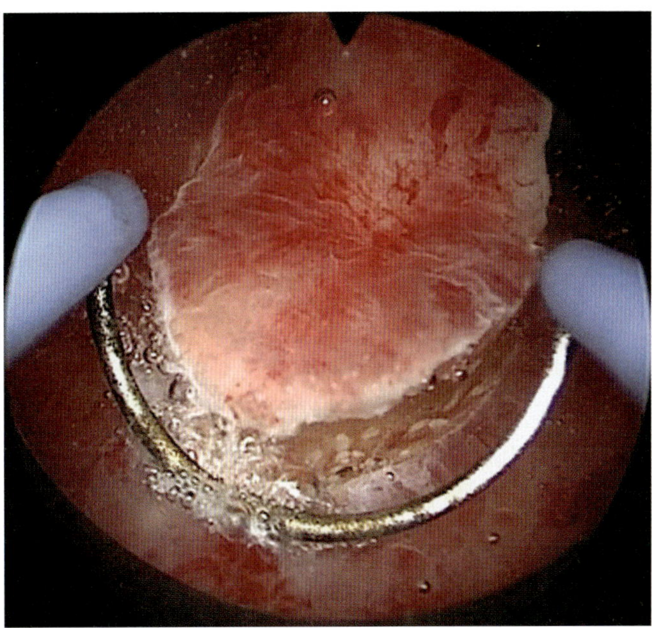

Figure 1.7 The endometrium over the myoma is resected to reveal the myoma.

unidirectional fashion (e.g., from left to right), with care to avoid tunneling in one place.

11. The pseudocapsule provides an excellent guide to the boundaries of the myoma. Using your inactive loop, extend it to gently tease out the edges of the cleavage plane of the pseudocapsule to release its fibers connecting it to the surrounding myometrium (Figure 1.8). Note the depth of the previous resections you have made with each swipe of the loop. Deeper resections can be attained by dropping your hand slightly toward the ground while bringing the loop toward the lens, keeping in mind that the consequence of going too deep is perforation (Figure 1.9). Also note that when encountering fibroids that are large, it may require that you move in a synchronized fashion in which you bring the entire scope toward you while simultaneously closing the handles of the working element to bring the loop toward the lens. In effect, you are able to successfully shave more surface area of the fibroid than when moving only the loop in isolation. Never resect with a motion that pushes forward with the loop activated, as this can result in perforation with significant damage to surrounding organs secondary to application of thermal energy.

12. During your resection, transected myometrial vessels will bleed into the cavity. If you are using a bipolar resectoscope, you can choose to selectively arrest the bleeding by approximating the edge of your loop to the bleeder and briefly activating the coagulation current (Figure 1.10).

13. You will encounter chips and air bubbles that compromise adequate visualization. When you encounter a bubble in front of your view, turn your entire scope 180°sideways quickly to see if this dislodges it. If you encounter a larger buildup of bubbles, turn off your inflow, rotate your entire

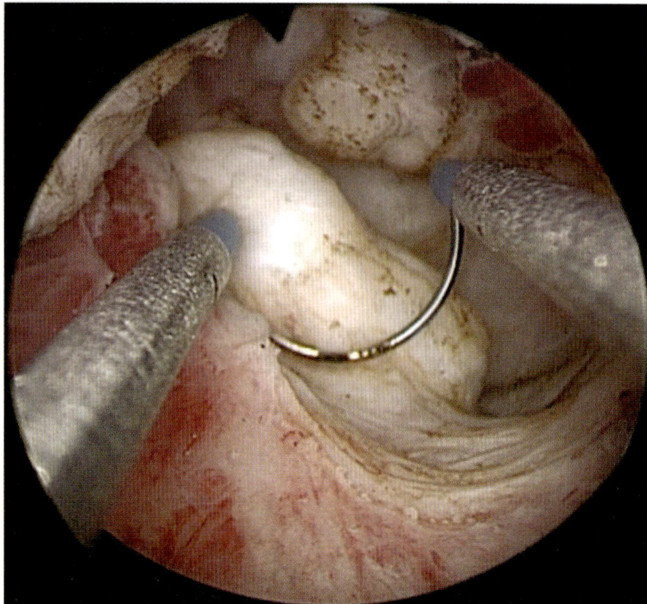

Figure 1.8 The pseudocapsule is identified by pushing up on the edge of the myoma with the resectoscope loop without applying current.

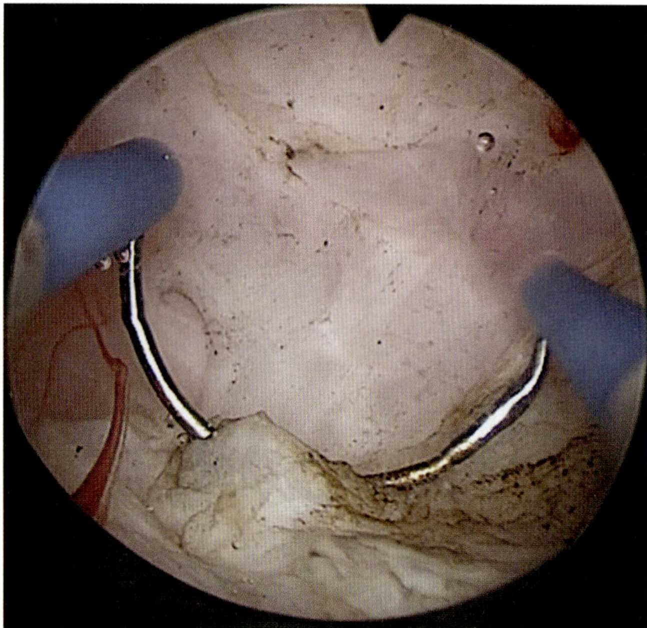

Figure 1.9 The myoma is resected with cutting current.

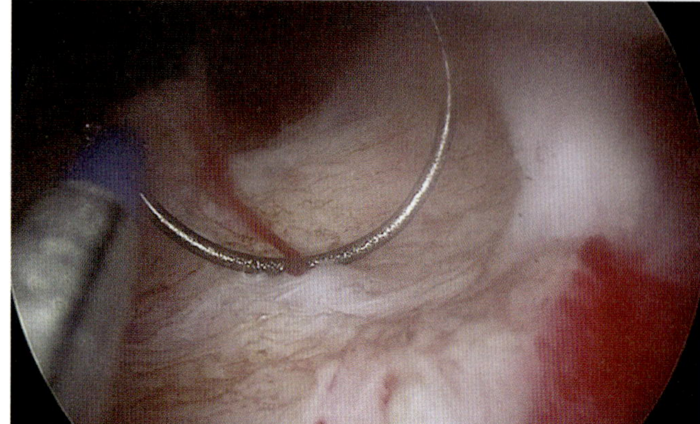

Figure 1.10 Bleeding vessels are sealed with coagulating current.

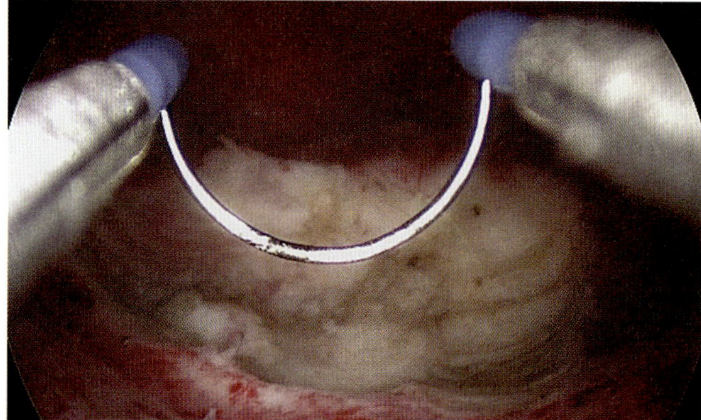

Figure 1.11 The myoma has been completely resected to normal myometrium.

surrounding, and activate the electrode of the loop to dislodge the chip.

14. When reinserting the scope after resection has begun, the cavity is often full of blood clots and visualization is hampered. Advancing the scope to the fundus allows for quick identification of this landmark as well as clearing of your view. Whenever the resectoscope is advanced through the cervix, the outflow should be on so as not to "piston" air into venous sinuses thus reducing the risk of air embolization.

15. You can consider the fibroid completely resected when only myometrial tissue is seen at the base of the surgical site (Figure 1.11).

16. While extracting the hysteroscope, evaluate the endocervical canal.

1.10.10 Postoperative Management

Long-term studies indicate that transcervical resection of myomas has a high rate of success, i.e., >94% [29]. Rates of requiring a second surgery are related to the overall size of the fibroid, depth of myometrial invasion, as well as location and number of fibroids. In addition, comorbid conditions such as adenomyosis can result in persistent abnormal uterine bleeding that may result in subsequent hysterectomy for definitive treatment.

scope 180°, and fully open your outflow in order to extract the bubbles. Chips should be removed by grasping them firmly in your loop as you close your hand and slowly extract the instrument. Be certain to directly visualize the chips in your loop as you extract the instrument to avoid losing the specimens in the cavity, as it is important to send chips to pathology for review. Many choose to keep the inflow running while extracting chips for sake of efficiency. If a chip is stuck onto your loop, bring your loop into the center of the cavity, ensure clear space

1.11 Complications of Operative Hysteroscopy

- Uterine perforation
- Fluid overload
- Heavy bleeding
- Infection
- Intrauterine adhesions

1.11.1 Uterine Perforation

The incidence of uterine perforation is 0.014% for hysteroscopic procedures. Known risk factors for uterine perforation due to traumatic entry are menopause, cervical stenosis, retroversion, and nulliparity. Signs and symptoms of uterine perforation include sudden increase in fluid deficit and loss of adequate intracavitary distention. It can result in bleeding and potentially significant injury to surrounding organs. Management of perforations is dependent on the location of the perforation and whether or not any energy (including mechanical shavers) was used. If thermal or mechanical injury of surrounding viscera is a possibility, a diagnostic laparoscopy is mandated. If the perforation is fundal and blunt as occurs during initial dilation of the cervix, then observation with discontinuation of the case is recommended. Lateral injuries incite concern for possible formation of broad ligament hematoma from vascular injury. If the perforation is anterior, hematuria may result and use of cystoscopy can aid in a thorough evaluation of the bladder.

1.11.2 Fluid Overload

The incidence of fluid overload is between 1.6% and 2.5%. Excess fluid absorption is one of the most common complications associated with hysteroscopic procedures. Careful observation of fluid deficit as well as thoughtful consideration of the distention media used is important for patient safety. Use of an electronic fluid management system is encouraged. See "Distention Media" section earlier for further details.

1.11.3 Heavy Bleeding

In the majority of cases, myometrial contraction is sufficient to arrest the bleeding postoperatively and heavy bleeding is uncommon after hysteroscopic surgery. Should it occur, prompt recognition and active management is essential. Intracervical injection of a prostaglandin F2α analog known as Carboprost or Hemabate can result in uterine contraction with subsequent decrease in uterine bleeding. If heavy bleeding persists, placement of a Foley catheter into the uterine cavity and inflating the balloon with 30 cc of saline can be used to effectively function as a tamponade. The balloon can be deflated and the Foley removed after the bleeding has subsided for 4 hours. In instances where bleeding persists despite the above interventions, consider consultation with interventional radiology for uterine artery embolization.

1.11.4 Infection

The incidence of infection is 0.01–1.6% of hysteroscopic cases. There is currently no established role for prophylactic antibiotic administration at this time.

1.11.5 Intrauterine Adhesions

When lesions on opposing sides of the uterine cavity (either the anterior, posterior, or lateral walls of the uterus) are resected simultaneously, adhesion formation has been noted in the postoperative period. Examining the cavity with office hysteroscopy 6 weeks after surgery in such instances can be useful both for diagnosis as well as treatment by bluntly lysing the adhesions with the tip of the hysteroscope.

References

1. Smith PP, Middleton LJ, Connor M, Clark TJ. Hysteroscopic morcellation compared with electrical resection of endometrial polyps: a randomized controlled trial. *Obstet Gynecol.* 2014;123(4):745–51.

2. Worldwide AAMIG, Munro MG, Storz K, Abbott JA, Falcone T, Jacobs VR, et al. AAGL practice report: practice guidelines for the management of hysteroscopic distending media. *J Minim Invasive Gynecol.* 2013;20(2):137–48.

3. El-Toukhy T, Sunkara SK, Coomarasamy A, Grace J, Khalaf Y. Outpatient hysteroscopy and subsequent IVF cycle outcome: a systematic review and meta-analysis. *Reprod Biomed Online.* 2008;16(5):712–9.

4. Di Spiezio Sardo A, Di Carlo C, Minozzi S, Spinelli M, Pistotti V, Alviggi C, et al. Efficacy of hysteroscopy in improving reproductive outcomes of infertile couples: a systematic review and meta-analysis. *Hum Reprod Update.* 2016;22(4):479–96.

5. Al-Fozan H, Firwana B, Al Kadri H, Hassan S, Tulandi T. Preoperative ripening of the cervix before operative hysteroscopy. *Cochrane Database Syst Rev.* 2015;(4):CD005998.

6. Oppegaard KS, Lieng M, Berg A, Istre O, Qvigstad E, Nesheim BI. A combination of misoprostol and estradiol for preoperative cervical ripening in postmenopausal women: a randomised controlled trial. *BJOG.* 2010;117(1):53–61.

7. Casadei L, Piccolo E, Manicuti C, Cardinale S, Collamarini M, Piccione E. Role of vaginal estradiol pretreatment combined with vaginal misoprostol for cervical ripening before operative hysteroscopy in postmenopausal women. *Obstet Gynecol Sci.* 2016;59(3):220–6.

8. Worldwide AAMIG. AAGL practice report: practice guidelines for management of intrauterine synechiae. *J Minim Invasive Gynecol.* 2010;17(1):1–7.

9. The American Fertility Society. The American Fertility Society classifications of adnexal adhesions, distal tubal occlusion, tubal occlusion secondary to tubal ligation, tubal pregnancies, mullerian anomalies and intrauterine adhesions. *Fertil Steril.* 1988;49(6):944–55.

10. Johary J, Xue M, Zhu X, Xu D, Velu PP. Efficacy of estrogen therapy in patients with intrauterine adhesions: systematic review. *J Minim Invasive Gynecol.* 2014;21(1):44–54.

11. Robinson JK, Colimon LM, Isaacson KB. Postoperative adhesiolysis therapy for intrauterine adhesions (Asherman's syndrome). *Fertil Steril.* 2008;90(2):409–14.

12. Practice Committee of the American Society for Reproductive Medicine. Uterine septum: a guideline. *Fertil Steril.* 2016;106(3):530–40.

13. Bosteels J, Weyers S, Kasius J, Broekmans FJ, Mol BW, D'Hooghe TM. Anti-adhesion therapy following operative hysteroscopy for treatment of female subfertility. *Cochrane Database Syst Rev.* 2015;(11):CD011110.

14. Hu R, Hilakivi-Clarke L, Clarke R. Molecular mechanisms of tamoxifen-associated endometrial cancer. *Oncol Lett*. 2015;9(4):1495–501.

15. Golan A, Cohen-Sahar B, Keidar R, Condrea A, Ginath S, Sagiv R. Endometrial polyps: symptomatology, menopausal status and malignancy. *Gynecol Obstet Invest*. 2010;70(2):107–12.

16. Revel A. Defective endometrial receptivity. *Fertil Steril*. 2012;97(5):1028–32.

17. Perez-Medina T, Bajo-Arenas J, Salazar F, Redondo T, Sanfrutos L, Alvarez P, et al. Endometrial polyps and their implication in the pregnancy rates of patients undergoing intrauterine insemination: a prospective, randomized study. *Hum Reprod*. 2005;20(6):1632–5.

18. American Association of Gynecologic Laproscopists. AAGL practice report: practice guidelines for the diagnosis and management of endometrial polyps. *J Minim Invasive Gynecol*. 2012;19(1):3–10.

19. Paradisi R, Rossi S, Scifo MC, Dall'O F, Battaglia C, Venturoli S. Recurrence of endometrial polyps. *Gynecol Obstet Invest*. 2014;78(1):26–32.

20. Yang JH, Chen CD, Chen SU, Yang YS, Chen MJ. Factors influencing the recurrence potential of benign endometrial polyps after hysteroscopic polypectomy. *PLoS One*. 2015;10(12):e0144857.

21. Spiewankiewicz B, Stelmachow J, Sawicki W, Cendrowski K, Wypych P, Swiderska K. The effectiveness of hysteroscopic polypectomy in cases of female infertility. *Clin Exp Obstet Gynecol*. 2003;30(1):23–5.

22. van Dongen H, de Kroon CD, Jacobi CE, Trimbos JB, Jansen FW. Diagnostic hysteroscopy in abnormal uterine bleeding: a systematic review and meta-analysis. *BJOG*. 2007;114(6):664–75.

23. Bosteels J, Kasius J, Weyers S, Broekmans FJ, Mol BW, D'Hooghe TM. Hysteroscopy for treating subfertility associated with suspected major uterine cavity abnormalities. *Cochrane Database Syst Rev*. 2015;(2):CD009461.

24. Vilos GA, Edris F, Abu-Rafea B, Hollett-Caines J, Ettler HC, Al-Mubarak A. Miscellaneous uterine malignant neoplasms detected during hysteroscopic surgery. *J Minim Invasive Gynecol*. 2009;16(3):318–25.

25. Tangsiriwatthana T, Sangkomkamhang US, Lumbiganon P, Laopaiboon M. Paracervical local anaesthesia for cervical dilatation and uterine intervention. *Cochrane Database Syst Rev*. 2013;(9):CD005056.

26. Ahmad G, O'Flynn H, Attarbashi S, Duffy JM, Watson A. Pain relief for outpatient hysteroscopy. *Cochrane Database Syst Rev*. 2010;(11):CD007710.

27. American Association of Gynecologic Laparoscopists: Advancing Minimally Invasive Gynecology W. AAGL practice report: practice guidelines for the diagnosis and management of submucous leiomyomas. *J Minim Invasive Gynecol*. 2012;19(2):152–71.

28. Munro MG, Critchley HO, Broder MS, Fraser IS, Disorders FWGoM. FIGO classification system (PALM-COEIN) for causes of abnormal uterine bleeding in nongravid women of reproductive age. *Int J Gynaecol Obstet*. 2011;113(1):3–13.

29. Polena V, Mergui JL, Perrot N, Poncelet C, Barranger E, Uzan S. Long-term results of hysteroscopic myomectomy in 235 patients. *Eur J Obstet Gynecol Reprod Biol*. 2007;130(2):232–7.

30. Casadio P, Youssef AM, Spagnolo E, Rizzo MA, Talamo MR, De Angelis D, et al. Should the myometrial free margin still be considered a limiting factor for hysteroscopic resection of submucous fibroids? A possible answer to an old question. *Fertil Steril*. 2011;95(5):1764–8 e1.

31. Ayus JC, Wheeler JM, Arieff AI. Postoperative hyponatremic encephalopathy in menstruant women. *Ann Intern Med*. 1992;117(11):891–7.

32. Phillips DR, Nathanson H, Milim SJ, Haselkorn JS. The effect of dilute vasopressin solution on blood loss during operative hysteroscopy. *J Am Assoc Gynecol Laparosc*. 1996; 3(4, Supplement):S38.

Adhesions in Reproductive Surgery: Treatment and Prevention

Kathryn D. Coyne and Steven R. Lindheim

2.1 Pathogenesis and Prevalence

Postoperative peritoneal adhesions are a physiologic response to surgical injury, peritonitis, or endometriosis. They serve to provide structural support, ward off infections, and deliver collateral circulation. Peritoneal trauma from surgical transection and ligation of vessels cause devascularization. Tissue ischemia, along with bleeding and lymphatic fluid drainage, stimulates a cascade of anaerobic metabolism, oxidative stress, and the formation of free radicals. When normal peritoneal and adhesion fibroblasts are exposed to free radicals such as superoxide, there is an increase in inflammatory mediators, histamines, cytokines, and growth factors. The impact of these mediators, including TNF-α, TGF-β, VEGF, IL-6, PAI-1, COX-2, type 1 collagen, fibronectin, and tissue inhibitors of metallproteinases (TIMP), is the formation of an impaired tissue plasminogen activator (tPA) system, resulting in decreased fibrinolysis and persistence of the early fibrinous adhesions (Figure 2.1). Continued fibrin deposition and capillary in-growth result in the development of permanent adhesions [1].

Adhesion phenotypes have been defined based on the biological characteristics of adhesion fibroblasts compared to normal peritoneal fibroblasts [2]. Extensive research has demonstrated that adhesion fibroblasts exhibit decreased NO, a decreased ratio of tPA/PAI-1, decreased apoptosis induced by hypoxia, and a greater production of TGF-β1 and extracellular membrane molecules [3]. There are two prominent types of adhesions: a thin filmy, avascular type and a thick cohesive, vascular type, with the former affording simple blunt lysis and the latter requiring careful sharp dissection to avoid injury to adjacent structures (Figure 2.2).

The sites, extent, and tenacity of adhesions can be quite variable and may involve the uterus, ovaries, fallopian tubes, peritoneum, omentum, or bowel and other organs. With respect to the fallopian tubes, this may result in agglutination of the fimbriae to complete occlusion with intraluminal damage, resulting in hydrosalpinges. Adhesions around the ovary or uterus can result in anatomic distortion due to adherence to adjacent organs and/or the pelvic sidewall. Adhesions can result in obliteration of the anterior and posterior cul-de-sacs.

Several risk factors have been directly associated with an increased risk of postoperative adhesion formation, including genetic polymorphisms of the IL-1 receptor antagonist, increased exposure to estrogen, and endometriosis [4]. Patients with endometriosis have been found to have increased levels of IL-6 and IL-8 in their peritoneal fluid and, moreover, the concentration of these cytokines has been correlated with the severity of adhesion formation [5]. The pro-inflammatory cytokines associated with endometriosis are believed to activate PAI-1, impairing fibrinolysis, and increased the propensity for adhesion formation in this population [6]. Factors that increase the risk of fibrosis are indirectly related to increased adhesion development, such as genetic polymorphisms in PAI-1, diabetes mellitus, metabolic syndrome, hyperglycemia, obesity, depression, binge alcohol consumption, anti-Parkinsonian therapy, oral hormone therapy, pregnancy, and malignancy [4].

Adhesions occur in up to 94% of patients following open abdominal or pelvic surgery. Laparoscopic abdominal or pelvic surgery may have comparable risk for adhesion related complications, including small bowel obstruction, impaired fertility, and abdominal or pelvic pain [7]. The extent of tissue injury is the predominant factor for adhesion development, rather than the surgical approach (laparotomy vs. laparoscopy), though the length of the abdominal incision is related to the risk for de-novo abdominal wall adhesions [8].

In order to facilitate patient management decisions by predicting outcomes such as pregnancy rates in cases of infertility caused by adhesions, numerous scoring systems have been developed; however, none have been clinically validated.

2.2 Clinical Consequences

The clinical implications and economic burden of intraperitoneal adhesions are significant, with an estimated $5 billion cost to the United States health care system annually [9]. A number of studies have examined the impact on health care including the inpatient burden of adhesiolysis. In one report of more than 350,000 hospitalizations, 23% were for primary adhesiolysis and almost 77% for secondary adhesiolysis with an average length of stay of 7.8 days [10]. In another study, approximately one-third of patients who had undergone laparotomy experienced an average of two hospital readmissions over the 10 years following initial surgery due to adhesions. In particular, ovarian surgery had the highest readmission rate as a direct result of adhesions (7.5/100 initial operations) [8].

There are a number of major consequences of adhesion formation (Box 2.1), including increased operative time and the risk of bowel-related injuries [11]. The distortion of normal anatomy, compromised exposure, and need for lysis of bowel

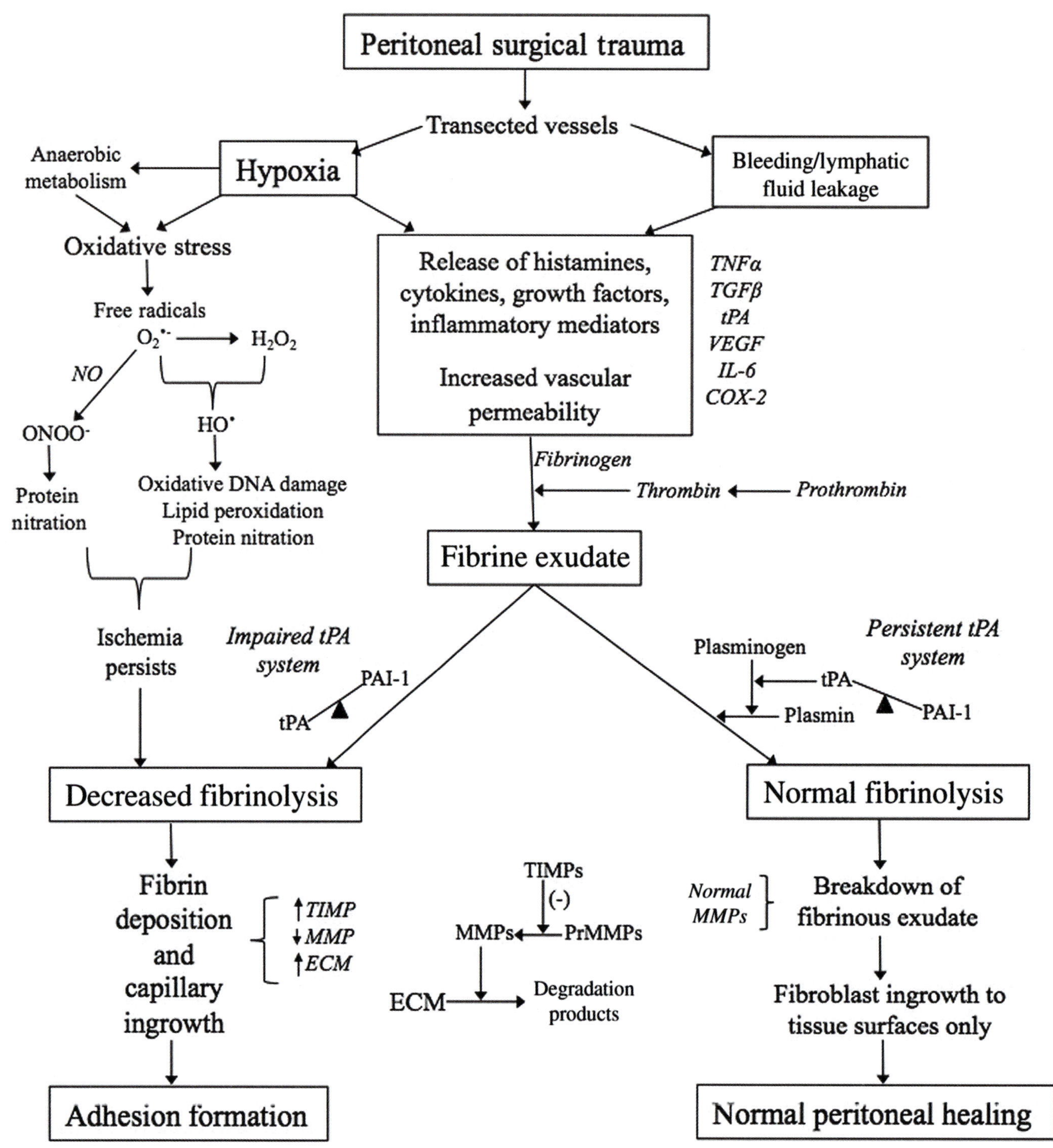

Figure 2.1 Pathogenesis of adhesion formation.

adhesions may lead to sharp or thermal injury to the bowel with resultant postoperative morbidity. Chronic abdominal or pelvic pain associated with adhesions has been attributed to visceral pain due to limited organ mobility, although the definitive relationship remains uncertain. Nerve fibers have been identified in pelvic adhesions, yet their prevalence and extent is not necessarily greater in those with more severe pain [8]. Fertility may be disturbed by peritoneal adhesions that distort the anatomic relationship between the tubes and ovaries, which compromise oocyte pickup. In addition, intrauterine adhesions may interfere with embryo implantation. Screening for uterine and tubal factor infertility may be accomplished through hysterosalpingography (HSG) or sonohysterosalpingography.

Postoperative intraabdominal adhesions are the most common cause of small bowel obstruction, responsible for 74% cases of bowel obstruction in 552 patients [12]. An

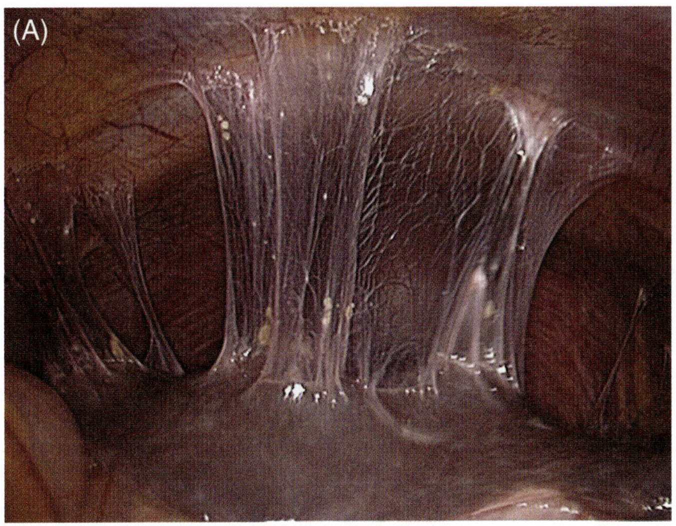

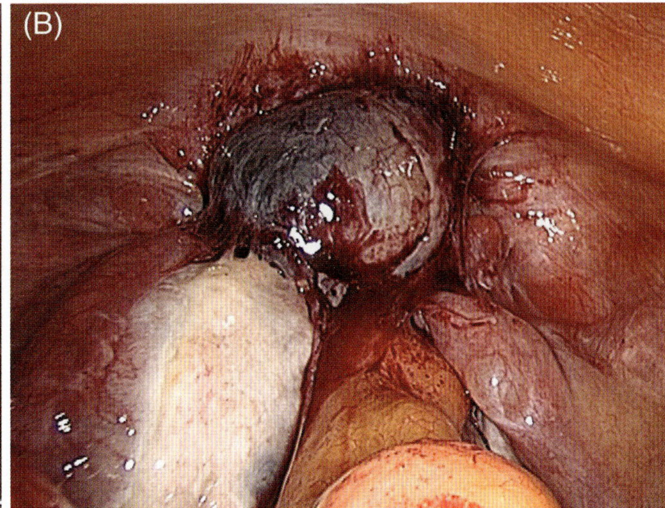

Figure 2.2 Thin filmy adhesions and dense cohesive adhesions.

> **Box 2.1** Major Consequences of Postoperative Adhesions
>
> Increased operating time in subsequent surgery
> Bowel injury
> Abdominal/pelvic pain
> Infertility
> Small bowel obstruction

often-unappreciated aspect is subsequent emergent cesarean section for fetal hypoxia. There are significant concerns related to delayed delivery due to difficult access to the uterus from adhesions resulting in lifelong morbidity including cerebral palsy, intraventricular hemorrhage, and respiratory distress syndrome [13].

2.3 Treatment Techniques

Surgical lysis of adhesions must begin with safely entering the abdominal or pelvic cavity (see Video 2.1). Even slow and methodical entry by laparotomy may result in injury to bowel that is densely adherent to the abdominal wall. Intraoperative recognition and repair is the key to preventing delayed complications. Access to the abdominal cavity during laparoscopic surgery with insertion of the trocar through the umbilicus carries a risk of injury due to bowel to abdominal wall adhesions. Primary trocar entry in the left upper quadrant (Palmer's point, 3 cm below the left costal margin in the mid-clavicular line) should be considered to minimize the risk of bowel perforation (Figure 2.3) [14]. Adhesions occurring at this point are less frequent, affording an assessment of the location and extent of adhesions for planning the sites for ancillary trocar insertions (see Video 2.2). As with all laparoscopic procedures, but especially with left upper quadrant trocar entry, it is essential that the stomach be decompressed with nasogastric tube suction to avoid injury to that organ.

If adhesions are observed, a structured approach can be undertaken with an initial step that includes lysis of adhesions along an avascular plane to ensure minimal bleeding. The

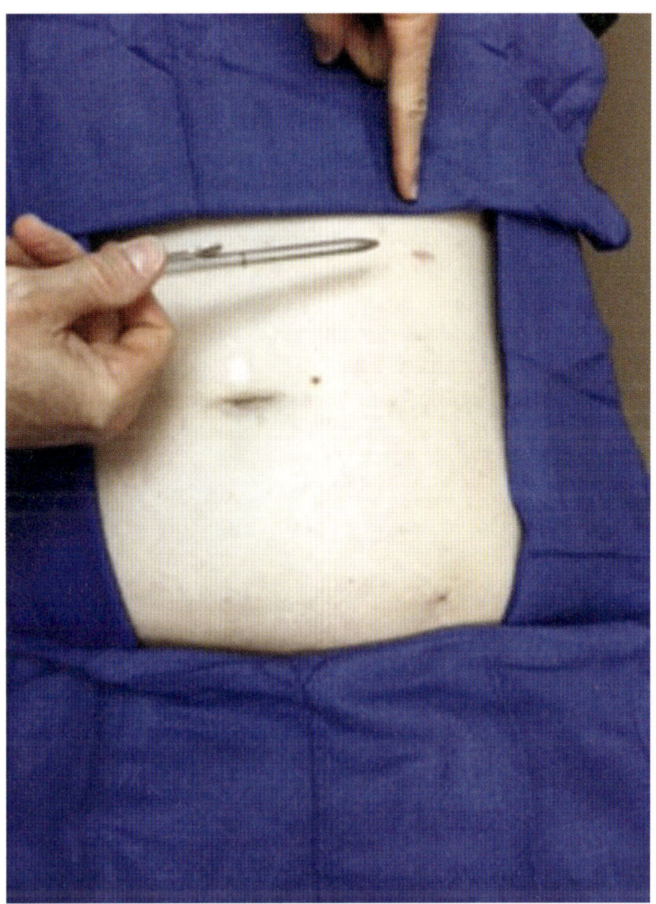

Figure 2.3 Palmer's point.

utilization of traction and countertraction creates tension and allows for clearer identification of an avascular plane. Adhesiolysis can be achieved by both sharp and blunt dissection techniques. Sharp dissection is the primary technique employed for dense adhesions but can by followed by blunt dissection for the remaining fine adhesions.

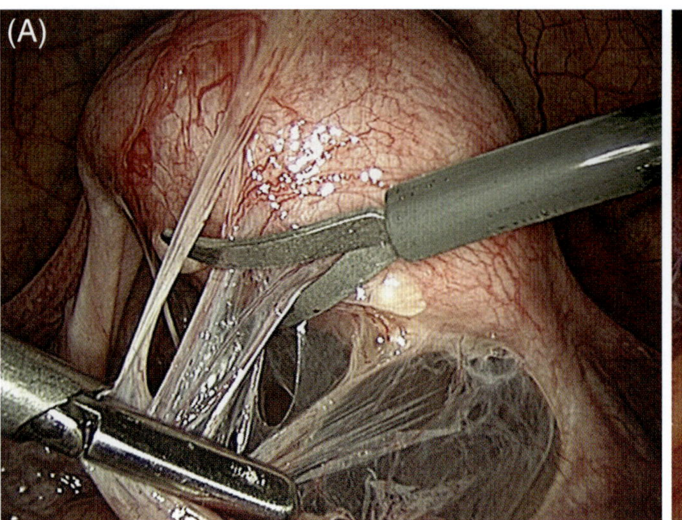
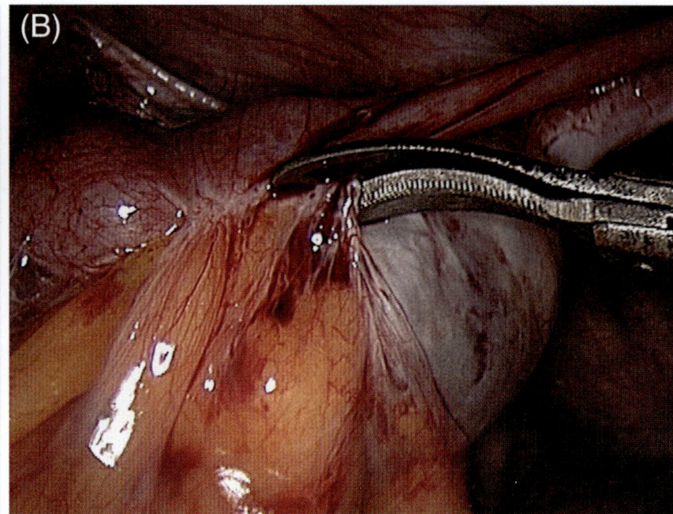

Figure 2.4 Dissection with rounded-tipped scissors while the adhesions are placed on traction.

Scissors are the preferred instrument to lyse adhesions. With the magnification of the laparoscope, most anterior abdominal wall, pelvic, and bowel adhesions can be clearly visualized and carefully divided with minimal bleeding. Scissors may aid in adhesiolysis not only through cutting but also via blunt mechanical tissue separation. Inserting scissors in a closed position and withdrawing it in the open position may separate loose fibrous tissue. Natural planes may be developed with the assistance of a partially open blunt scissor tip while pushing the tissue. Blunt or rounded-tip scissors with one stable blade and one moveable blade may be used to sharply divide thin and thick bowel adhesions (Figure 2.4).

Aquadissection has also been employed in the dissection of adhesions where instillation of pressurized fluid displaces the tissue to create planes in the path of least resistance. Aquadissection can produce edematous, distended tissue when instilled into closed spaces behind peritoneum or adhesions, which may allow for safer tissue division with blunt scissor dissection, laser, or electrosurgery after surgical planes are developed.

If anatomic planes are not evident, or vascular adhesions are anticipated, electrosurgery and lasers enable both dissection and hemostasis. Monopolar electrosurgical current can be used provided all vital structures are safely out of the way to avoid injury from electrical and thermal spread. If working on the bowel, bipolar desiccation may be employed, as it causes less spread. It is also more effective for larger vessel hemostasis [15]. Various types of lasers have been employed including argon, potassium-titanyl-phosphate (KTP-532), neodymium:yttrium-aluminum-garnet (Nd:YAG), and carbon dioxide, though none have been shown to be superior to scissors or electrocautery to justify the increased cost.

The harmonic scalpel has the ability to grasp, cut, and cauterize simultaneously utilizing ultrasonic energy, which avoids electrical injury and limits thermal spread. However, there are no studies demonstrating better clinical outcomes or reduced complications compared to other surgical modalities. Both robotic and conventional laparoscopy may be utilized effectively, with robotics affording greater visualization and articulation, and conventional laparoscopy allowing haptic feedback. Comparative studies reported longer operative times and greater cost with robotic surgery for benign gynecologic procedures with no offsetting benefit in terms of long- or short-term clinical outcomes.

2.4 Surgical Results

The effectiveness of lysis of bowel or adnexal adhesions on pain control has yet to be reliably demonstrated. A randomized study of laparotomy with adhesiolysis versus laparotomy alone in patients with chronic pelvic pain revealed an impact only in those having dense adhesions involving the bowel [16]. Another randomized control trial (RCT) evidenced relief of pain with laparoscopic lysis of mild abdominal adhesions, but with no greater improvement than placebo surgical intervention [17]. Regarding infertility, only one small retrospective study evaluated lysis of adnexal adhesions at laparotomy in women with otherwise-unexplained infertility. Cumulative pregnancy rates at 1 and 2 years were higher in those who underwent lysis compared to untreated controls [18]. As such, adhesiolysis in and of it itself is associated with a risk of intraoperative complications, including inadvertent bowel, bladder, ureter, and vascular injury [14] and prevention strategies are of paramount importance.

2.5 Prevention

Preventive methods that are currently accepted in the management and reduction of postoperative adhesions include adherence to microsurgical principles, peritoneal instillate with Icodextrin 4% (ADEPT), and surgical barriers such as Interceed (see Video 2.3), Gore-Tex, and Seprafilm (Box 2.2). There is no current evidence to support the effectiveness of peritoneal irrigation with anti-inflammatories or heparin, antibiotic peritoneal instillates, hyaluronic acid solution, or fibrin sealant/sheets in the prevention or reduction of postoperative adhesions.

Box 2.2 Prevention of Postoperative Adhesions

Microsurgical techniques	Careful atraumatic tissue handling
	Meticulous hemostasis
	Prevention of tissue desiccation
	Use of fine nonreactive sutures without undue tension
	Avoiding unnecessary foreign bodies (e.g., packs, sponges, sutures)
Surgical barriers	Oxidized regenerated cellulose (Interceed)
	Expanded polytetrafluoroethylene (Gore-Tex)
	Modified hyaluronic acid and carboxymethylcellulose film (Seprafilm)
Peritoneal instillate	Icodextrin 4% (ADEPT)

The basic principles of microsurgical technique to avoid or limit peritoneal damage are to be essentially followed during all abdominal and pelvic surgical procedures. The employment of peritoneal closure is controversial and is not currently recommended. Data suggest increased incidence of adhesions at the site of closure after laparotomy with peritoneal closure (22%) compared to without peritoneal closure (16%) [19]. This is likely due to tissue ischemia at the suture line and foreign body reaction from the suture material. However, conflicting evidence purports a reduction in dense and filmy adhesions with parietal peritoneal closure at primary cesarean delivery [20].

Numerous systemic and intraperitoneal agents have been tried over the past century including gonadotropin-releasing hormone agonist, reteplase plasminogen activator, steroids and non-steroidal anti-inflammatory agents, promethazine noxytioline, and heparin with no significant reduction in post-operative peritoneal adhesions [21].

Intraoperative peritoneal irrigation is recommended to avoid tissue desiccation in the prevention of postoperative adhesions. However, there is no current evidence to support the effectiveness of peritoneal irrigation with anti-inflammatory agents, heparin, antibiotics, or hyaluronic acid solution in the prevention or reduction of postoperative adhesions [21]. In addition, leaving large volumes of crystalloid irrigation fluid or 32% dextran 70 (Hyscon) in the peritoneal cavity is also without clinical benefit.

ADEPT® Adhesion Reduction Solution is the only FDA-approved antiadhesion product for laparoscopic gynecologic surgery [7]. It is easy to instill laparoscopically and provides a temporary hydroflotation effect allowing for the retention of a reservoir of fluid within the peritoneal cavity for 3–4 days. However, its clinical effectiveness is marginal at best.

Numerous mechanical adhesion barriers such as amnion and peritoneal grafts have been tried unsuccessfully over the past century to cover the surgical site and prevent other structures from adhering to it. Interceed was the first FDA-approved

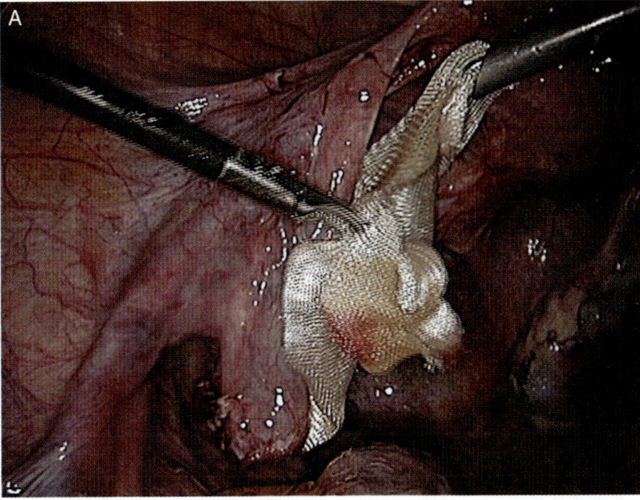

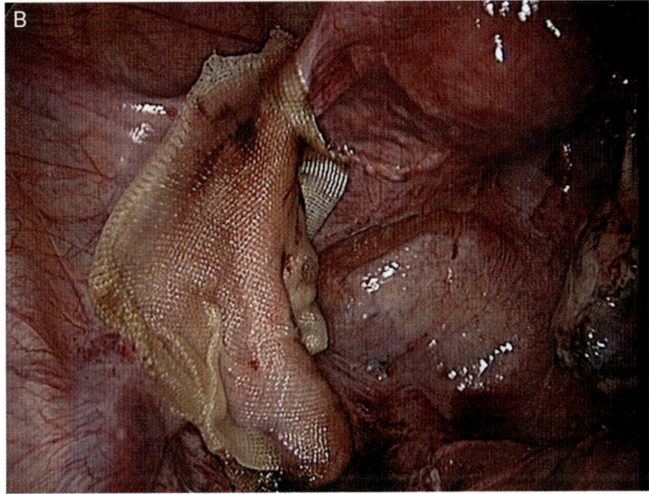

Figure 2.5 Interceed application: The device is being wrapped around the ovary. A few drops of irrigation fluid hold the fabric in place without sutures.

device for adhesion reduction in open gynecologic pelvic surgery in 1989 [7]. In a study of 13 RCTs of Interceed versus no treatment at laparoscopy or laparotomy, the incidence of re-formed adhesions was found to be lower in the intervention group for both laparoscopy and laparotomy [22]. Clinical applications in gynecology include myomectomy, ovarian cyst-ectomy, tuboplasty, and to cover peritoneal defects resulting from extensive lysis of adhesions. Interceed is an absorbable fabric made of oxidized regenerated cellulose, which is similar to Surgicel, the hemostatic material, but with a tighter weave. They have different physical properties and cannot be used interchangeably. It is placed over the operative site and adheres to the site with a few drops of irrigation solution. It is imperative that the site is completely hemostatic as blood renders the device ineffective (Figure 2.5).

Gore-Tex, or expanded polytetrafluoroethylene (ePTFE), is another surgical membrane approved by the FDA for peritoneal, as well as pericardial, adhesion prevention [7]. It is a 0.1 mm thick nonabsorbable sheet and must be sutured in to place until peritoneal healing is accomplished, at which point the membrane may be removed if desired [7]. A RCT of Gore-Tex versus no treatment at gynecological surgery demonstrated reduction in new adhesion formation, and two RCTs of Gore-Tex versus Interceed at gynecological surgery found no difference between groups in adhesion reduction [22]. Since Gore-Tex must be sutured in place, it is more difficult to apply than Interceed, especially during laparoscopic surgery.

Seprafilm is a modified hyaluronic acid and carboxymethylcellulose film adhesion barrier that was approved by the FDA in 1996 [7]. Use of Seprafilm is indicated in abdominal or pelvic laparotomy to reduce the incidence, extent, and severity of postoperative peritoneal adhesions [7]. A RCT of Seprafilm versus no treatment at gynecological surgery evidenced that Seprafilm was associated with a lower adhesion score at second-look laparoscopy [22]. The Seprafilm sheet is thin, brittle, and sticky, making it difficult to handle even during laparotomy and impractical for laparoscopic use.

Although the use of surgical barriers during intra-abdominal and pelvic surgeries may reduce postoperative adhesion development, they have not been shown to be effective in improving fertility, decreasing adhesion-associated pain, nor reducing the incidence of postoperative bowel obstruction [22]. Insufficient evidence and data on pelvic pain, fertility outcomes, and quality of life or safety precludes any conclusions on the impact of anti-adhesion agents in gynecological surgery [21]. Further research is required to establish more definitive and effective management and prevention of postoperative peritoneal adhesions and the associated consequences.

2.6 Intrauterine Adhesions

Intrauterine adhesions may present with hypo- or amenorrhea, infertility, and/or recurrent miscarriage. They typically result from dilation and curettage, especially for control of postpartum hemorrhage, as the hypoestrogenemic state does not allow for repair by rapid endometrial proliferation. Removal of submucosal myomas by hysteroscopy, laparoscopy, or laparotomy is also a frequent cause of intrauterine adhesions.

Intrauterine adhesions run the gamut from a single filmy adhesion to complete obliteration of the cavity. The more severe cases are referred to as Asherman's syndrome. Treatment consists of hysteroscopic adhesiolysis, with the goal of restoring the uterine cavity's size and shape, as well as endometrial function and fertility [23]. Blind dilation and curettage for adhesiolysis is not appropriate. Intrauterine adhesiolysis is begun by placing the hysteroscope at the internal os and lysing adhesions with sharp dissection using scissors. The use of electrosurgical energy devices should be avoided as they may cause a bowel burn in the event of uterine perforation. The risk of perforation is high with a contracted cavity devoid of the normal anatomic landmarks. Transabdominal ultrasonographic guidance should be considered to facilitate orientation and avoid complications.

Strategies to prevent adhesion formation or reformation include avoiding hyteroscopic myomectomy as a single procedure for large myomas on opposing uterine walls, placing a pediatric Foley balloon or special uterine stent for a few days, administering high-dose estrogen postoperatively for several weeks, and performing early second-look office hysteroscopy

to easily lyse the adhesions before they become organized and dense.

2.7 Conclusion

Postoperative adhesions occur as a result of trauma that induces inflammation and local suppression of peritoneal fibrinolysis, which supports the invasion of fibroblasts, fibrin deposition, and capillary ingrowth. Adhesions are present in up to 94% of patients following open abdominal or pelvic surgery, but the sites, extent, and tenacity of adhesions can be quite variable. The major consequences include small bowel obstruction, increased operating time, and risk of bowel injury in subsequent surgery, abdominal/pelvic pain, and subfertility or infertility. Intrauterine adhesions specifically represent an adversity to fertility. The consequences of both abdominal/pelvic adhesions and intrauterine adhesions in the gynecological setting are significant and warrant appropriate prevention and treatment.

Adhesiolysis carries intraoperative risks and must be performed with meticulous attention to pelvic anatomy. The prevention methods that are currently approved in the management and reduction of postoperative adhesions include adherence to microsurgical principles, peritoneal instillate with Icodextrin 4% (ADEPT), and surgical barriers such as Interceed, Gore-Tex, and Seprafilm. Further research is required to establish more effective prevention and treatment modalities to avoid the consequences of postoperative peritoneal adhesions.

References

1. Diamond MP, El-Mowafi DM. Pelvic adhesions. *Surg Technol Int.* 1998;VII: 273–83.

2. Saed GM, Diamond MP. Molecular characterization of postoperative adhesions: the adhesion phenotype. *J Am Assoc Gynecol Laparosc.* 2004;11(3):307–14.

3. Braun KM, Diamond MP. The biology of adhesion formation in the peritoneal cavity. *Semin Pediatr Surg.* 2014;23:336–43.

4. Fortin CN, Saed GM, Diamond MP. Predisposing factors to post-operative adhesion deveopment. *Hum Reprod Update.* 2015; 21(4):536–51.

5. Barcz E, Milewski Ł, Dziunycz P, Kamiński P, Płoski R, Malejczyk J. Peritoneal cytokines and adhesion formation in endometriosis: an inverse association with vascular endothelial growth factor concentration. *Fertil Steril.* 2012;6:1380–6.e1.

6. Dong J, Fujii S, Imagawa S, et al. IL-1 and IL-6 induce hepatocyte plasminogen activator inhibitor-1 expression through independent signaling pathways converging on C/EBPdelta. *Am J Physiol Cell Physiol.* 2007;292:C209–15.

7. Bolnick A, Bolnick J, Diamond MP. Postoperative adhesions as a consequence of pelvic surgery. *J Min Invasive Gynecol.* 2015;22(4):549–63.

8. Practice Committee of ASRM and SRS. Pathogenesis, consequences, and control of peritoneal adhesions in gynecologic surgery: a committee opinion. *Fertil Steril.* 2013;99(6):1550–5.

9. Butureanu SA, Butureanu TAS. Pathophysiology of adhesions. *Gen Rep Chirurgia.* 2014; 109:293–8.

10. Sikirica V, Bapat B, Candrilli SD, et al. The inpatient burden of abdominal and gynecological adhesiolysis in the US. *BMC Surg.* 2011;11:13.

11. Coleman MG, McLain AD, Moran BJ. Impact of previous surgery on time taken for incision and division of adhesions during laparotomy. *Dis Colon Rectum.* 2000; 43:1297–9.

12. Miller G, Boman J, Shrier I, Gordon PH. Etiology of small bowel obstruction. *Am J Surg.* 2000;180:33–6.

13. Awonuga AO, Fletcher NM, Saed GM, Diamond MP. Postoperative adhesion development following cesarean and open intra-abdominal gynecological operations: a review. *Reproduc Sci.* 2011; 18(12):1166–85.

14. Herrmann A, De Wilde RL. Adhesions are the major cause of complications in operative gynecology. *Best Pract Res Clin Obstet Gynaecol.* 2015;pii: S1521-6934(15)00193-5. doi: 10.1016/j.bpobgyn.2015.10.010. [Epub ahead of print]

15. Reich H, Vancaillie T, Soderstrom R. Electrical techniques. Operative laparoscopy. In Martin DC, Holtz GL, Levinson CJ, Soderstrom RM, eds. *Manual of Endoscopy.* Santa Fe Springs: American Association of Gynecologic Laparoscopists, 1990:105.

16. Peters AA, Trimbos-Kemper GC, Admiraal C, Trimbos JB, Hermans J. A randomized clinical trial on the benefits of adhesiolysis in patients with intraperitoneal adhesions and chronic pelvic pain. *Br J Obstet Gynaecol.* 1992;99:59–62.

17. Swank DJ, Swank-Bordewijk SC, Hop WC, et al. Laparoscopic adhesiolysis in patients with chronic abdominal pain: a blinded randomised controlled multi-centre trial. *Lancet.* 2003;361:1247–51.

18. Tulandi T, Collins JA, Burrows E, et al. Treatment-dependent and treatment-independent pregnancy among women with periadnxal adhesions. *Am J Obstet Gynecol.* 1990;162:354–7.

19. Roset E, Boulvain M, Irion O. Nonclosure of the peritoneum during caesarean section: long-term follow-up of a randomised controlled trial. *Eur J Obstet Gynecol Reprod Biol.* 2003;108:40–4.

20. Lyell DJ, Caughey AB, Hu E, Daniels K. Peritoneal closure at primary cesarean delivery and adhesions. *Obstet Gynecol.* 2005;106:275–80.

21. Hindocha A, Beere L, Dias S, Watson A, Ahmad G. Adhesion prevention agents for gynaecological surgery: an overview of Cochrane reviews. *Cochrane Database Systemat Rev.* 2015, Issue 1. Art. No.: CD011254. DOI: 10.1002/14651858.CD011254.pub2.

22. Ahmad G, O'Flynn H, Hindocha A, Watson A. Barrier agents for adhesion prevention after gynaecological surgery. *Cochrane Database Systemat Rev.* 2015, Issue 4. Art. No.: CD000475. DOI: 10.1002/14651858.CD000475.pub3

23. Yu D, Wong YM, Cheong Y, et al. Asherman syndrome – one century later. *Fertil Steril.* 2008; 89:759.

Müllerian Anomalies

Samantha M. Pfeifer

3.1 Introduction

Müllerian anomalies are disorders of development of the female reproductive organs, specifically involving the uterus, cervix, and vagina. These anomalies may be asymptomatic, but some typically present during puberty or adolescence with symptoms such as pain or amenorrhea. Alternatively, müllerian anomalies may be detected during the reproductive years either incidentally on exam or imaging, or during an evaluation for infertility or reproductive loss. Surgical intervention is often performed either to treat symptoms or with the intention of decreasing the risk of potential adverse reproductive outcomes in future. This chapter will address the surgical treatment of uterine anomalies in the adult female.

3.2 Incidence

Müllerian anomalies are rare and the incidence is difficult to ascertain as it may vary depending on the specific anomaly and, in addition, many of these anomalies are asymptomatic. There are several classification systems to characterize müllerian anomalies [1–4]. There is no universally accepted classification system. All classification systems have advantages and disadvantages. The oldest and most widely used system is the American Fertility Society (now known as the American Society for Reproductive Medicine [ASRM]) classification (Figure 3.1) [1].

3.3 Reproductive Issues and Uterine Anomalies

Patients with uterine malformations have a higher incidence of abortions, preterm birth, and lower live birth rates [5]. The most common uterine malformations seen in reproductive age women include arcuate, septate, bicornuate, and didelphic uteri [5]. Arcuate uterus is felt, in some studies, to contribute to poor reproductive outcomes; however, in most studies it is believed to be clinically irrelevant and should not be corrected [6]. This discrepancy may be related to the classification of some septate uteri as arcuate as there is no universally accepted definition of these anomalies.

Traditionally, the poorest reproductive outcomes were seen with septate and bicornuate uteri [5] and these anomalies were corrected surgically by laparotomy. Treatment of septate uterus was revolutionalized with the advent of hysteroscopy and hysteroscopic septum resection, a much safer and less invasive surgical alternative when compared to an abdominal metroplasty. Advances in obstetrical and neonatal management of pregnancy with a bicornuate uterus have improved over time and as the methods to correct this anomaly are challenging, the surgery is not performed as frequently. Uterus didelphys, although associated with preterm delivery, is considered to be best managed by optimizing prenatal and neonatal care for the mother and baby. Surgical correction is rarely performed.

3.4 Septate Uterus

Septate uterus describes a uterus with a normal convex exterior and an endometrial cavity that is divided by fibromuscular tissue. This anomaly results from failure of resorption of the tissue connecting the paramesonephric (müllerian) ducts prior to the 20th week of fetal development. Its prevalence is difficult to ascertain as many of these anomalies are asymptomatic, but ranges vary between 1–2 per 1,000 and 15 per 1,000 [7]. Septate uterus may be viewed as part of a spectrum of the developmental uterine anomalies including arcuate, septate, bicornuate, and didelphys. A uterine septum may be further classified as being partial or complete. A partial septate uterus refers to a single convex external uterine fundus with a septum extending from the top of the endometrial cavity toward, but not including, the cervix. A complete septate uterus refers to a single outer uterine fundus with a septum that extends internally from the top on the endometrial cavity through the cervix, dividing both into two separate cavities, and is often associated with a longitudinal vaginal septum. Alternatively this anomaly may be associated with a duplicated cervix and longitudinal vaginal septum, similar to a uterus didelphys. Although traditionally believed to be a fibrous tissue, biopsy specimens and magnetic resonance imaging (MRI) imaging have shown that the septum is actually composed primarily of muscular tissue [8,9].

3.4.1 Diagnosis

As a septate uterus may be confused with a normal, arcuate, or bicornuate uterus or uterus didelphys, diagnostic evaluation should include an assessment of the outer uterine contour as well as the endometrial cavity so as to differentiate this anomaly from a bicornuate or didelphic uterus. The gold standard for the diagnosis of septate uterus had traditionally been laparoscopy with hysteroscopy. However, as radiologic techniques have improved ultrasound, 3-dimensional (3D) ultrasonography, with or without saline infusion, and MRI have largely replaced

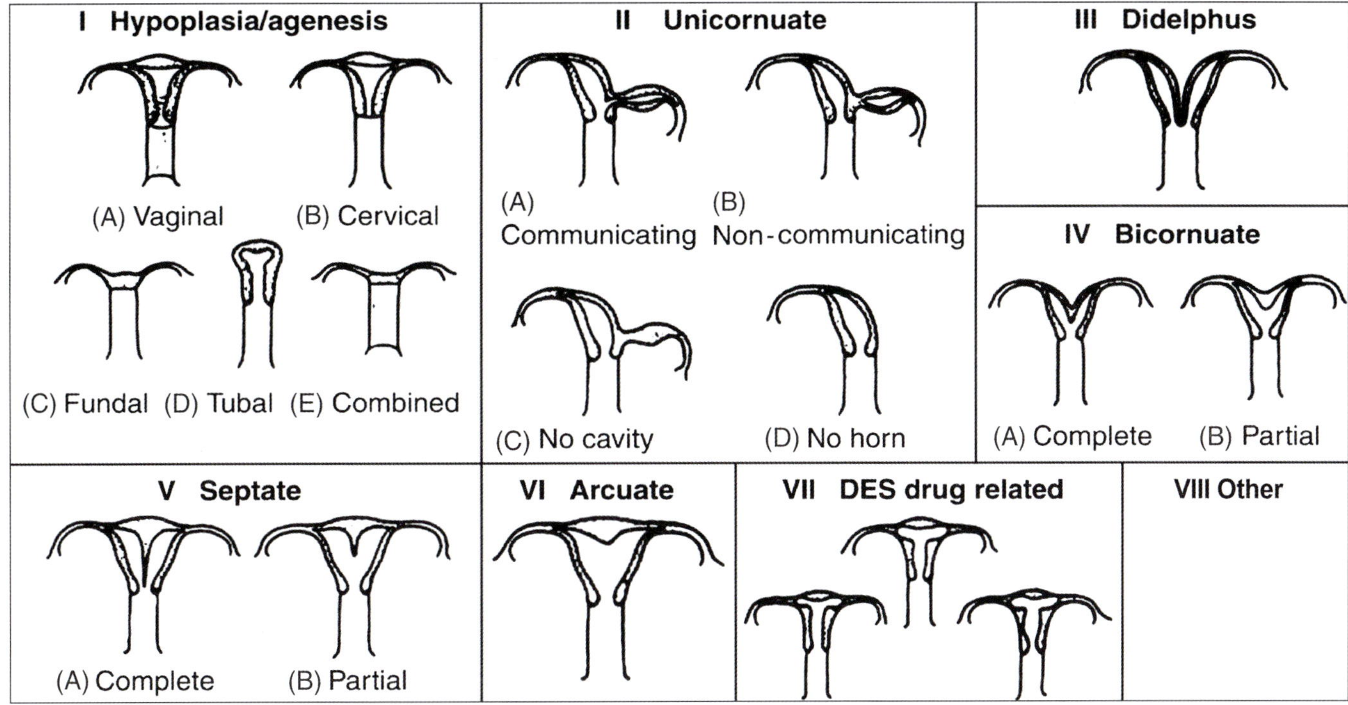

Figure 3.1 ASRM classification of müllerian anomalies [1].

the more invasive surgical diagnostic methods [9–15]. 3-D ultrasonography alone [10,11] or in combination with saline infusion [11] has been shown to have 88% and 100% accuracy respectively when compared to laparoscopy or hysteroscopy in the diagnosis of septate uterus. MRI is also a valuable tool to diagnose septate uteri [9,13–15]. Hysteroscopy, when combined with imaging of the outer uterine contour, is also an effective and less invasive method. Hysterosalpingography or hysteroscopy alone are not adequate for the diagnosis of septate uterus as these techniques only assess the endometrial cavity.

3.4.2 Partial Septate Uterus

A partial septate uterus has a septum that divides the endometrial cavity but does not involve the cervix. The septum may vary in length, width, and vascularity. Although many classification systems exist, there is no single strict universally accepted definition of septate uterus. A standard definition would be helpful in many ways to differentiate septate from arcuate uterus, an anomaly that is not considered clinically relevant, to better characterize anomalies for research studies and also to help direct which patients would benefit from surgical correction. The widely used and accepted AFS classification [1], now referred to as the ASRM classification system, provides a pictorial depiction of the septate uterus with no strict parameters to differentiate it from an arcuate or bicornuate uterus. Proposed modifications to this classification suggest that a partial septum be defined as having the central point of the septum at an acute angle and the length to be greater than 1.5 cm, which differentiates it from an arcuate uterus, which has a broad obtuse fundal indentation and a depth between 1.0 and 1.5 cm [6,16,17]. In contrast, the European Society of Human Reproduction and Embryology and the European Society for Gynecological Endoscopy (ESHRE-ESGE) define a septate uterus as having an internal indentation extending >50% of the myometrial wall thickness [4] and there is no definition of arcuate uterus. When these two classification systems are compared, ESHRE-ESGE system classifies a uterus as septate rather than normal more frequently when the ASRM criteria are used (16.9% vs 6.1% respectively, RR 2.74, 95% CI 1.6–4.72, $P<0.01$) [18]. This difference in diagnosis leads to more potentially unnecessary surgeries being performed to correct a septum when the ESHRE-ESGE criteria are used.

3.4.3 Indication for Treatment

Many women with a septate uterus experience no adverse reproductive issues. However, septate uterus has been implicated in miscarriage, recurrent pregnancy loss, as well as preterm birth and other adverse pregnancy outcomes. These may be due to reduced sensitivity to steroids, defect of VEGF receptors, uncoordinated muscle contractions, and poor vascularization with poor placentation. A recent guideline by the ASRM evaluated and graded the literature regarding reproductive outcomes with, and following correction of, a uterine septum [6]. Overall, the studies assessing this topic are limited and comprised of generally small descriptive studies. Surgical correction of a uterine septum has been associated with a reduction in miscarriage rates and improvement in live birth rates in women with a history of miscarriage or recurrent pregnancy loss. Hysteroscopic septoplasty has also been show to improve clinical pregnancy rates in cases of otherwise unexplained infertility [6]. Thus, even in a patient with primary infertility, it may be reasonable to consider surgical correction given the potential to improve fertility and reduce poor reproductive outcomes with a simple procedure having minimal invasiveness and risk.

3.4.4 Treatment

Hysteroscopic techniques for correcting uterine septum have replaced the more invasive procedures such as the Jones wedge resection or Tompkins metroplasty.

3.4.4.1 Preoperative Considerations

- Confirmation of septate configuration should be performed prior to surgery with imaging of external fundal contour as well as internal contour to avoid operating on a bicornuate uterus. If there are any concerns regarding the correct diagnosis, then intraoperative use of ultrasound or laparoscopy should be planned.
- Surgery should be performed in the early follicular phase of the cycle or with medical suppression to achieve a thin endometrial lining for better visualization.
- Preoperative hormonal manipulation to thin the endometrial lining may be achieved with combined oral contraceptive pills or progestin-only medication such as medroyprogesterone acetate or norethindrone acetate. However, these medications have not been systematically evaluated in the literature.
- Preoperative treatment with danazol or GnRH agonists have been shown to have similar rates of bleeding, complications, adhesions, and residual septa [19]. These medications have a higher rate of side effects compared to combined hormonal contraceptives or progestins, and are no longer typically used for this indication.

3.4.4.2 Intraoperative Procedure

Hysteroscopic septoplasty divides a uterine septum using a variety of instruments including cold scissors, unipolar or bipolar cautery electrodes, or laser (see Video 3.1). No tissue is removed. Hysteroscopic distending media should be dictated by the technique or energy source with saline used for cold scissors or bipolar energy and nonconducting media such as glycine for unipolar cautery.

- This procedure is typically performed in an operating room setting with sedation or general anesthesia. However, this may also be performed as an office hysteroscopic procedure with appropriate patient selection, surgeon experience, and equipment.
- Dilation of the cervical canal may be necessary depending on the size of hysteroscope utilized. If a 5 mm scope is used, then dilation is often not necessary.
- The hysteroscope is introduced through the cervical canal and advanced under direct visualization into both uterine horns, assessing the length and width of the septum as well as the presence of other pathology (Figure 3.2). Any adhesions, myomas, or polyps should be corrected during the same procedure.
- There are different approaches to septum incision and the technique utilized depends on the size of the septum. Usually the septum is incised starting at the leading edge of

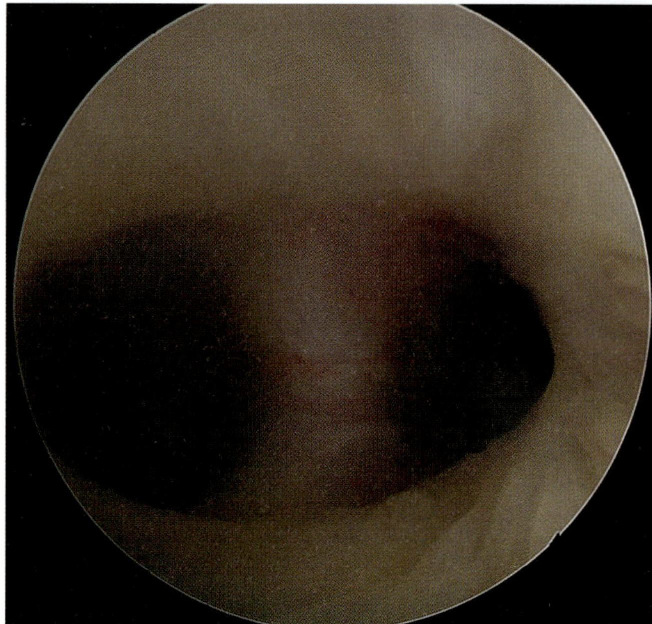

Figure 3.2 Hysteroscopic view of a uterine septum.

the septum, typically just superior to the internal cervical os. The incision is then carried up toward the fundal region. As the septum gets wider toward the fundal region, the septum may be thinned by incising the lateral edges.

- As septal tissue is predominantly fibrous, it retracts when incised and effectively disappears (Figure 3.3).
- Care should be taken to have good visualization of the cavity at all times to ensure the line of incision is in the correct plane in the middle of the septum and not deviating anteriorly or posteriorly entering the myometrium and risking uterine perforation. Continually looking at the tubal ostia and visualizing the plane connecting them can be helpful.
- If scissors are used, bleeding may occur, preventing good visualization. Cautery may be used to point cauterize the bleeding areas. Incising the septum with cautery reduces areas of bleeding, but cautery may cause damage beyond the incised area due to thermal spread.
- Although there are several instruments available to surgically correct a uterine septum, one method has not been shown to be superior to another [6]. Scissors have the advantage of more control, lack of potential thermal damage, and the ability to uncover and detect and avoid blood vessels more easily. Cautery methods may be faster, but carry the risk of damage to the tissue beyond the area incised due to thermal spread. Reproductive outcomes following septum incision with available techniques are not significantly different although there are few randomized controlled trials comparing the methods.
- It may be difficult to determine when the septum has been completely divided. The septum is traditionally incised until bleeding is encountered. However, this may not result in complete removal of the septum as, although mostly fibrous tissue, it may contain muscle

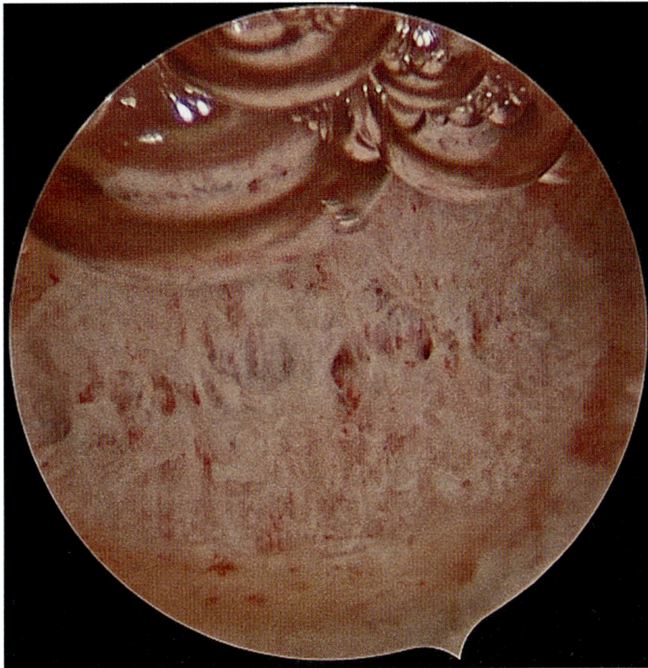

Figure 3.3 Hysteroscopic view of septum after incision. Note the septal tissue retracts and is no longer visible.

and vascular tissue. Typically visual inspection is used to judge when the septum incision is complete. The hysteroscope should pass from one tubal ostia to the other without any intervening septal tissue visible. It may be difficult to accurately assess as the cornual regions of the endometrial cavity are often closer to the outer uterine contour than the fundal region, and if the septum is taken up too far, this may lead to incising and thinning the fundal myometrium. It is often best to err on the side of not incising the tissue as far up in the midline at the fundus to create a gentle curve to the fundal contour of the endometrial cavity. Alternative methods to assess adequate septal incision include simultaneous transabdominal ultrasonography or laparoscopy. Transabdominal ultrasonography is a noninvasive method that allows visualization of both the cavity and the outer uterine contour to assess when septal incision is complete and to avoid uterine perforation. Simultaneous laparoscopy has the advantage of allowing assessment and treatment of other pelvic pathologies but is more invasive than ultrasound and because it only provides visualization of the outer uterine contour, it is better suited to avoiding uterine fundal perforation rather than assessing whether the septal resection is adequate.

- Care should be taken to avoid resection beyond the septal tissue. In addition to the obvious consequence of intraoperative uterine perforation, there is concern regarding delayed uterine perforation during subsequent pregnancy or delivery. Although rare, there have been 18 cases reported in the literature [7]. The risk of uterine rupture during a subsequent pregnancy is correlated with excessive septal incision, penetration of the myometrium,

uterine wall perforation, and excessive use of cautery or laser energy during the procedure.

3.4.4.3 Postoperative Considerations

Postoperative adhesions are a concern following any hysteroscopic procedure, but are relatively rare following septum incision with an incidence of approximately 7% [20]. Methods proposed to decrease the risk of adhesions following septum incision include placement of an intrauterine balloon or device and postoperative estrogen therapy. These methods have not been adequately evaluated in the literature and no method has been proven to be superior to another or no treatment for this indication [6]. However, postoperative adhesion prevention strategies are often utilized.

- Typically estrogen is used postoperatively for a period of 3–4 weeks. The rationale is to help proliferation of the endometrium over the recently incised septum. Doses used are typically higher than given to a postmenopausal female and include:
  - conjugated equine estrogens 0.625–1.25 mg orally twice daily;
  - 17 β-estradiol 1–2 mg orally twice daily;
  - 17 β-estradiol transdermal system 0.05–0.1 mg patch apply one to two patches, twice weekly.
- Typically a progestin is given for the last 7–10 days of the estrogen therapy using either medroxy-progesterone acetate 5–10 mg, norethindrone acetate 1–5 mg, or oral micronized progesterone 100–200 mg.
- An intrauterine balloon is often used to separate the walls of the endometrial cavity. A pediatric Foley catheter 8–12 French is ideal for this purpose with the balloon filled with 1.5–5 ml of sterile water. The Foley can be left in place for 2–7 days and then removed in the office. During this time antibiotics are usually prescribed to prevent infection.
- Assessing for postoperative adhesions can be done by saline infusion ultrasonography (SIS), hysterosalpingography, or hysteroscopy. SIS is more sensitive than hysterosalpingography for detecting intrauterine adhesions. Hysteroscopy has the advantage of diagnosing and simultaneously treating any adhesions encountered and can be performed in an office setting with no anesthesia.
- It is recommended to assess for the formation of postoperative adhesions and presence of residual septum following surgical correction, especially if the initial septum was large. This can be performed by 3-D ultrasound, SIS, hysterosalpingography, or hysteroscopy. 3-D ultrasonography can evaluate if there is a residual septal tissue present, but cannot assess for intrauterine adhesions. Hysteroscopy has the advantage of allowing for simultaneous surgical correction, but may be more invasive or involved, especially if performed in an operating room. The decision whether to correct a residual septum may be controversial. A large residual septum should be resected, especially in the setting of prior poor reproductive history. However,

there are no strict guidelines regarding the definition of, or the clinical significance of, a small residual septum or whether it should undergo additional surgical intervention. The risks and benefits of an additional surgery should be considered in the context of the clinical situation of the individual patient.

- There are a few studies evaluating the length of time from septum resection until pregnancy may be attempted. By 8 weeks postoperatively the uterine cavity has been shown to be morphologically normal and the endometrium normal as well [21]. In another study the endometrial cavity was shown to be healed in 100% of patients by 2 months postoperatively [22]. A study of 282 women who underwent in vitro fertilization (IVF) or intracytoplasmic sperm injection (ICSI) demonstrated that pregnancy and miscarriage rates were no different at <9, 10–16, or >17 weeks following septum resection [23]. While the uterine cavity appears to be healed by 2 months, there is no strict time frame recommended for when to allow a patient to conceive. Most advocate not less than 2 months following surgery.
- A vaginal delivery is feasible in women who have undergone hysteroscopic uterine septum incision.

3.4.5 Complete Uterine Septum

A complete septum extends from the fundal region down through the cervix, creating a septated or duplicated cervix. Both may be seen in combination with a longitudinal vaginal septum. A complete septate uterus may be confused with a uterus didelphys, as both have a duplicated endometrial cavity, cervix, and a longitudinal vaginal septum. The difference is that the complete septate uterus had a single uterine fundus externally while with the didephys, the two hemi-uterine horns are distinct and often very disparate. Imaging is most helpful is distinguishing these anomalies, with 3-D ultrasound and MRI providing better evaluation [14,15].

When clinical outcomes are evaluated, complete septate uterus and partial septate uterus are associated with similar rates of first-trimester losses, second-trimester losses, and term deliveries [24]. As with a partial septate uterus, many women with a complete septate uterus have no reproductive issues. Indications for surgically correcting a complete septate uterus are similar to those for a partial septate uterus. The preoperative and postoperative considerations are similar for complete and partial septate uteri. The only difference is that a complete septate uterus is often associated with a longitudinal vaginal septum. Indications for removal of the vaginal septum are dyspareunia, desire to use tampons effectively, desire for a single vaginal canal, and for religious reasons to simplify detection of menstrual blood. In theory, it may improve fertility as the chance for conception may be reduced during cycles where intercourse occurs in the hemi-vagina contralateral to the ovulating ovary. Although a longitudinal vaginal septum is not a contraindication for a vaginal delivery, it increases the risk of complications.

3.4.5.1 Intraoperative Considerations

- If there is a longitudinal vaginal septum, it is easier to resect the vaginal septum prior to resecting the uterine septum to allow better visualization and access to the cervices. Unlike the uterine septum, the vaginal septum needs to be removed to avoid redundant vaginal tissue that may prolapse out through the introitus. In addition, the vaginal septum is vascular. The septum may be removed by first separating the septum from the anterior vaginal wall starting at the introitus and progressing up to the level of the cervix. Techniques include successive bites with a clamp such as hemostat then cutting the vaginal tissue, or alternatively using a device such as a ligature, which cuts and cauterizes. The vaginal septum is then separated from the posterior vaginal wall in a similar fashion. Care should be taken to avoid damage to the adjacent rectum and bladder, which are often closer than they appear. The incisions can then be sutured in interrupted or running fashion to assure hemostasis.
- There are two approaches for correcting a complete septate uterus. One is to preserve the cervical septum and just incise the uterine portion of the septum. The other is to divide both the cervical and uterine septae at the same time. The advantage of removing just the uterine septum and preserving the cervical septum is that cervical integrity is preserved. Cervical incompetence has been described in patients following unification of the cervical portion [25]. However, it can be a more challenging procedure. The advantage of resecting both cervical and uterine septa is that it is an easier and therefore quicker procedure. The decision is usually based on the thickness of the cervical septum. Thin septae are divided, whereas thick septae are left untreated.
- The uterine septum can then be addressed. As for partial septum, the hysteroscope is passed through the cervical os, but both cervices need to be cannulated. The endometrial cavities are assessed as with a partial septate uterus. A tenaculum is placed on the anterior lip of both cervices. These hemi-cervices are typically small and tear easily.
- If the cervical septum is to be preserved, a window is made in the uterine septum at the level of the internal cervical os and then the uterine septum is incised just as with the partial septum. Making a window from one endometrial canal to the other through the septum is the challenging part of the procedure. It is best to traverse the septum at the thinnest part, which is usually around the level of the internal cervical os. To identify the correct location and facilitate making the initial incision through the septum, a uterine sound, dilator, a Crile Bozeman, or other similar long-curved clamp placed in one uterine horn serves to tent the septum (Figure 3.4) [26,27]. With the hysteroscope in the other uterine horn, the tented septum can be easily visualized and an incision is made in the septum to communicate with the other side. An alternative

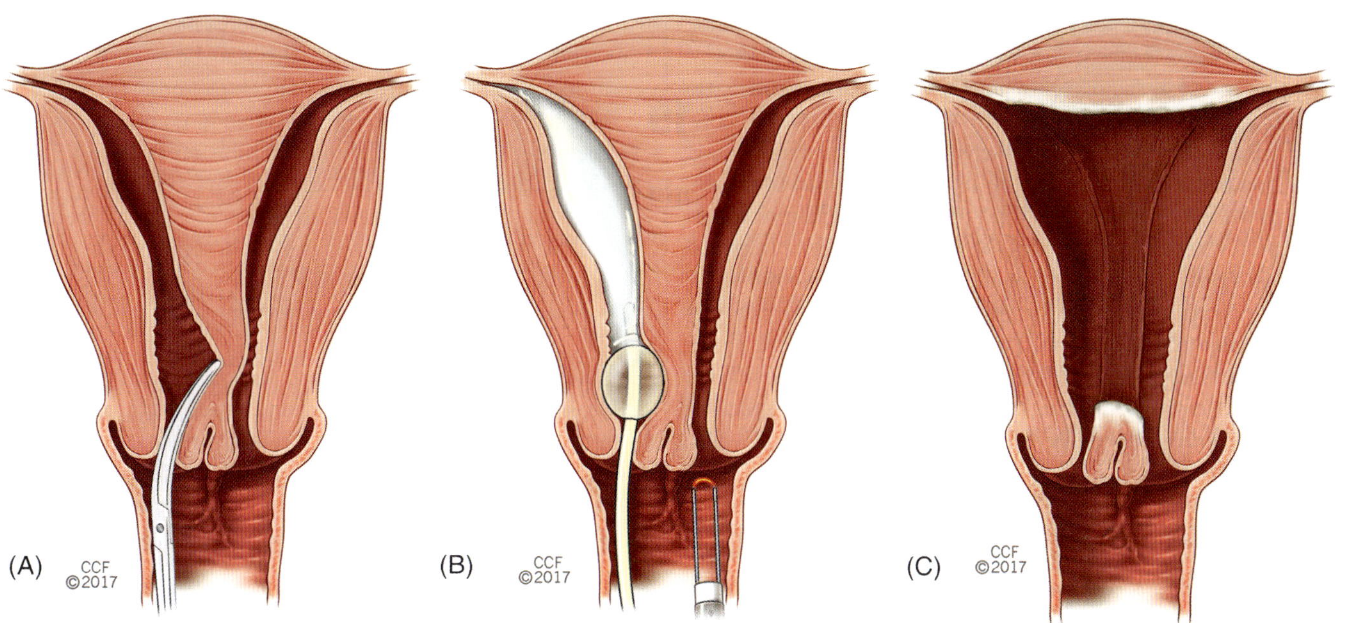

Figure 3.4 Technique for incision of complete uterine septum preserving the cervical septum. Instrument is placed in one cervical canal to tent septum to facilitate creating an opening in the septum from the other side [26].

technique is to place a pediatric Foley catheter in one uterine horn and distend it with saline while viewing with transabdominal ultrasonography. The relationship between the resectoscope and the septum is easy to see.

- Once there is a communication between the two cavities, the hysteroscopic fluid drains out through the cervix not occluded by the hysteroscope and uterine distention is lost. There are several options to occlude this outflow channel. As the external hemi-cervix is usually small, it can usually be clamped closed with an Allis or ring forceps. Alternatively a stitch can be placed through the external cervix to effectively occlude the outflow tract. Another option is to use a pediatric Foley balloon to occlude the cervical canal, especially if the Foley was used to facilitate creating an opening through the septum to join the two cavities.
- Once a window is made in the septum, the hysteroscope is advanced through the window to evaluate both cavities and confirm correct location. The septum is then incised starting at the window just created incising the septum up to the fundus just as with the partial septum. The only difference is that the procedure is performed with the hysteroscope in one of the cervical canals so the approach is not directly in the midline.
- If the cervical septum is resected at the same time as the uterine septum, the cervical septum may be cut using either heavy scissors or a monopolar electrode, or hysteroscopically using scissors or energy. The cervical septum is resected starting at the leading edge at the external cervical os and taken up through to the uterine septum and fundus utilizing the same techniques as with a partial septum. The external cervical os may be occluded using a clamp or suture if not sufficiently occluded with the hysteroscope.

3.5 Bicornuate Uterus

A bicornuate uterus is relatively common, representing 10–25% of uterine anomalies [5,14]. The bicornuate uterus results from incomplete fusion of the müllerian ducts at the level of the fundus leading to a fundal cleft and a divided endometrial cavity. The fundal cleft is variable in size and the outer contour of the uterus can appear as single fundus with a small indention or two separate uterine horns. There are various suggested criteria for distinguishing a septate from a bicornuate uterus based on the extent of the external fundal indentation but no standard objective definition. Internally the endometrial cavities can be completely separate or partially communicating at some level above the internal cervical os. Although the fundal cavity is duplicated, there is a typically a solitary cervix (bicornuate unicollis) and less commonly a duplicated cervix (bicornuate bicollis). Longitudinal vaginal septum has also been reported with a bicornuate uterus [14]. It is important to differentiate this anomaly from a partial septate uterus as the indications for surgical correction are different and mistakenly incising the "septum" of a bicornuate uterus will result in uterine perforation. Diagnosis can be made by ultrasound, 3-D ultrasound, sonohysterography, MRI, or hysteroscopy combined with imaging of the external uterine fundus [9,12,14,15]. As with a septate uterus, hysteroscopy or hysterosalpingogram alone are not effective for diagnosis as the external uterine fundus is not evaluated.

3.5.1 Indication for Treatment

Many women with a bicornuate uterus are asymptomatic and have no reproductive issues. For these individuals surgical correction is not indicated. Bicornuate uterus may be diagnosed incidentally at the time of pelvic imaging, or detected during evaluation for abnormal bleeding, expulsion of an intrauterine device (IUD), or pregnancy with an IUD in place [28]. Bicornuate uterus has been implicated in second-trimester loss, preterm delivery, and fetal malpresentation [5,28–31]. In patients with an untreated bicornuate uterus, term delivery occurred in 31%, preterm delivery in 22% with the majority occurring during 29–37 weeks, and miscarriage in 46%, the majority of which were in the first trimester [5]. The standard surgical procedure to correct a bicornuate uterus is the Strassman metroplasty. As this is an invasive and complicated procedure, efforts should be focused on confirming that the bicornuate uterus is the cause of the nonviable preterm delivery while excluding all other causes. In addition, optimizing obstetrical management should be considered before performing metroplasty. In one retrospective cohort study, cervical cerclage has been shown to result in a significant improvement in term pregnancy rates in women with a bicornuate uterus [32]. In the 26 women who had a cervical cerclage, term delivery rate was 76.2% compared to 27.3% in the 14 women who did not have a cerclage [32].

3.5.2 Treatment

Surgical treatment of a bicornuate uterus involves opening the two separate uterine horn and combining them to make a single uterus with a larger unified cavity. The most common procedure is the Strassman metroplasty.

3.5.2.1 Preoperative Considerations

- The procedure should be performed during the first portion of the follicular phase so the endometrium is thin and the patient is not pregnant. The endometrium may be thinned using combined oral contraceptive or progestins.
- Confirmation of anatomy should be confirmed with imaging. If there is concern about the anatomy then laparoscopy and hysteroscopy may be performed for confirmation prior to surgical correction.

3.5.2.2 Intraoperative Considerations

- This procedure should be performed by surgeons who have expertise or experience in uterine reconstructive procedures.
- The Strassman metroplasty has traditionally been performed at laparotomy, but with advances in laparoscopic and robotic techniques, a minimally invasive approach is feasible [33].
- Hemostasis may be facilitated by using either vasopressin injected along the proposed uterine incision lines (20 mIU in 40 ml of sterile saline 10 ml, or 5 mIU in 100 ml 20 ml). Alternatively, if performed at laparotomy, a tourniquet may be applied, preferably around the uterine vessels by placing the tourniquet through a window through the broad ligament, sparing the ovarian vessels, and left in place for no more than 2 hours. The tourniquet may be placed around the ovarian and uterine vessels, but this application occludes blood flow to the ovaries and may contribute to ovarian damage and decrease in ovarian reserve.
- An incision is then made transversely from 1 cm to the right cornua to 1 cm to the left cornua along the medial

aspects of the uterine horns and perpendicular to the cleft between the two horns. This may be made using unipolar cautery, harmonic scalpel, or knife. The incision is taken down through the endometrium and the cavity is entered and opened along this incision (Figure 3.5). Unification of the uterine cavity is performed by suturing the incision vertically, i.e., anterior to anterior and posterior to posterior. The endometrium is not sutured, but may be approximated by suturing the subendometrial layer with a running stitch of 4-0 vicryl. The myometrium may be approximated with interrupted stitches, or a continuous stitch with 0, 2-0, or 3-0 delayed absorbable suture depending on the size of the uterus and the surgical technique. This may be done in one or more layers. The serosa is then approximated with a running stitch with 4-0 delayed absorbable suture. In this manner, the cavity is unified and all myometrium is utilized and none resected.

- Microsurgical principles are utilized during this procedure, including careful tissue handling, meticulous hemostasis, and avoiding desiccation during open procedures. Adhesion barriers may be applied at the completion of the procedure.
- Intraoperative risks include bleeding, damage to the uterus and other adjacent organs, and infection.

3.5.2.3 Postoperative Considerations

- Prevention of intrauterine adhesions is a concern. There are no data addressing this issue with this procedure. As there is an incision from the anterior uterine wall extending over the fundus and extending posteriorly, adhesions may form within the cavity between these areas. A pediatric Foley can be placed at the end of the repair and the balloon inflated to separate the anterior and posterior endometrial walls, but care should be taken to not inflate to the point of placing tension on the uterine incision. Alternatively, the cavity may be packed with plain, noniodonized, ¼-inch sterile packing tape with the one end advanced through the cervical canal and into the vagina for easy removal postoperatively. Antibiotics should be continued while there is a Foley or packing in the endometrial cavity and the vagina to decrease the risk of infection. Postoperative estrogen therapy is not necessary if the woman has endogenous ovarian estrogen production, but may be utilized if the patient is hypoestrogenic either from ovarian dysfunction or due to preoperative ovarian suppression.
- The patient may attempt pregnancy after a period of 3–6 months following the surgery.
- The patient should be counseled that a C-section is advised for delivery in the future.
- The success of Strassman metroplasty has been evaluated in several small, heterogeneous observational cohort studies. Some of the studies have included patients with bicornuate, septate, and arcuate uteri in the analysis, while some have evaluated bicornaute uterus alone. Some have evaluated patients with a history of poor

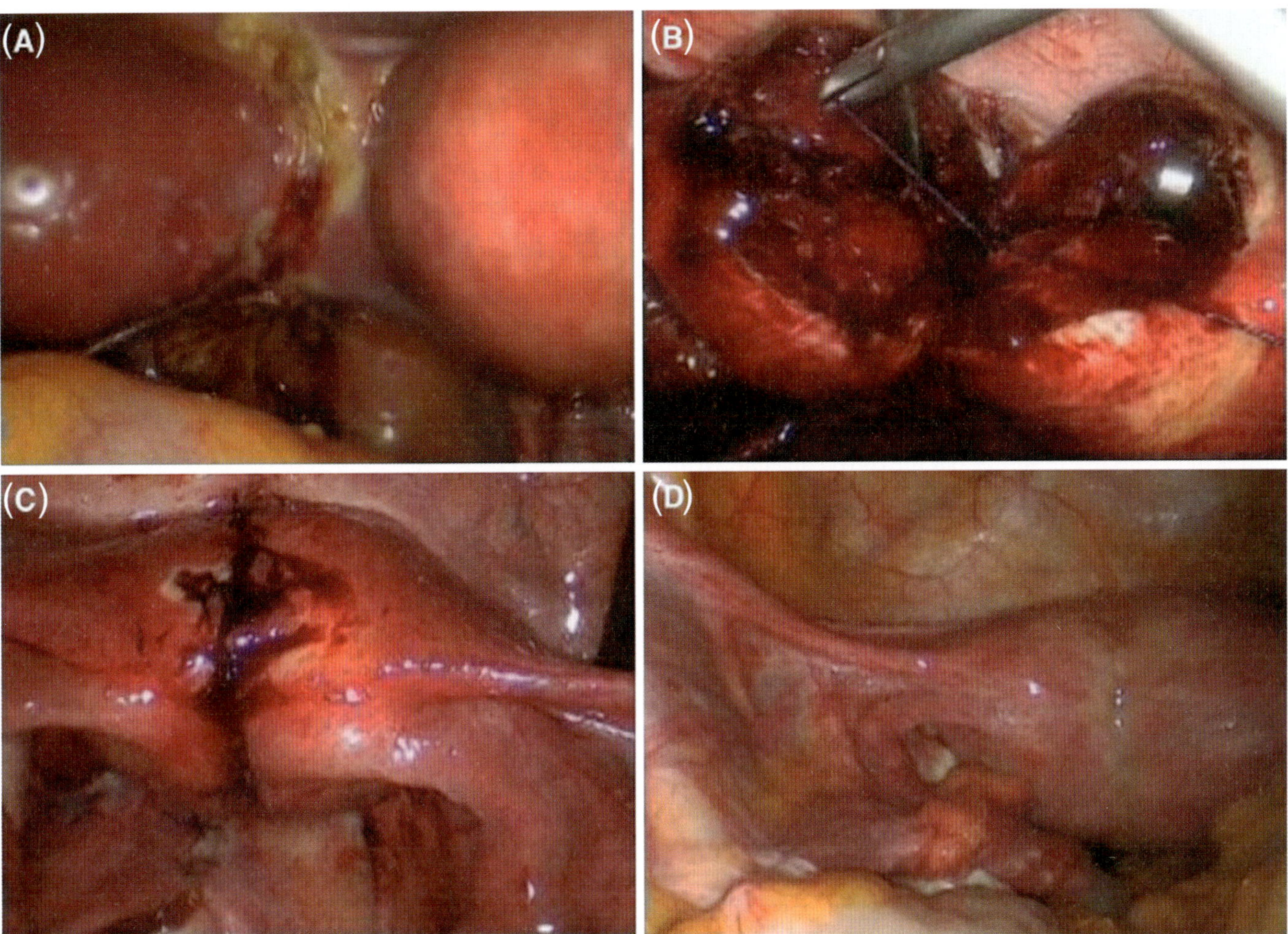

Figure 3.5 Technique for Strassman metroplasty [33]. (A) Didelphic uterus, two horns identified. (B) Both horns opened, sewing posterior uterine wall. (C) Approximation of second layer. (D) Second-look laparoscopy showing unified uterus.

reproductive outcome, while others have included patients with infertility. Most have reported a live birth rate presurgery of 0–5% and post metroplasty live birth incidence of 75–85% [33–37]. If a patient has a history of preterm birth or late miscarriage, with no other identifiable cause and which is unresponsive to medical or obstetrical management, then the patient may be a candidate for a Strassman metroplasty.

- Postoperative concerns include adhesion formation in the endometrial cavity and involving the uterine serosa and adnexa that may lead to infertility. Uterine rupture during subsequent pregnancy appears rare and has been reported in one study with 2 patients out of 89 who had undergone metroplasty for septate or bicornuate uterus [36]. However, most studies have not reported this complication [33–35,37].

3.6 Obstructed Uterine Horn

A unicornuate uterus occurs in approximately 1 in 1,000 to 1 in 5,400 women, and 74–90% of those women have an associated contralateral rudimentary uterine horn [38]. The appearance of the unicornuate uterus and associated rudimentary horn is variable and reflects the disruption of the normal development process during which the two müllerian ducts come together and fuse to form the single uterus. As such, the spectrum of observed anomalies ranges from a rudimentary uterine horn that is distinct and separate from the unicornuate uterus aligned with the opposite pelvic side wall and connected by a fibrous band, or it may be closely associated so that the outer uterine contour has an appearance similar to a bicornuate uterus. The rudimentary horn may be cavitated, with an endometrial cavity with a functional endometrium, or noncavitated. Further, the cavitated horn may communicate with the unicornuate uterus or be noncommunicating. The majority of the rudimentary horns are right sided. Approximately 30–40% are associated with an ipsilateral renal ageneis or other anomaly [38]. Although many present with dysmenorrhea during adolescence, the median age at presentation is 23 ±7.4 years, and 78% of the patients present with this condition during or after the third decade of life [38]. A noncommunicating rudimentary horn with functional endometrium may lead to pelvic pain, retrograde menstruation with development of endometriosis, pelvic adhesions, and subsequent infertility [39]. These obstructive anomalies have been identified in women with secondary infertility. This chapter addresses the diagnosis and surgical management of an obstructed uterine horn in the reproductive age woman.

3.6.1 Diagnosis

A noncommunicating cavitated rudimentary uterine horn will typically cause lateral pain during menses due to outflow obstruction. As menstruation occurs normally from the nonobstructed unicornuate uterus, symptoms are typically attributed to primary or secondary dysmenorrhea. These müllerian anomalies are rare and as such are usually not considered in the differential diagnosis, especially in a reproductive or parous woman, leading to a delay in diagnosis. With an obstructed cavitated horn, the dysmenorrhea is typically focal rather than diffuse and worsens with time. A delay in diagnosis may lead to severe complications such as development of endometriosis, hematosalpinx, ovarian endometrioma, adhesions, infertility, and chronic pelvic pain. Diagnosis may be made by ultrasound, but 3-D ultrasound or MRI is more effective in sorting out the correct anatomy. With these complex anomalies, MRI displays the anatomic relationship between the unicornuate uterus and the remnant and may identify presence of endometrium within the remnant and may be more beneficial when planning a surgical approach. It is important to review all images with a radiologist who is experienced in imaging of müllerian anomalies. Simultaneous hysteroscopy and laparoscopy is a more invasive test and is reserved for those in whom MRI could not provide diagnostic information.

3.6.2 Indication for Treatment

Noncavitated uterine remnants do not require treatment but patients should be informed of the risk for ectopic pregnancy in the blind ending tube. While cavitated remnants that communicate with the unicornuate uterus do not cause symptoms from outflow obstruction, excision may be considered due to the risk of late uterine rupture. Treatment of a cavitated noncommunicating rudimentary horn is indicated for symptom relief, prevention of endometriosis from retrograde menstruation, and the risk of uterine rupture in pregnancy. If the patient is not ready to conceive, she should be on continuous oral contraceptives in order to halt the progression of endometriosis from retrograde menstruation.

There is concern for ectopic pregnancy occurring in the fallopian tube associated with a noncavitated uterine horn remnant. The fallopian tube and fimbriae usually develop normally on the side of the remnant horn and pick up and fertilization of an oocyte can occur with migration of sperm from the patent unicornuate uterus and fallopian tube [40]. Pregnancies have also been reported in cavitated noncommunicating uterine horns with a patent fallopian tube [41]. These pregnancies are associated with a 50% rupture rate due to late diagnosis, but fetal survival may be as high as 15% [41].

Prophylactic removal of the fallopian tube ipsilateral to the remnant is not routine, although the patient should be counseled regarding the low risk of ectopic pregnancy in this situation and for some a prophylactic salpingectomy may be indicated. In the case of an ectopic pregnancy diagnosed in the ipsilateral fallopian tube to the remnant, the fallopian tube should be removed due to the risk of recurrence unless effective contraception is subsequently utilized.

3.6.3 Treatment

The mainstay of treatment for a symptomatic cavitated noncommunicating uterine horn is surgical removal. As discussed earlier, it does not have to be removed until the patient is ready to conceive as long as amenorrhea is induced with continuous hormonal suppression.

3.6.3.1 Preoperative Considerations

- Surgery should be performed in the follicular phase of the menstrual cycle to avoid the presence of corpus luteum or pregnancy.
- If not performed in the follicular phase then agents to prevent ovulation and thin the endometrium, such as norethindrone acetate, should be used or combined with oral contraceptive pills.
- To plan the removal of the symptomatic blind uterine horn, MRI is very helpful to determine the extent and the location of the connection between the rudimentary horn and the unicornuate uterus.
- Two things need to be assessed:
  - The location of the rudimentary horn in relation to the unicornuate uterus. The horn may be located far away connected by a fibrous band or be an integral part of the unicornuate uterus. If the rudimentary horn is closely associated with the unicornuate uterus, and especially if the connection is low down at the level of the cervix, then the bladder needs to be dissected off the cervix to identify the inferior portion of the horn and any vessels supplying the structure. The location of the vessels supplying the rudimentary horn is variable; unlike the uterine vessels, it is easily identified with a normal uterus.
  - The degree of retrograde menstruation and presence of endometriosis or ovarian endometrioma and hematosalpinx. As the diagnosis of these anomalies is often delayed, there may be significant adhesions and endometriosis present when there is retrograde menstruation. In these cases the endometriosis is often limited to the side of the rudimentary horn and obstruction. Surgical planning involves assessing the extent of disease, consideration regarding feasibility of salvage of the ipsilateral ovary, and laparoscopic access and possible need for laparotomy.

In addition, it is important to establish if there is renal agenesis and whether there is a ureter on the side of the rudimentary uterine horn, as removal of the horn may require dissection in the ipsilateral retroperitoneum. The placement of ureteral stents may be considered in these cases.

3.6.3.2 Intraoperative Considerations

The principles and the technique for performing the procedure at laparotomy or laparoscopy are the same. For a laparoscopic approach, the operative port placement depends on the anatomy and operator preference. For laparotomy, the incision should be planned to accommodate the surgery effectively while considering the medical and surgical history of the patient.

- If the procedure is performed laparoscopically, then a uterine manipulator is helpful to move the uterus, identify the endometrial cavity, and identify a perforation into the cavity. If the procedure is performed at laparotomy, a uterine manipulator may still be beneficial. Alternatively, the cavity may be identified by injecting dye (methylene glue) via a 22-guage needle placed through the myometrium from the external fundus and into the endometrial cavity.
- Once the abdominal cavity is entered, the anatomy of the uterus and rudimentary horn is assessed. Evaluation by inspection should be correlated with the anatomy, as defined by imaging. The size and location are typically variable. An assessment of the ovaries, fallopian tubes, and other pathologies should be performed. If there is endometriosis present, then it is often better to resect or ablate prior to addressing the rudimentary horn.
- Resection of rudimentary horn distant from unicornuate uterus (Figures 3.6–3.10).
  - In this situation, the rudimentary horn is isolated and relatively easy to access. The ureter is identified if present. The round ligament is cauterized and transected and the retroperitoneum opened lateral to the ovary. The anterior broad ligament is opened and the bladder taken down off the uterus as necessary. The utero-ovarian ligament is isolated and then cauterized and transected. If the ovary is normal, there is no need to remove it and the ovarian blood supply should be preserved. The rudimentary horn is then dissected from the surrounding tissue and vessels are identified and cauterized and transected as necessary. The vessels supplying the remnant uterine horn are not in a particular standard location and there may be many. The fibrous band is then transected.
  - The ipsilateral fallopian tube is removed with the uterine remnant or after it has been resected to avoid a subsequent ectopic pregnancy.
- Resection of rudimentary horn closely associated with the unicornuate uterus (Figures 3.11–3.14).
  - If the rudimentary horn is closely associated with the unicornuate uterus, then resection of the horn should be performed with the thought of avoiding damage to the unicornuate uterus. In some cases this will involve preserving enough myometrium from the rudimentary horn to reinforce the defect created by resecting it from the unicornuate uterus. The entire endometrial cavity of the remnant and any associated adenomyosis should be removed.
  - The procedure starts in the same fashion as a distant rudimentary horn. The horn is isolated from the lateral pelvic wall, round and utero-ovarian ligaments, and feeding vessels. Again, there is no need to remove a normal ovary and its blood supply should be preserved. If the ipsilateral ureter is present then it should be identified. Once the horn is isolated, an incision is made on the myometrium a few centimeters from the connection between the

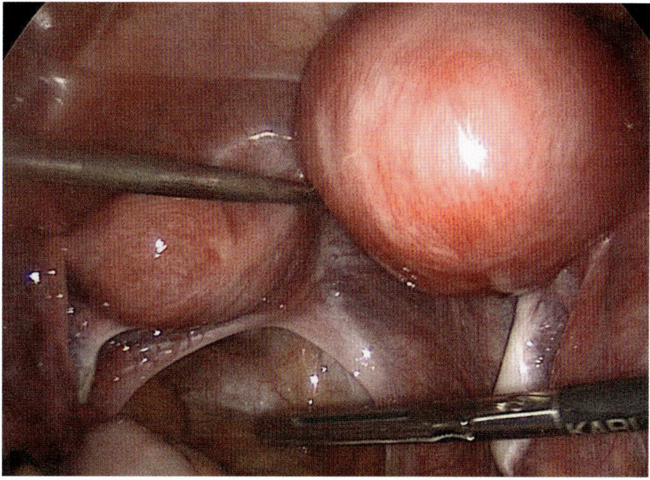

Figure 3.6 Blind separate right uterine horn.

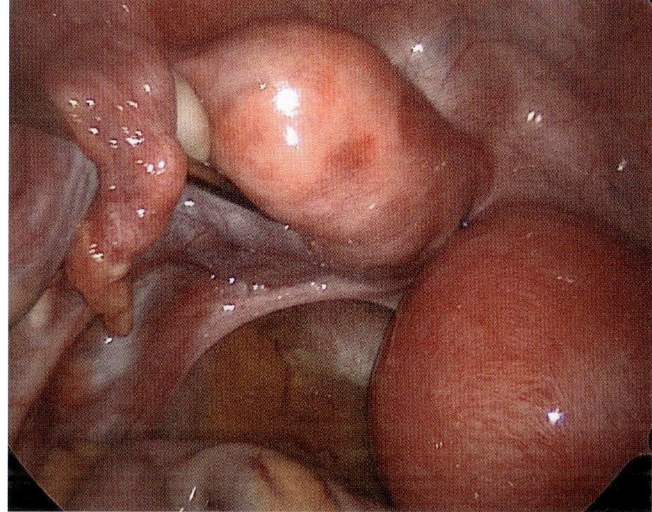

Figure 3.7 Normal left unicornuate uterus.

two. The endometrial cavity of the rudimentary horn is then resected from the surrounding myometrium using monopolar or bipolar cautery, harmonic scalpel, or a knife. Any endometrium or adenomyosis, typically having a yellowish or brownish hue, should also be resected along with the specimen to be excised. If endometrial tissue or adenomyosis is left behind, then the patient will continue to experience pain with menstruation at this site. Care should be taken to avoid entering the endometrial cavity of the unicornuate uterus. This can be identified by palpation of the specimen, palpation of the uterine manipulator within the endometrial canal, or by dye staining the endometrium. Once the rudimentary horn is removed, the myometrial defect is closed by reinforcing the area with the redundant myometrium left from the resection of the rudimentary horn. This should be reinforced in a few layers using 3-0 or 2-0 delayed absorbable suture in an interrupted or continuous fashion depending on the size of the defect. If the endometrial cavity of the unicornuate

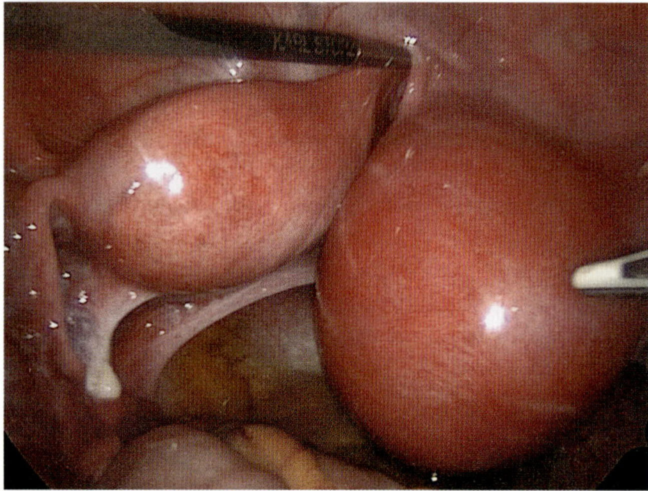

Figure 3.8 Fibrous band between right rudimentary uterine horn and left unicornuate uterus.

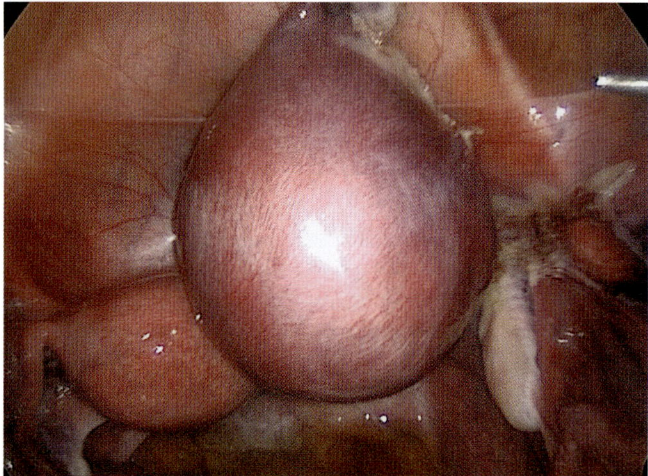

Figure 3.9 Isolating right rudimentary uterine horn.

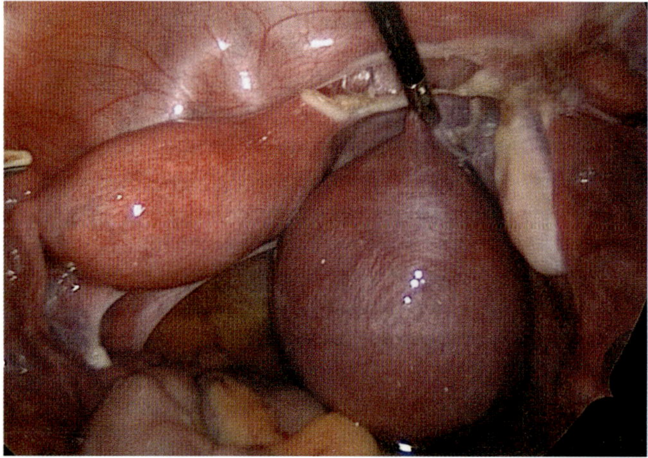

Figure 3.10 Right separate rudimentary horn resected.

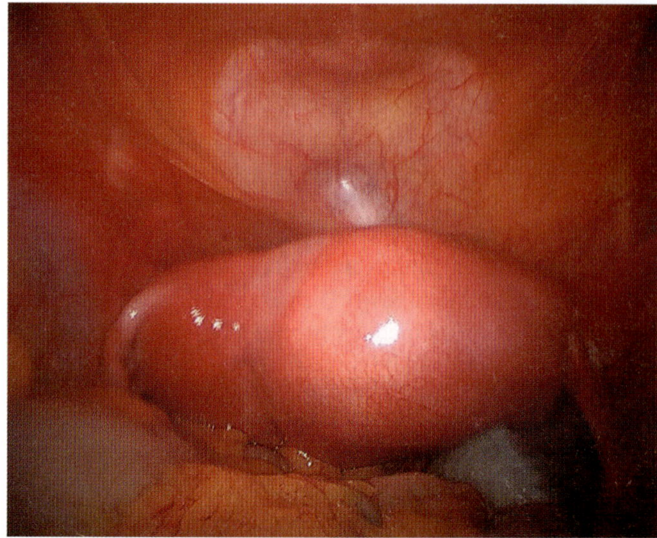

Figure 3.11 Blind uterine horn closely associated with unicornuate uterus.

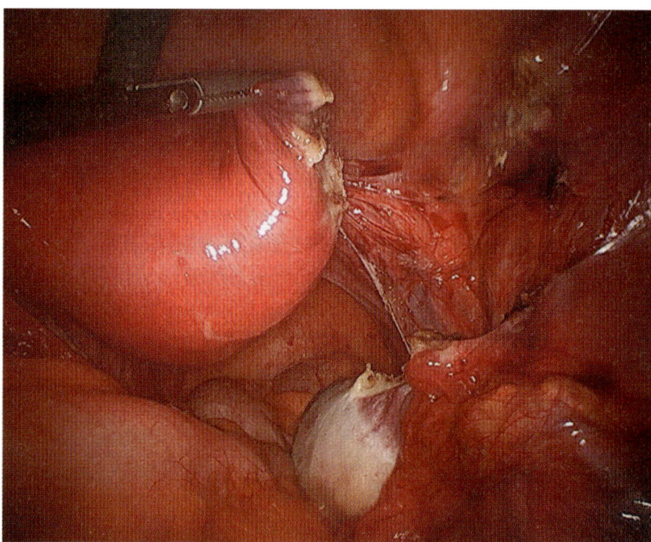

Figure 3.12 Separating the rudimentary horn from right pelvic side wall transecting round ligament and utero-ovarian anastomosis.

uterus is entered, it needs to be closed and the myometrium closed in several layers over the defect reinforcing with the excess myometrium left from the resection of the rudimentary horn. Bleeding is usually not significant as the blood supply to the rudimentary horn is occluded prior to resection from the unicornuate uterus. Dilute vasopressin may be injected within the myometrium to reduce bleeding. A tourniquet is usually not helpful in these anomalies.

- The ipsilateral fallopian tube is removed with the uterine remnant or after it has been resected to avoid a subsequent ectopic pregnancy.
- Resection of rudimentary horn with hematosalpinx or endometrioma.
  - Retrograde menstruation from outflow obstruction may lead to severe endometriosis with ovarian endometriomas, hematosalpinges, and significant pelvic and bowel adhesions. These cases can be very challenging as it is often difficult to identify the anatomy. If the endometrioma is very large and the anatomy is very distorted, the ovary may have to be removed en bloc with the fallopian tube and rudimentary uterine

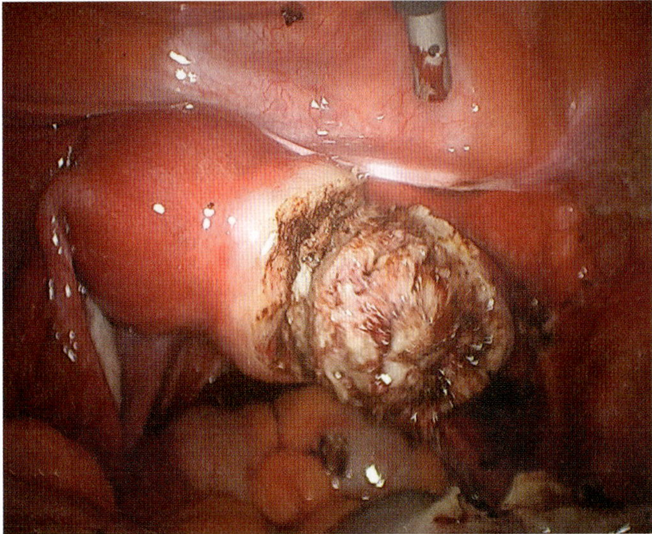

Figure 3.13 Resecting blind right uterine horn with adenomyosis from normal left hemiuterus leaving some myometrium from the rudimentary horn.

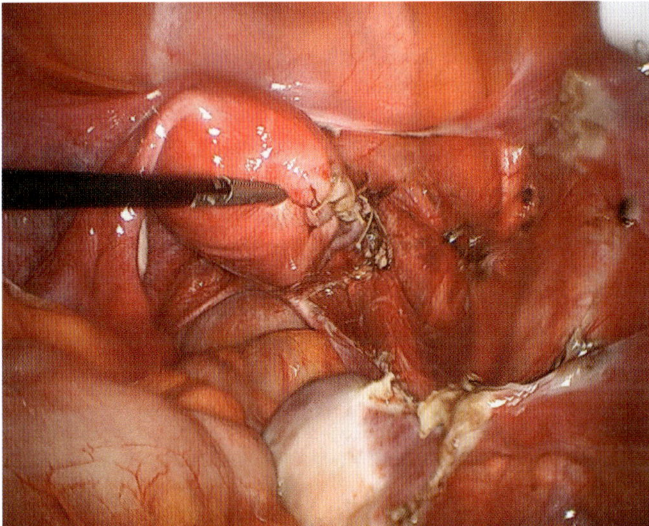

Figure 3.14 Closing the defect in several layers using myometrium from right rudimentary horn to reinforce the defect on left hemiuterus. Note the right fallopian tube has been removed.

horn. However, the endometriosis in these cases has been shown to spontaneously regress following relief of the outflow obstruction [39]. Consideration may therefore be given to excision of the rudimentary horn only as above, especially in young patients.

3.6.3.3 Postoperative Considerations

- The patient needs to be counseled regarding the likelihood of conception based on the evaluation of the pelvis at the time of the surgery including presence of endometriosis and pelvic adhesions.
- If IVF is necessary, elective single embryo transfer should be performed and residual embryos cryopreserved.
- Patients should be followed closely during pregnancy as a unicornuate uterus is associated with an increased risk of preterm delivery, reported in one study to be 16.2% [5].

- If the uterine horn is closely associated with the unicornuate uterus, or if the endometrial cavity of the unicornuate uterus is entered during the procedure, the patient should be counseled to delivery by C-section to reduce the risk of uterine rupture.

3.7 Conclusion

Uterine anomalies may go undetected and are associated with uncomplicated reproductive history. Some are detected incidentally during pelvic imaging or during an evaluation for infertility or reproductive issues. However, they may also cause symptoms such as pain, infertility, and reproductive loss. It is important to know when it is appropriate to surgically correct these anomalies as well as how to accomplish the surgery in order to best preserve reproductive function.

References

1. American Fertility Society. Classification of adnexal adhesions, distal tubal occlusion, tubal occlusion secondary to tubal ligation, tubal pregnancies, Mullerian anomalies, and intrauterine adhesions. *Fertil Steril.* 1988;49:944–55.

2. Acien P, Acien MI. The history of female genital tract malformation classifications and proposal of an updated system. *Hum Reprod Update.* 2011;17:693–705.

3. Oppelt P, Renner SP, Brucker S, et al. The VCUAM (Vagina Cervix Uterus Adnex-associated Malformation) classification: a new classification for genital malformations. *Fertil Steril.* 2005; 84:1493–7.

4. Grimbizis GF, Gordts S, Di Spiezio Sardo A, et al. The ESHRE/ESGE consensus on the classification of female genital tract congenital anomalies. *Hum Reprod.* 2013;28:2032–44.

5. Grimbizis GF, Camus M, Tarlatzis BC, Bontis JN, Delvoy P. Clinical implications of uterine malformations and hysteroscopic treatment results. *Hum Reprod Update.* 2001;7:161–74.

6. Practice Committee of the American Society for Reproductive Medicine. Uterine septum: a guideline. *Fertil Steril.* 2016;106:530–40.

7. Valle RF, Ekpo GE. Hysteroscopic metroplasty for the septate uterus: review and meta-analysis. *J Min Invas Gynecol.* 2013;20:22–42.

8. Dabirashrafi H, Bahadori M, Mohammad K, et al. Septate uterus: new idea on the histologic features of the septum in this abnormal uterus. *Am J Obstet Gynecol.* 1995;172:105–7.

9. Pellerito JS, McCarthy SM, Doyle MB, Glickman MG, DeCherney AH. Diagnosis of uterine anomalies: relative accuracy of MR imaging, endovaginal sonography, and hysterosalpingography. *Radiology.* 1992;183:795–800.

10. Moini A, Mohammadi S, Hosseini R, Eslami B, Ahmadi F. Accuracy of 3-dimensional sonography for diagnosis and classification of congenital uterine anomalies. *J Ultrasound Med.* 2013;32:923–7.

11. Ludwin A, Pityński K, Ludwin I, Banas T, Knafel A. Two- and three-dimensional ultrasonography and sonohysterography versus hysteroscopy with laparoscopy in the differential diagnosis of septate, bicornuate, and arcuate uteri. *J Minim Invasive Gynecol.* 2013;20:90–9.

12. Alborzi S, Dehbashi S, Parsanezhad ME. Differential diagnosis of septate and bicornuate uterus by sonohysterography eliminates the need for laparoscopy. *Fertil Steril.* 2002;78:176–8.

13. Mueller GC, Hussain HK, Smith YR, et al. Müllerian duct anomalies: comparison of MRI diagnosis and clinical diagnosis. *AJR Am J Roentgenol.* 2007;189:1294–302.

14. Troiano RN, McCarthy SM. Müllerian duct anomalies: imaging and clinical issues. *Radiology.* 2004;233:19–34.

15. Bermejo C, Martínez Ten P, Cantarero R, et al. Three-dimensional ultrasound in the diagnosis of Müllerian duct anomalies and concordance with magnetic resonance imaging. *Ultrasound Obstet Gynecol.* 2010;35:593–601.

16. Woelfer B, Salim R, Banerjee S, Elson J, Regan L, Jurkovic D. Reproductive outcomes in women with congenital uterine anomalies detected by three-dimensional ultrasound screening. *Obstet Gynecol.* 2001;98:1099–103.

17. Ludwin A, Ludwin I, Banas T, Knafel A, Miedzyblocki M, Basta A. Diagnostic accuracy of sonohysterography, hysterosalpingography and diagnostic hysteroscopy in diagnosis of arcuate, septate and bicornuate uterus. *J Obstet Gynaecol Res.* 2011;37:178–86.

18. Ludwin A, Ludwin I. Comparison of the ESHRE-ESGE and ASRM classifications of Müllerian duct anomalies in everyday practice. *Hum Reprod.* 2015;30:569–80.

19. Fedele L, Bianchi S, Gruft L, Bigatti G, Busacca M. Danazol versus a gonadotropin-releasing hormone agonist as preoperative preparation for hysteroscopic metroplasty. *Fertil Steril.* 1996;65:186–8.

20. March CM. Asherman's syndrome. *Sem Reprod Med.* 2011;29:83–94.

21. Candiani GB, Vercellini P, Fedele L, Carinelli SG, Merlo D, Arcaini L. Repair of the uterine cavity after hysteroscopic septal incision. *Fertil Steril.* 1990;54:991–4.

22. Yang JH, Chen MJ, Chen CD, Chen SU, Ho HN, Yang YS. Optimal waiting period for subsequent fertility treatment after various hysteroscopic surgeries. *Fertil Steril.* 2013;99:2092–6.e3.

23. Berkkanoglu M, Isikoglu M, Arici F, Ozgur K. What is the best time to perform intracytoplasmic sperm injection/embryo transfer cycle after hysteroscopic surgery for an incomplete uterine septum? *Fertil Steril.* 2008;90:2112–5.

24. Zlopasa G, Skrablin S, Kalafatić D, Banović V, Lesin J. Uterine anomalies and pregnancy outcome following resectoscope metroplasty. *Int J Gynaecol Obstet.* 2007;98:129–33.

25. Grynberg M, Gervaise A, Faivre E, Deffieux X, Frydman R, Fernandez H. Treatment of twenty-two patients with complete uterine and vaginal septum. *J Minim Invasive Gynecol.* 2012;19:34–9.

26. Wang J, Xu K, Lin J, Chen X. Hysteroscopic septum resection of complete septate uterus with cervical duplication, sparing the double cervix in patients with recurrent spontaneous abortions or infertility. *Fertil Steril.* 2009;91:2643–9.

27. Rock JA, Roberts CP, Hesla JS. Hysteroscopic metroplasty of the Class Va uterus with preservation of the cervical septum. *Fertil Steril.* 1999;72:942–5.

28. Rackow BW, Arici A. Reproductive performance of women with müllerian anomalies. *Curr Opin Obstet Gynecol.* 2007;19(3):229–37.

29. Raga F, Bauset C, Remohi J, Bonilla-Musoles F, Simon C, Pellicer A. Reproductive impact of congenital müllerian anomalies. *Hum Reprod.* 1997;12:2277–81.

30. Hua M, Odibo A, Longman R, Macones G, Roehl K, Cahill A. Congenital uterine anomalies and adverse pregnancy outcomes. *AJOG.* 2011;6:558.

31. Acien P. Reproductive performance of women with uterine malformations. *Hum Reprod.* 1993;8:122–6.

32. Yassaee F, Mostafaee L. The role of cervical cerclage in pregnancy outcome in women with uterine anomaly. *J Reprod Infertil.* 2011;12(4):277–9.

33. Alborzi S, Asefjah H, Amini M, et al. Laparoscopic metroplasty in bicornuate and didelphic uteri: feasibility and outcome. *Arch Gynecol Obstet.* 2015;291:1167–71.

34. Papp Z, Mezei G, Gavai M, Hupuczi P, Urbancsek J. Reproductive performance after transabdominal metroplasty: a review of 157 cases. *J Reprod Med.* 2006;51:544–52.

35. Rechberger T, Monist M, Bartuzi A. Clinical effectiveness of Strassman operation in the treatment of bicornuate uterus. *Ginekol Pol.* 2009;80:88–92.

36. Ayhan A, Yucel I, Tuncer ZS, Kisnisci HA. Reproductive performance after conventional metroplasty: an evaluation of 102 cases. *Fertil Steril.* 1992;57:1194–6.

37. Helm P, Sorensen SS. Pregnancy outcome after metroplasty in women with mullerian anomalies. *Acta Obstet Gynecol Scand.* 1988;67:215–18.

38. Jayasinghe Y, Rane A, Stalewski H et al. The presentation and early diagnosis of the rudimentary uterine horn. *Obstet Gynecol.* 2005;105:1456–67.

39. Sanfilippo JS, Wakim NG, Schikler KN et al. Endometriosis in association with uterine anomaly. *Am J Obstet Gynecol.* 1986;154:39–43.

40. Nahum GG, Stanislaw H, McMahon C. Preventing ectopic pregnancies:how often does transperitoneal transmigration of sperm occur in effecting human pregnancy? *BJOG.* 2004;111:706–14.

41. Nahum GG. Rudimentary uterine horn pregnancy: the 20th-century worldwide experience of 588 cases. *J Reprod Med.* 2002;47:151–63.

Chapter 4

Ovarian Surgery with a Focus on Reproduction

Nigel Pereira and Samantha M. Pfeifer

4.1 Introduction

Ovarian surgery is an important skill in the field of reproductive surgery. The ovary is a unique organ essential to female reproduction. It contains a finite number of eggs that decreases over time and cannot be regenerated. The challenge of ovarian surgery is to maintain or enhance reproductive function by preserving the eggs and minimizing trauma and the risk of adhesive disease. The most common ovarian procedure performed is ovarian cystectomy, with treatment of ovarian torsion, and laparoscopic ovarian drilling is done less frequently.

4.2 Ovarian Cystectomy

Ovarian cysts are one of most commonly encountered gynecologic pathologies in women of reproductive age. Women may choose to undergo surgical management of ovarian cysts to reduce symptoms such as pain or prevent potential complications such as rupture. In such scenarios, the benefits of surgical management must be weighed against the risks of nonvital reduction of ovarian tissue or reserve [1].

4.2.1 Differential Diagnosis and Diagnosis

Ovarian cysts can be divided into two main categories: functional (physiologic) or pathologic. Functional cysts refer to ovarian cysts that develop as part of the normal ovulatory function of the ovary. Thus, depending on where a woman is during her menstrual cycle, functional cysts can include follicular or corpus luteum cysts. Almost all women will develop a functional cyst during their lifetime. Theca-lutein cysts are also functional cysts that can develop during pregnancy as a result of exposure to increasing levels of human chorionic gonadotropin. In contrast, pathologic ovarian cysts are not related to the menstrual cycle and are further subcategorized into benign or malignant entities [2,3] (Box 4.1). In women of reproductive age, almost all ovarian cysts are either functional or benign. The overall incidence of malignant transformation of benign ovarian cysts in premenopausal women is 1:1,000, increasing to 3:1,000 after age 50 [3].

Any evaluation of ovarian cysts must include a detailed medical history and thorough physical examination. Specific attention must be paid to any family history of endometriosis, breast or ovarian cancer. Symptoms such as nonspecific bloating, abdominal distention, unintentional weight loss, early satiety, or increased urinary frequency should alert the physician to the possibility of malignancy. Personal symptoms suggestive of endometriosis should also be accounted for. The physical examination should include palpation of the cervical, supraclavicular, axillary, and groin lymph nodes [2]. In addition to an abdominal and pelvic examination, a rectovaginal examination should be considered in women with symptoms of endometriosis. Of note, pelvic examination has a very poor sensitivity (<50%) for detecting ovarian cysts [4], and this is further reduced in patients with a body mass index (BMI) >30 kg/m^2.

Transvaginal ultrasonography (TVUS) of the pelvis is perhaps the single most effective modality for diagnosing ovarian cysts [3]. Ultrasonographic examination assesses the size, laterality, and characteristics of the cysts, including the presence or absence of papillary excrescences, septations, mural nodules, or pelvic ascites [2]. Benign cysts are typically simple in appearance, have thin smooth walls, lack solid components, are septated, demonstrate internal blood flow on color Doppler, and do not have a definitive cut-off for size [5]. Common benign

---

Box 4.1 Differential Diagnosis of Pathologic Ovarian Cysts

Benign ovarian
Endometrioma
Tubo-ovarian abscess
Mature cystic teratoma
Serous cystadenoma
Mucinous cystadenoma

Benign nonovarian
Paratubal cyst
Hydrosalpinx
Tubo-ovarian abscess
Diverticular abscess
Appendiceal abscess
Pelvic kidney

Malignant ovarian
Epithelial cancer
Germ cell tumor
Sex-cord or stromal cell tumor
Metastatic cancer

Malignant nonovarian
Gastrointestinal cancer
Metastatic cancer

Table 4.1 Diagnostic Accuracy of Transvaginal Ultrasonography of the Pelvis to Diagnose Ovarian Cysts

Diagnosis	Sensitivity (%)	Specificity (%)	Positive Predictive Value (%)	Negative Predictive Value (%)
Functional ovarian cyst	94	92	83	97
Endometrioma	78	88	78	88
Mature cystic teratoma	80	92	63	97

cysts encountered in reproductive age women include simple cysts, serous or mucinous cystadenomas, endometriomas, and mature cystic teratomas. Endometriomas are characterized by ground glass echogenicity and one to four compartments without any papillary structures [6]. Mature cystic teratomas are associated with fat-fluid levels, diffuse high-amplitude echoes, and shadowing echogenicity [7]. Table 4.1 summarizes the sensitivity, specificity, positive predictive value, and negative predictive value of TVUS to diagnose functional ovarian cysts, endometriomas, and mature cystic teratomas [8].

Other imaging modalities such as computed tomography (CT) or magnetic resonance imaging (MRI) are not indicated for the initial evaluation of ovarian cysts but may occasionally be helpful to further elucidate the nature of the cysts after ultrasound imaging [2]. Finally, laboratory testing for tumor markers such as CA-125, lactate dehydrogenase, alpha-fetoprotein, or human chorionic gonadotropin are generally not indicated when ovarian cysts are simple, thin-walled, and <5 cm in diameter [9].

4.2.2 Management of Ovarian Cysts – See Ovarian Cystectomy Video

Simple ovarian cysts measuring <5 cm can be managed expectantly, as more than two-thirds of these cysts will regress spontaneously within three menstrual cycles [5,10]. Alternatively, combined oral contraceptives may be used to facilitate cyst regression and prevent new cyst formation [11]. Other medical adjuncts that can be used include progestins, gonadotropin-releasing hormone agonists, and antagonists. Ovarian cysts persisting after expectant and medical management may not be functional.

The decision to proceed with surgery depends on a number of factors. If the cyst is benign in appearance by imaging and asymptomatic, then expectant management may be pursued with close follow-up. If the cyst is >10 cm then surgery is typically recommended. Other considerations for surgical intervention include symptom relief and reducing the possibility of ovarian torsion, which would place the patient at risk of losing the ovary. Any cyst that has features indicative of malignancy by imaging and/or laboratory results should be addressed surgically by an appropriately trained surgeon.

Laparoscopic ovarian cystectomy is the preferred approach for the surgical management of benign ovarian cysts (see Video 4.1). Three 5 mm ports are commonly used – one in the umbilicus, one in the right lower quadrant, and one in the left lower quadrant. A 10 mm umbilical port may be used to facilitate removal of the specimen. The ovary is stabilized using graspers and dilute vasopressin (20 U/100 ml of injectable saline) is injected between the ovarian cortex and cyst wall to help develop the surgical plane by hydrodissection (Figure 4.1). This step also serves to aid hemostasis and minimize the need for electrocautery with potential thermal injury to the cortex.

The ovarian cortex is incised down to the cyst wall with cold scissors, unipolar energy, or laser on the anti-mesenteric aspect to avoid damaging the vascular hilum (Figure 4.2). The incision should also be placed to avoid damage to the fimbria. It is important to preserve all of the ovarian cortex, even if it is stretched thin across a large cyst so as not to diminish the ovarian reserve. An elliptical incision that allows a portion of the ovarian cortex to be removed with the cyst should never be used. The incision should be made large enough to allow removal of the cyst from the ovary. It is important to recognize that all the oocytes are located in the ovarian cortex so care should be taken to avoid damage to the cortex by using excessive cautery or energy. After the cyst is identified, the cyst wall is separated from the ovary using a combination of blunt and sharp dissection. Blunt dissection is preferred and is easy if one is in the correct plane. Blunt dissection is accomplished by applying traction and countertraction with grasping instruments on the ovarian tissue and/or cyst wall to facilitate peeling the ovarian cortex off the cyst wall (Figures 4.3 and 4.4). Hydrodissection may also be helpful. Other techniques include grasping the ovarian cortex and rolling the instrument to roll the cortex off the cyst like a sardine can.

Care should be taken to keep the cyst intact in most cases (Figure 4.5). If the cyst ruptures, then trying to contain the cyst fluid in the posterior cul-de-sac is important, especially with a dermoid cyst, as postoperative chemical peritonitis may result. Copious irrigation with saline or lactated ringers should be used to remove all the cyst fluid. The fatty cyst contents will float to the surface of the irrigation used and are fairly easy to identify. Performing cystectomy within a containment system has been advocated to avoid spilling the cyst contents. In cases of very large cysts, decompressing the cyst by aspirating its contents can facilitate separating the cyst from the ovary. Simple cysts can be aspirated with a laparoscopic injection needle. To aspirate the thick contents of an endometrioma or dermoid cyst, a 5 mm opening is created to allow the suction or irrigator tube to be inserted into the cyst cavity.

Once the cyst is excised from the ovary (Figure 4.6), it is placed into an endoscopic retrieval bag through a 10 mm umbilical port and decompressed by suction aspiration if still intact (Figure 4.7). Enlarging the lateral ports requires facial closure with the risk of entrapment of the ilio-inguinal or ilio-hypogastric nerves leading to postoperative pain. Incisional

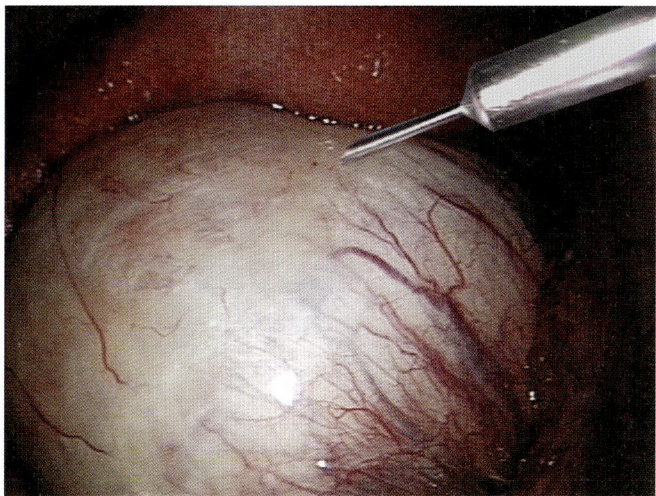

Figure 4.1 Dilute vasopressin is injected between the ovarian cortex and cyst wall.

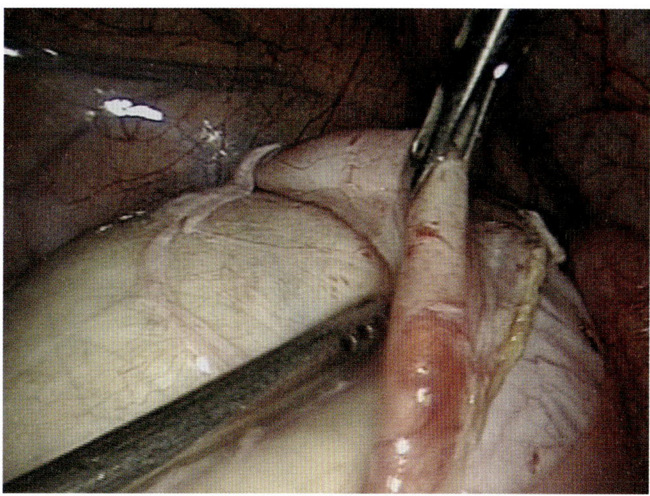

Figure 4.4 The edge of the cortex is everted and held with the Allis as blunt dissection continues.

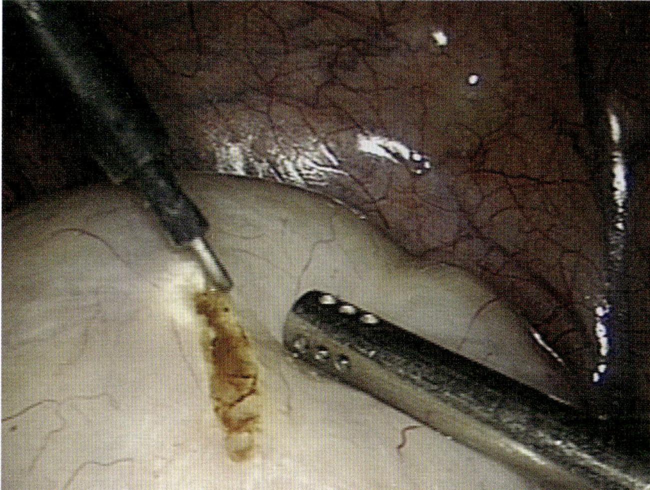

Figure 4.2 The ovarian cortex is incised with the unipolar hook to the cyst wall.

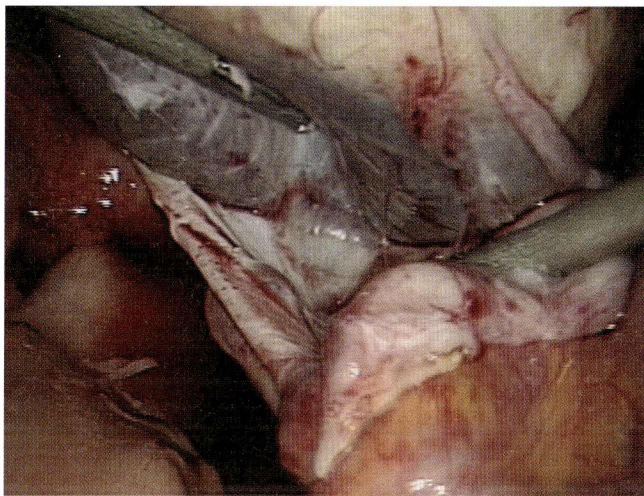

Figure 4.5 The last attachments between the cyst and the ovary are bluntly separated.

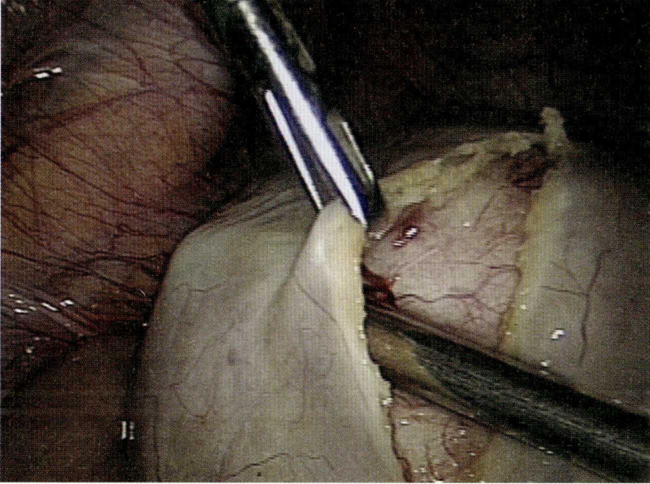

Figure 4.3 One edge of the ovarian cortex is grasped with an Allis while another Allis grasper is used to bluntly develop the plane between the ovary and the cyst.

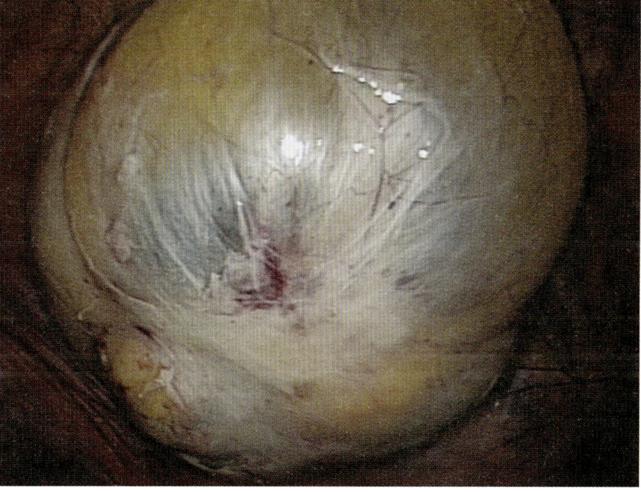

Figure 4.6 The cyst has been removed intact.

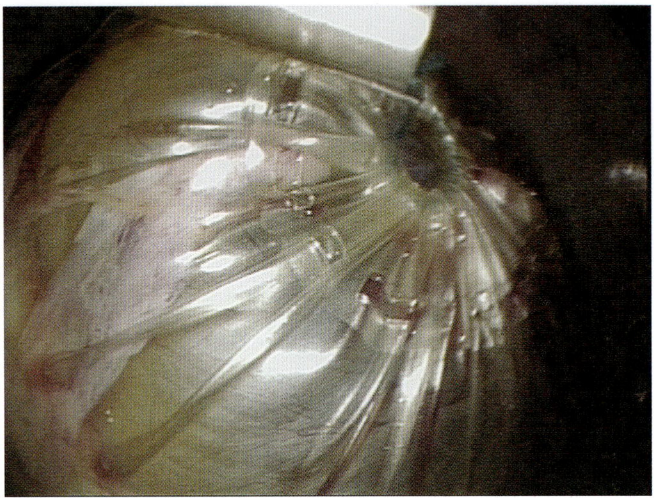

Figure 4.7 The cyst is placed in an endo-catch bag for removal through the 10 mm umbilical port.

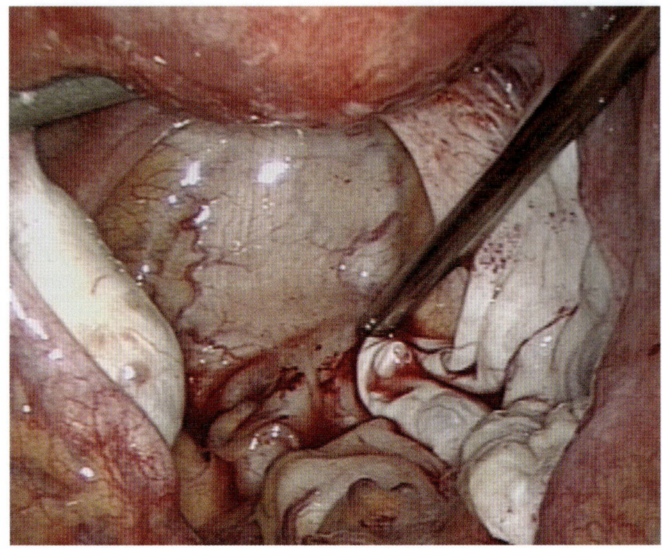

Figure 4.8 After complete hemostasis is assured, the ovary is left to heal without suturing.

hernias are also more common in lateral ports. A suprapubic port is a cosmetic location for tissue removal and the incision can be easily enlarged if needed. Care should be taken to avoid damage to the bladder.

It is important to achieve excellent hemostasis following ovarian cystectomy. Excessive cautery of the ovary to achieve hemostasis post cystectomy risks damage to the ovary with diminished ovarian reserve and should be avoided. A key step during the cystectomy is to find the correct plane between the cyst and ovary. Dissecting in the correct plane during cyst removal decreases bleeding and ovarian trauma. Alternatively cauterizing bleeding vessels encountered during cystectomy can minimize need for use of cautery following removal.

To achieve hemostasis, bipolar energy is preferred over monopolar energy as it causes less thermal damage [1]. Coagulation should be used as sparingly as possible. If there is significant bleeding, typically seen at the base of the ovarian defect, then suture may be utilized to achieve hemostasis rather than cautery. If suture is used, then whole defect does not need to be closed, but only enough to achieve hemostasis. Studies that assessed AMH levels with bipolar cautery versus suturing for cystectomy yielded conflicting results with some studies showing a greater decline with cautery while others found no difference. Various hemostatic agents may also be utilized to limit the use of cautery.

The ovarian defect heals well without suture closure (Figure 4.8). Consideration should be given to reducing post-operative adhesion formation. Interceed is an absorbable sheet of oxidized regenerated cellulose which can be wrapped around the ovary at the completion of the case. It has been shown to result in significantly fewer adhesions and more adhesion-free ovaries following cystectomy for endometriomas. Unlike other anti-adhesion barriers such as Seprafilm and Gore-Tex, it is easy to apply laparoscopically, adheres without sutures, and is not permanent. Its limitation is that complete hemostasis must be achieved since blood renders the device ineffective. Icodextrin 4% solution is the only product approved by the FDA for adhesion prevention by laparoscopy. Unfortunately, it is minimally effective at best and may cause labial edema for several days as well as rare case reports of icodextrin leading to disseminated intravascular coagulopathy, pleural effusions, and peritoneal fibrosis.

While the cystectomy procedure described earlier applies to cysts of all types, cystectomy for endometriomas may be more difficult as the cyst wall tends to be adherent to the ovary. In addition, dense ovarian adhesions to the uterus, bowel, and pelvic sidewall further increase the level of difficulty and surgical risk. For these reasons laparoscopic drainage with electrocoagulation or laser ablation of the cyst wall has been advocated as a simpler technique. A Cochrane review and subsequent meta-analysis indicated that laparoscopic cystectomy is associated with decreased recurrence of the endometrioma, decreased recurrence of pain, as well as higher rates of spontaneous conception compared to laparoscopic drainage and ablation of the cyst wall. However, cystectomy is associated with a significant reduction in ovarian reserve. The reduction is greater with bilateral and larger cysts. It is also greater for endometriomas compared to other benign cysts. This is likely due to endometriomas being more adherent to the ovary as mentioned above. As a result, significantly more normal ovarian tissue is removed during cystectomy for endometriomas vs non-endometrioma cysts. Furthermore, ovaries containing endometriomas have been shown to have a lower follicle density compared with non-endometrioma cysts. In fact, preoperative anti-müllerian hormone levels are lower in women with endometriomas. Another reason to favor cystectomy for endometriomas is to obtain a definitive tissue diagnosis as women with endometriomas have a significantly higher incidence of ovarian cancer, especially clear cell and endometrioid adenocarcinomas.

Some have proposed removing endometriomas prior to in vitro fertilization (IVF) to improve the ovarian response to stimulation, facilitate follicle monitoring and oocyte retrieval, reduce the risk of abscess if the endometrioma is punctured with the aspiration needle, and to avoid contamination of the endometrioma contents with follicular fluid. However, systematic reviews found no significant differences in the number of mature oocytes or the clinical pregnancy rates whether the endometriomas were removed or not prior to IVF. The practice guidelines from the American Society for Reproductive Medicine and the European Society of Human Reproductive and Embryology state that endometriomas, particularly those with a mean diameter below 4 cm, should not be systematically removed before IVF.

4.3 Ovarian Torsion

Ovarian torsion is defined as the partial or complete twisting of an ovary about its vascular axis [34]. Torsion of an ovary may occur in isolation, or with the fallopian tube, i.e., adnexal torsion. Impairment of blood flow to the ovary can occur during torsion, thereby increasing the risk of transient or even permanent ischemic damage; thus, ovarian torsion is considered a gynecologic emergency that requires prompt recognition and treatment [34].

Ovarian torsion may occur in girls or women of any age; however, it is much more common in women of reproductive age [35]. Studies indicate that the annual prevalence of ovarian torsion may range between 2.7% and 6% [34,35]. However, the true incidence of ovarian torsion is unknown because its definitive diagnosis is made in an operating room, and patients who are misdiagnosed may not be brought to the operating room [35]. Torsion occurs commonly with moderately enlarged ovaries, most often due to cysts [35]. In general, ovaries with benign cysts such as follicular cysts, cystic teratomas, or cystadenomas that are >5 cm increase the risk for torsion [36,37]. Interestingly, more than 50% of premenarchal patients with ovarian torsion will have normal-appearing ovaries [38]. Torsion of the right ovary is more common than the left ovary due to the hypermobility of the cecum and ileum on the right in comparison to the fixed sigmoid colon on the left [34]. Also, the right mesosalpinx and utero-ovarian ligament is thought to be longer than the left, predisposing the ovary and fallopian tube to torsion. Pregnancy, particularly after assisted reproductive techniques (ART) involving ovarian stimulation, increases the risk and recurrence of ovarian torsion [39]. Additional risk factors for ovarian torsion include paratubal cysts and tubal ligation [37].

4.3.1 Diagnosis

The diagnosis of ovarian torsion is a clinical diagnosis made by assessing the patient's history, physical exam, laboratory findings, and imaging. One cannot rely purely on imaging to make the diagnosis. Definitive diagnosis is made at laparoscopy. If the diagnosis is missed, the ovary may necrose with loss of function and potential negative implications for fertility. The key is to make the diagnosis before the blood flow to the ovary is compromised.

During torsion, compression of the ovarian vessels occurs. Venous and lymphatic outflow are compromised first, resulting in ovarian edema, which can then compress the thicker arterial walls [34]. Once arterial blood flow is compromised, the ovary undergoes progressive ischemia leading to possible necrosis, hemorrhage, infection, or peritonitis [34]. Depending on the progression of ovarian edema and/or ischemia, patients may present with acute unilateral abdominal or pelvic pain. The pain may radiate to the lumbo-sacral region and increase in duration and severity [37]. In up to 70% of the cases, ovarian torsion may be associated with nausea and vomiting [40]. Fever, flank pain, or generalized peritoneal signs can be present in a subset of patients. Given these signs and symptoms, a broad differential diagnosis, including appendicitis, nephrolithiasis, pelvic inflammatory disease, ectopic pregnancy, mesenteric lymphadenitis, and gastroenteritis, should be considered [35].

Physical examination may reveal a low-grade fever and mild tachycardia [35,37]. A unilateral palpable and tender adnexal mass may indicate ovarian torsion [37]. Abdominal exam may reveal peritoneal signs such as guarding or rebound. Most routine laboratory tests are normal, although occasional leukocytosis or sterile pyuria may be noted. Pelvic ultrasound is the most commonly utilized diagnostic modality in patients with suspected ovarian torsion [34,41]. Unilateral ovarian enlargement is generally seen in most patients with ovarian torsion. Other ultrasonographic signs include ovarian edema, pelvic-free fluid, and peripheral follicles in the torsed ovary [35,41]. The affected ovary may deviate to the side of the torsion and can lie medially and above its usual location [35]. Doppler imaging is frequently used in conjunction with US to improve its diagnostic accuracy. Studies have indicated that ovarian enlargement and the absence of ovarian venous Doppler flow are perhaps the most precise indicators of ovarian torsion [41,42]. Yet, most patients with ovarian torsion actually have ovarian enlargement with arterial and venous Doppler flow [41]. Thus, normal Doppler flow studies cannot exclude the diagnosis of ovarian torsion as they may reflect partial torsion [37,41]. It is also important to note that the diagnostic accuracy of US and Doppler imaging is largely affected by the ultrasound operator as well [42]. The use of CT and MRI have also been described in some special circumstances [43].

4.3.2 Treatment Considerations and Methods

Definitive diagnosis and treatment of ovarian torsion is achieved surgically, most often via laparoscopy [37]. Concomitant treatment of ovarian pathology should be considered during the definitive treatment of ovarian torsion as well.

4.3.2.1 Preoperative Considerations

Age, preservation of future fertility, and evidence of concomitant ovarian disease are important factors that should be considered prior to the surgical management of ovarian torsion [34]. In general, surgical treatments for ovarian torsion belong to two main categories – conservative and radical [35,37]. Conservative treatment entails de-torsing the ovary, followed by aspiration or removal of any ovarian cysts. In contrast, radical treatment involves oophorectomy with or without salpingectomy. As expected, conservative treatment strategies are favored in women of reproductive age.

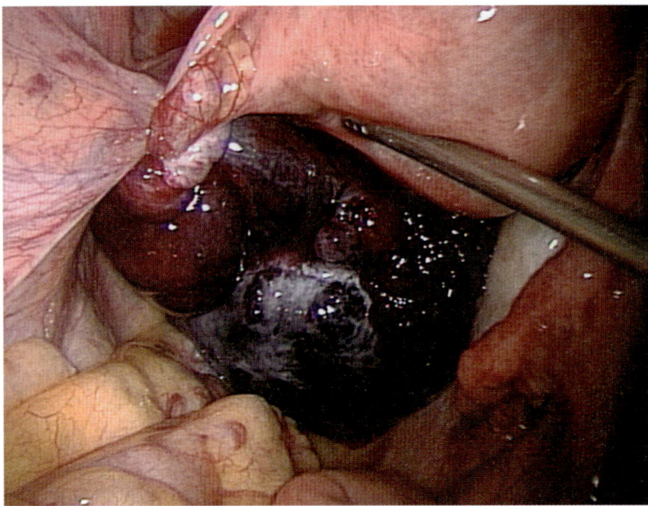

Figure 4.9 The left fallopian tube and ovary are torsed.

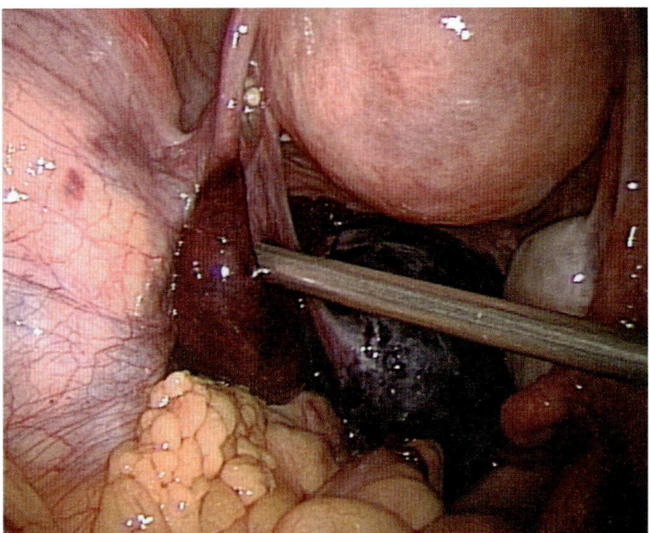

Figure 4.10 Detorsion was performed with the suction-irrigator probe.

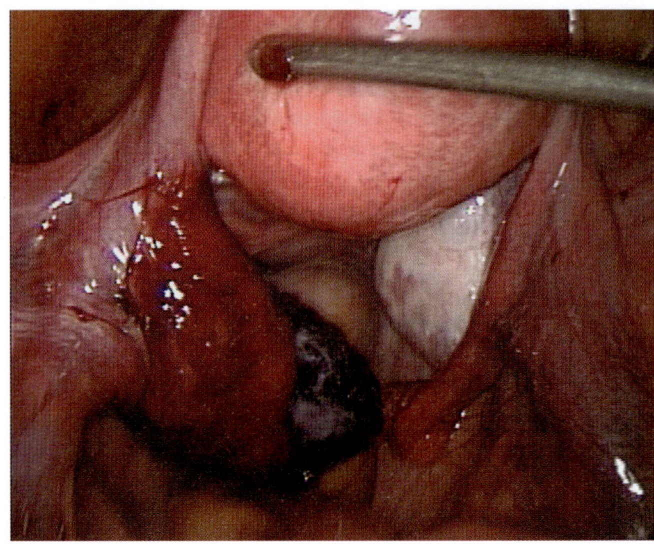

Figure 4.11 The adnexa is beginning to reperfuse.

Thus, most providers concur that ovarian cystectomy at the time of de-torsion is the ideal treatment strategy, albeit loss of tissue planes may occur due to ovarian edema [34,35,37].

Ovarian de-torsion with oophoropexy is the treatment of choice in the pediatric population [48,49], and such surgeries can be accomplished with a single-site approach [50]. Oophoropexy can be accomplished by shortening the utero-ovarian ligament, or fixing the ovary to the uterosacral ligament or pelvic sidewall using permanent suture. One concern about fixing the ovary to the uterosacral ligament is the risk of dyspareunia following the surgery. Care should be taken to avoid injury to the ureter if the ovary is affixed to the side wall.

In any pediatric, adolescent, or reproductive age female every effort should be made to preserve the ovary. In a postmenopausal woman with ovarian torsion, oophorectomy with or without salpingectomy is a reasonable option [34].

4.3.2.3 Postoperative Considerations

Long-term outcomes after laparoscopic de-torsion have been well documented [51]. In one study of 102 de-torsions, ultrasonography showed normal follicular development in 93% of patients after de-torsion. Furthermore, oocytes were successfully retrieved from the untwisted ovaries of infertile patients requiring ART at a later date [52]. A second-look laparoscopy is generally unwarranted after laparoscopic de-torsion given that ovarian structure and function are preserved in 88–100% of patients who are assessed at a later date [37].

4.4 Laparoscopic Ovarian Diathermy

Laparoscopic ovarian diathermy or drilling (LOD) is a surgical technique used to promote ovulation in women with polycystic ovary syndrome (PCOS) who remain anovulatory in response to oral ovulation-inducing agents such as clomiphene citrate and letrozole, with or without the addition of metformin. It has advantages over the alternative gonadotropin therapy, as will be discussed later. The procedure is a less invasive version of the ovarian wedge resection, which was the method to treat

4.3.2.2 Intraoperative Procedure

Treatment of ovarian torsion begins with diagnostic laparoscopy. Depending on the size of ovary and surgeon preference, a conventional three-port setup (5–12 mm) can be used. Simple untwisting of an ovary and/or fallopian tube can be performed with a blunt probe or nontraumatic laparoscopic instrument (Figures 4.9–4.11). Although initial adopters of this technique were concerned about the theoretical risk of dislodging and spreading vascular emboli [35,37], studies have shown that the risk of pulmonary emboli associated with de-torsion is approximately 0.2% [45]. Of note, many gynecologic surgeons may be dissuaded from simply untwisting a dark-blue or necrotic-looking ovary. However, most ischemic-appearing ovaries are found to have normal appearance, Doppler flow, and follicular development 6 weeks after de-torsion [34,46]. Although simple de-torsion with ovarian cyst aspiration has been described in some situations, such a management strategy is associated with higher rate of recurrence and surgical re-intervention [47].

anovulatory infertility from 1930 until the availability of clomiphene citrate and gonadotropins in the late 1960s. In the ovarian wedge resection, one-third to half of each ovary was removed by laparotomy. Ovulation was restored in approximately 80–90% of women and pregnancy rates following the procedure ranged from 25% to almost 90% [53]. However, postoperative adnexal adhesions were discovered to be a significant issue and responsible for failure to conceive, even when microsurgical techniques were utilized [53]. Ovarian atrophy was also described following ovarian wedge resection [53].

With the advent of laparoscopic surgery, techniques were described that intended to emulate the effect of ovarian wedge resection by a minimally invasive approach. Compared to laparotomy, the laparoscopic approach meant less invasive surgery with quicker recovery and a decreased risk of postoperative adhesions. As with bilateral ovarian wedge resection, the mechanism by which LOD restores ovulation in women with PCOS is still not clearly understood. The prevailing theory is that excision, or thermal destruction, of the ovarian stromal component leads to a reduction in ovarian androgens, restoring the normal estrogen and testosterone intraovarian milieu, enabling resumption of follicular maturation and ovulation. LOD has been shown to significantly reduce circulating levels of testosterone, LH, inhibin, and AMH as well as normalization of the ovarian morphology with improved blood flow to the ovary.

4.4.1 Technique

There is no consensus regarding the optimal technique for LOD as far as the number of punctures, energy settings, duration of application, and whether one or both ovaries should be treated. While LOD has been performed using multiple punch biopsies, bipolar cautery, and various lases, the unipolar needle remains the most common modality (see Video 4.2).

The ovary may be stabilized by grasping the utero-ovarian ligament. The punctures should be evenly distributed over the ovary avoiding the hilum, which could cause bleeding and/or compromise of the ovarian vascular supply. Care should be taken not to damage the fallopian tubes. The needle should be applied to the surface of the ovary at a right angle and current applied after the needle is in the stroma to avoid damage to the oocytes in the cortex (Figure 4.12).

The effect of LOD depends on the energy delivered to the ovary and the depth of penetration. The energy (Joules) is measured by the power (Watts) × duration (seconds) × number of punctures. In the literature, the amount of thermal energy delivered via monopolar cautery has ranged from 3 to 25 punctures per ovary at 30–400 W [54–58]. Four to five punctures with 40 W of current for 4 seconds seems to strike a good balance between high efficacy and minimizing excessive cautery [54] (Figure 4.13). Again, it remains to be determined whether one or both ovaries should be treated as some studies showed comparable results.

4.4.2 Complications

Incidence of periovarian adhesions following LOD is hard to determine as few studies have performed second-look

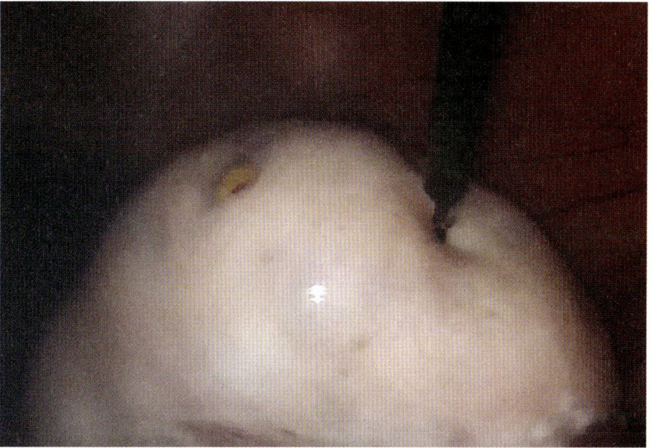

Figure 4.12 The enlarged polycystic ovary is placed on the retroverted uterus for support and the unipolar needle is inserted perpendicular to the ovarian surface. Current is then applied. Four to five punctures are made in each ovary.

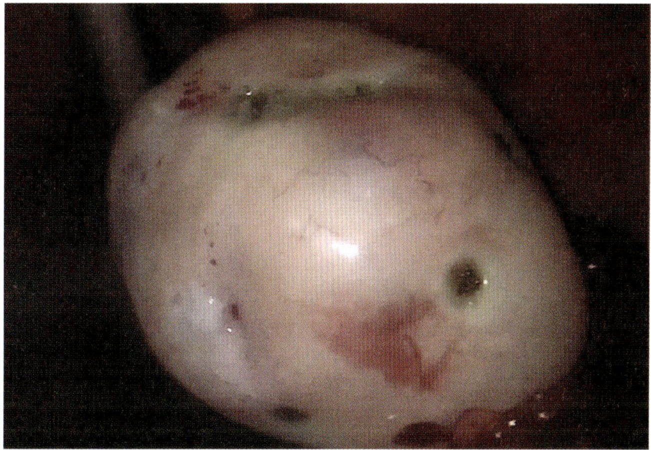

Figure 4.13 This is the appearance following the drilling procedure.

laparoscopy to evaluate. In those studies the incidence of adhesions ranged from 0% to 100% [56,60,61]. However, the adhesions were not clinically significant and were independent of the number of punctures. The application of Interceed as an anti-adhesion barrier was of no benefit.

Damage to ovarian reserve is a concern when surgery is performed on the ovary. This has also been a concern with LOD. Only a single case report of ovarian atrophy was published following excessively high-energy application (eight penetrations at 400 W for 5 seconds) [58]. Subsequent studies have evaluated ovarian reserve markers pre- and post-LOD [63]. These studies measured ovarian reserve by many different markers including day 3 FSH, Clomiphene citrate challenge test, inhibin B, antral follicle count, and anti-müllerian hormone. Overall no concrete evidence for decreased ovarian reserve or premature ovarian failure was noted. Antral follicle count was significantly decreased following LOD, but was still significantly higher when compared to normal ovulatory controls. The reduction in anti-müllerian hormone, inhibin, and antral follicle count should be viewed as normalization from the PCOS condition and not as diminished ovarian reserve.

4.4.3 Outcomes

The effectiveness of LOD in achieving spontaneous pregnancies has been evaluated in several case studies. In one meta-analysis, ovulation and pregnancy rates in women with PCOS treated with LOD by electrocautery was reported to be 79.7% (95% CI 78–87%) and 63.6% (95% CI 44–62%) [64], respectively. LOD has been compared to gonadotropin therapy in women with PCOS who are resistant to CC. A meta-analysis of randomized controlled trials and a separate systematic review observed that ovulation and pregnancy rates after LOD are similar to those achieved by treatment with gonadotropin therapy but the risk of multiple pregnancy is significantly lower with LOD compared to gonadotropin treatment (1% versus 16%). In addition, the cost to achieve a live birth was significantly lower with LOD and that didn't include the costs for managing multiple pregnancies or ovarian hyperstimulation, or the fact that some spontaneous pregnancies occurred in the LOD group following closure of the study. The benefits do not appear to be transient, with decreases in LH, testosterone, androstenedione, and PCO-appearing ovaries maintained for over 3 years. There are limited data showing that LOD may also reduce the increased miscarriage rates associated with PCOS as well as improve acne and hirsutism.

4.5 Conclusions

Ovarian surgery should be done only after careful consideration of the indications. The goal should include preservation of the ovary and reproductive function. Every effort should be made to minimize trauma to the ovary and preserve all of the ovarian cortex. Care should be taken to minimize use of cautery and if cautery is used, bipolar is the preferred modality. Ovarian torsion is a clinical diagnosis and making the diagnosis before the ovary is no longer viable is important. LOD is a modality that can facilitate ovulation in women with PCOS who are CC-resistant.

References

1. Legendre G, Catala L, Morinière C, et al. Relationship between ovarian cysts and infertility: what surgery and when? *Fertil Steril.* 2014;101(3):608–14.

2. American College of Obstetricians and Gynecologists. ACOG Practice Bulletin. Management of adnexal masses. *Obstet Gynecol.* 2007;110(1):201–14.

3. Royal College of Obstetricians and Gynaecologists, British Society of Gynaecologic Endoscopists. Management of suspected ovarian masses in premenopausal women. RCOG Green-Top Guideline; 2011:62. www.rcog.org.uk/en/guidelines-research-services/guidelines/gtg62/ (accessed on October 12, 2016).

4. Padilla LA, Radosevich DM, Milad MP. Accuracy of the pelvic examination in detecting adnexal masses. *Obstet Gynecol.* 2000;96(4):593–8.

5. American College of Obstetricians and Gynecologists Practice Bulletin. Evaluation and management of adnexal masses. Number 174, November 2016.

6. Van Holsbeke C, Van Calster B, Guerriero S, et al. Endometriomas: their ultrasound characteristics. *Ultrasound Obstet Gynecol.* 2010;35(6):730–40.

7. Patel MD, Feldstein VA, Lipson SD, Chen DC, Filly RA. Cystic teratomas of the ovary: diagnostic value of sonography. *AJR Am J Roentgenol.* 1998;171(4):1061–5.

8. Theodoridis TD, Zepiridis L, Mikos T, et al. Comparison of diagnostic accuracy of transvaginal ultrasound with laparoscopy in the management of patients with adnexal masses. *Arch Gynecol Obstet.* 2009;280(5):767–73.

9. Im SS, Gordon AN, Buttin BM, et al. Validation of referral guidelines for women with pelvic masses. *Obstet Gynecol.* 2005;105(1):35–41.

10. MacKenna A, Fabres C, Alam V, Morales V. Clinical management of functional ovarian cysts: a prospective and randomized study. *Hum Reprod.* 2000;15(12):2567–9.

11. Grimes DA, Jones LB, Lopez LM, Schulz KF. Oral contraceptives for functional ovarian cysts. *Cochrane Database Syst Rev.* 2014;(4):CD006134.

12. Hart RJ, Hickey M, Maouris P, Buckett W. Excisional surgery versus ablative surgery for ovarian endometriomata. *Cochrane Database Syst Rev.* 2008;(2):CD004992.

13. Psaroudakis D, Hirsch M, Davis C. Review of the management of ovarian endometriosis: paradigm shift towards conservative approaches. *Curr Opin Obstet Gynecol.* 2014;26(4):266–74.

14. Dan H, Limin F. Laparoscopic ovarian cystectomy versus fenestration/coagulation or laser vaporization for the treatment of endometriomas: a meta-analysis of randomized controlled trials. *Gynecol Obstet Invest.* 2013;76:75–82.

15. Kobayashi H, Kajihara H, Yamada Y, et al. Risk of carcinoma in women with ovarian endometrioma. *Front Biosci.* 2011;3:529–39.

16. Kalampokas T, Kamath MS, Kalampokaset E. AMH after laparoscopic surgery of the ovaries: a review. *Gynecol Endocrinol.* 2013;29:408–11.

17. Iwase A, Nakamura T, Nakahara T, Goto M, Kikkawa F. Assessment of ovarian reserve using anti-Müllerian hormone levels in benign gynecologic conditions and surgical interventions: a systematic narrative review. *Reprod Biol Endocrinol.* 2014;12:125.

18. Chang HJ, Han SH, Lee JR, et al. Impact of laparoscopic cystectomy on ovarian reserve: serial changes of serum anti-Müllerian hormone levels. *Fertil Steril.* 2010;94:343–9.

19. Chen Y, Pei H, Chang Y, et al. The impact of endometrioma and laparoscopic cystectomy on ovarian reserve and the exploration of related factors assessed by serum anti-Mullerian hormone: a prospective cohort study. *J Ovarian Res.* 2014;7:108.

20. Kuroda M, Kuroda K, Arakawa A, et al. Histological assessment of impact of ovarian endometrioma and laparoscopic cystectomy on ovarian reserve. *Obstet Gynaecol Res.* 2012;38:1187–93.

21. Goodman LR, Goldberg JM, Flyckt RL, et al. Effect of surgery on ovarian reserve in women with endometriomas, endometriosis and controls. *Am J Obstet Gynecol.* 2016;215:589.e1–6.

22. Somigliana E, Benaglia L, Paffoni A, Busnelli A, Vigano P, Vercellini P. Risks of conservative management in women with ovarian endometriomas undergoing IVF. *Hum Reprod Update.* 2015;21:486–99.

23. Benschop L, Farquhar C, van der Poel N, Heineman MJ. Interventions for women with endometrioma prior to assisted reproductive technology (Review). *Cochrane Database Syst Rev.* 2010;CD008571.

24. ESHRE guideline: management of women with endometriosis. *Hum Reprod.* 2014;29:400–12.

25. Practice Committee of the American Society for Reproductive Medicine. Endometriosis and infertility: a committee opinion. *Fertil Steril.* 2012;98:591–8.

26. Tsoumpou I, Kyrgiou M, Gelbaya TA, Nardo LG. The effect of surgical treatment for endometrioma on in vitro fertilization outcomes: a systematic review and meta-analysis. *Fertil Steril.* 2009;92:75–87.

27. Keckstein J, Ulrich U, Sasse V, Roth A, Tuttlies F, Karageorgieva E. Reduction of postoperative adhesion formation after laparoscopic ovarian cystectomy. *Hum Reprod.* 1996;11:579–82.

28. Uncu G, Kasapoglu I, Ozerkan K, Seyhan A, Oral Yilmaztepe A, Ata B. Prospective assessment of the impact of endometriomas and their removal on ovarian reserve and determinants of the rate of decline in ovarian reserve. *Hum Reprod.* 2013;28(8):2140–5.

29. Benaglia L, Candotti G, Busnelli A, Paffoni A, Vercellini P, Somigliana E. Antral follicle count as a predictor of ovarian responsiveness in women with endometriomas or with a history of surgery for endometriomas. *Fertil Steril.* 2015;103(6):1544–50.e1–3.

30. Jang WK, Lim SY, Park JC, Lee KR, Lee A, Rhee JH. Surgical impact on serum anti-Müllerian hormone in women with benign ovarian cyst: a prospective study. *Obstet Gynecol Sci.* 2014;57(2):121–7.

31. Cagnacci A, Bellafronte M, Xholli A, et al. Impact of laparoscopic cystectomy of endometriotic and non-endometriotic cysts on ovarian volume, antral follicle count (AFC) and ovarian doppler velocimetry. *Gynecol Endocrinol.* 2016;32(4):298–301.

32. Mohamed AA, Al-Hussaini TK, Fathalla MM, El Shamy TT, Abdelaal II, Amer SA. The impact of excision of benign nonendometriotic ovarian cysts on ovarian reserve: a systematic review. *Am J Obstet Gynecol.* 2016;215(2):169–76.

33. Raffi F, Metwally M, Amer S. The impact of excision of ovarian endometrioma on ovarian reserve: a systematic review and meta-analysis. *J Clin Endocrinol Metab.* 2012;97(9):3146–54.

34. Pergialiotis V, Prodromidou A, Frountzas M, Bitos K, Perrea D, Doumouchtsis SK. The effect of bipolar electrocoagulation during ovarian cystectomy on ovarian reserve: a systematic review. *Am J Obstet Gynecol.* 2015;213(5):620–8.

35. Ata B, Turkgeldi E, Seyhan A, Urman B. Effect of hemostatic method on ovarian reserve following laparoscopic endometrioma excision: comparison of suture, hemostatic sealant, and bipolar dessication. A systematic review and meta-analysis. *J Minim Invasive Gynecol.* 2015;22(3):363–72.

36. Spinelli C, Piscioneri J, Strambi S. Adnexal torsion in adolescents: update and review of the literature. *Curr Opin Obstet Gynecol.* 2015;27(5):320–5.

37. Sasaki KJ, Miller CE. Adnexal torsion: review of the literature. *J Minim Invasive Gynecol.* 2014;21(2):196–202.

38. Huchon C, Staraci S, Fauconnier A. Adnexal torsion: a predictive score for pre-operative diagnosis. *Hum Reprod.* 2010;25(9):2276–80.

39. Huchon C, Fauconnier A. Adnexal torsion: a literature review. *Eur J Obstet Gynecol Reprod Biol.* 2010;150(1):8–12.

40. Ganer Herman H, Shalev A, Ginat S, Kerner R, Keidar R, Bar J, Sagiv R. Clinical characteristics of adnexal torsion in premenarchal patients. *Arch Gynecol Obstet.* 2016;293(3):603–8.

41. Ginath S, Shalev A, Keidar R, et al. Differences between adnexal torsion in pregnant and nonpregnant women. *J Minim Invasive Gynecol.* 2012;19(6):708–14.

42. McWilliams GD, Hill MJ, Dietrich CS 3rd. Gynecologic emergencies. *Surg Clin North Am.* 2008;88(2):265–83.

43. Shadinger LL, Andreotti RF, Kurian RL. Preoperative sonographic and clinical characteristics as predictors of ovarian torsion. *J Ultrasound Med.* 2008;27(1):7–13.

44. Mashiach R, Melamed N, Gilad N, Ben-Shitrit G, Meizner I. Sonographic diagnosis of ovarian torsion: accuracy and predictive factors. *J Ultrasound Med.* 2011;30(9):1205–10.

45. Rha SE, Byun JY, Jung SE, et al. CT and MR imaging features of adnexal torsion. *Radiographics.* 2002;22(2):283–94.

46. Cohen SB, Wattiez A, Seidman DS, et al. Laparoscopy versus laparotomy for detorsion and sparing of twisted ischemic adnexa. *JSLS.* 2003;7(4):295–9.

47. McGovern PG, Noah R, Koenigsberg R, Little AB. Adnexal torsion and pulmonary embolism: case report and review of the literature. *Obstet Gynecol Surv.* 1999;54(9):601–8.

48. Shalev E, Bustan M, Yarom I, Peleg D. Recovery of ovarian function after laparoscopic detorsion. *Hum Reprod.* 1995;10(11):2965–6.

49. Pansky M, Smorgick N, Herman A, Schneider D, Halperin R. Torsion of normal adnexa in postmenarchal women and risk of recurrence. *Obstet Gynecol.* 2007;109(2 Pt 1):355–9.

50. Celik A, Ergün O, Aldemir H, et al. Long-term results of conservative management of adnexal torsion in children. *J Pediatr Surg.* 2005;40(4):704–8.

51. Geimanaite L, Trainavicius K. Ovarian torsion in children: management and outcomes. *J Pediatr Surg.* 2013;48(9):1946–53.

52. Lacher M, Kuebler JF, Yannam GR, et al. Single-incision pediatric endosurgery for ovarian pathology. *J Laparoendosc Adv Surg Tech A.* 2013;23(3):291–6.

53. Oelsner G, Cohen SB, Soriano D, Admon D, Mashiach S, Carp H. Minimal surgery for the twisted ischaemic adnexa can preserve ovarian function. *Hum Reprod.* 2003;18(12):2599–602.

54. Oelsner G, Bider D, Goldenberg M, Admon D, Mashiach S. Long-term follow-up of the twisted ischemic adnexa managed by detorsion. *Fertil Steril.* 1993;60(6):976–9.

55. Donesky BW, Adashi EY. Surgically induced ovulation in the polycystic ovary syndrome: wedge resection revisited in the age of laparoscopy. *Fertil Steril.* 1995;63:439–63.

56. Gjönnaess H. Polycystic ovarian syndrome treated by ovarian electrocautery through the laparoscope. *Fertil Steril.* 1984;41:20–5.

57. Seow KM, Juan CC, Hwang JL, Ho LT. Laparoscopic surgery in polycystic ovary syndrome: reproductive and metabolic effects. *Semin Reprod Med.* 2008;26:101–110.

58. Fernandez H, Morin-Surruca M, Torre A, Faivre E, Deffieux X, Gervaise A. Ovarian drilling for surgical treatment of polycystic ovarian syndrome: a comprehensive review. *Reprod Biomed Online.* 2011;22:556–68.

59. Amer SAK, Li TC, Cooke ID. A prospective dose-finding study of the amount of thermal energy required for laparoscopic ovarian diathermy. *Hum Reprod.* 2003;18:1693–8.

60. Dabirashrafi H. Complications of laparoscopic ovarian cauterization. *Fertil Steril.* 1989;52:878–9

61. Armar NA, McGarrigle HHG, Honour J, Holownia P, Jacobs HS, Lachelin GCL. Laparoscopic ovarian diathermy in the management of anovulatory infertility in women with polycystic ovaries:endocrine changes and clinical outcome. *Fertil Steril.* 1990;53:45–9.

62. Gurgan T, Urman B, Aksu T, Yarali H, Develioglu O, Kisnisci HA. The effect of short-interval laparoscopic lysis of adhesions on pregnancy rates following Nd-YAG laser photocoagulation of polycystic ovaries. *Obstet Gynecol.* 1992;80:45–7.

63. Greenblatt EM, Casper RF. Adhesion formation after laparoscopic ovarian cautery for polycystic ovarian syndrome: lack of correlation with pregnancy rates. *Fertil Steril.* 1993;60:766–70.

64. Mercorio F, Mercorio A, Di Spiezio Sardo A, Barba GV, Pellicano M, Nappi C. Evaluation of ovarian adhesion formation after laparoscopic ovarian drilling by second look minilaparoscopy. *Fertil Steril.* 2008;89:1229–33.

65. Api M. Is ovarian reserve diminished after laparoscopic ovarian drilling? *Gynecol Endocrinol.* 2009;25:159–65

66. Campo S. Ovulatory cycles, pregnancy outcomes and complications after surgical treatment of polycystic ovary syndrome. *Obstet Gynecol Surv.* 1998;53:297–308.

67. The Thessaloniki ESHRE/ASRM-Sponsored PCOS Consensus Workshop Group. Consensus on infertility treatment related to polycystic ovary syndrome. *Fertil Steril.* 2008;89:505–22.

68. Farquhar C, Brown J, Marjoribanks J. Laparoscopic drilling by diathermy or laser for ovulation induction in anovulatory polycystic ovary syndrome. *Cochrane Database Syst Rev.* 2012;6. Art. No:CD001122.

69. Abu Hashim H, El Lakany N, Sherief L. Combined metformin and clomiphene citrate versus laparoscopic ovarian diathermy for ovulation induction in clomiphene-resistant women with polycystic ovary syndrome: a randomized controlled trial. *J Obstet Gynaecol Res.* 2011;37:169–77.

70. Abu Hashim H, Foda O, Ghayaty E. Combined metformin-clomiphene in clomiphene resistant polycystic ovary syndrome: a systematic review and meta-analysis of randomized controlled trials. *Acta Obstet Gynecol Scand.* 2015;94:921–30.

Surgical Management of Proximal and Distal Tubal Disease

Linnea R. Goodman and Jeffrey M. Goldberg

5.1 Background

In the workup of infertility, tubal disease comprises up to one-third of female factor etiologies [1]. In the current era of increasing in-vitro fertilization (IVF) success rates, the clinician must decide how best to manage tubal factor infertility – surgical repair or bypassing the fallopian tubes and proceeding directly to IVF.

Risk factors for compromised tubal function include pelvic inflammatory disease, endometriosis, ectopic pregnancy, and prior pelvic surgery. Subsequent deleterious outcomes of tubal disease include primary or secondary infertility and increased risk for ectopic pregnancy. The location and extent of tubal disease influence the treatment plan and, therefore, it is essential to make an accurate diagnosis for effective management.

5.1.1 Diagnosis

Hysterosalpingogram (HSG) is the first-line diagnostic test to assess tubal patency [2]. The hysteroscopic features of hydrosalpinges, such as size and the presence of mucosal folds, help to estimate the potential for performing a neosalpingostomy. A distally dilated tube with free spill is consistent with fimbrial phimosis, which may be managed by fimbrioplasty. The loculation of contrast after spilling from the tube is suspicious for peritubal adhesions.

The negative predictive value of HSG is relatively high [3]. However, a finding of proximal tubal occlusion is usually due to functional spasm of the utero-tubal ostium as over 60% of patients will be patent on a repeat HSG 1 month later [4]. Similarly, over half of the patients will have normal fill and spill of dye during chromopertubation at the time of laparoscopy [3]. While direct visualization during laparoscopy is the gold standard, it is not absolutely definitive, as spontaneous pregnancies have occurred after bilateral tubal occlusion was reported [5].

Other forms of diagnostic evaluation have been used to investigate risks for tubal occlusion including sonohysterosalpingography and transvaginal hydrolaparoscopy with chromotubation; however, these have not become widespread and positive and negative predictive values remain suboptimal [6–8]. Testing for chlamydia antibodies can provide additional information to help rule out likelihood of tubal disease. It, however, has a high incidence of false-positives and cannot provide information regarding actual tubal patency [9].

At the present time, HSG remains the least invasive, first-line diagnostic tool for investigating tubal patency in the infertile patient. It also provides a therapeutic effect, presumably from clearing mucus and/or debris from the proximal tubal lumen, as higher pregnancy rates have been reported in the first few months following the procedure [10].

5.1.2 Treatment Considerations

The primary question regarding the infertile patient with a tubal factor diagnosis is to proceed with attempting surgical correction versus immediate IVF. Treatment options depend on a number of factors including pathology and clinic site-specific factors. The patient's age, desired number of children, treatment preference, and religious beliefs, as well as ovarian reserve and semen parameters should be considered. The potential for a good reproductive outcome following tubal repair based on the surgeon's experience should be compared to the success rates of the IVF clinic, taking financial considerations into account.

Throughout the United States, IVF success rates are tracked through a uniform registry (SART.org) and in 2013 patients with tubal factor infertility had a live-birth rate of just over 32% for all age groups per cycle initiated [11]. Unfortunately, there is no comparable registry for tubal surgery outcomes. Surgical results are all gathered from retrospective studies, many of them older than 20 years. They are heterogeneous with variable follow-up intervals and report success as cumulative pregnancy rates. Thus, pregnancy rates are based on the percentage of patients conceiving within a given time interval as opposed to IVF pregnancy rates per cycle.

Because it is difficult to directly compare the ultimate outcome of pregnancy success rates, it is imperative to evaluate and discuss potential risks and benefits of each procedure with the patient. The benefits of IVF include high chances of pregnancy, particularly in the short term, and a less invasive procedure. However, it can be considerably more expensive as insurance coverage is less pervasive in this area and more than one cycle may be necessary to achieve the desired number of children. IVF also requires a more medically intensive experience with daily injections and frequent monitoring, and carries the risk of multiple gestations and ovarian hyperstimulation syndrome. Fetal risks associated with IVF have also been reported, including pre-term delivery, low birth weight, and congenital malformations [13–15].

Tubal surgery is generally a one-time, minimally invasive outpatient procedure. In experienced hands, it has minimal risks; however, there are always risks of surgical complications and postoperative discomfort and pain. Corrective tubal surgery allows for repeated attempts at conception and has the potential of multiple conceptions without medical intervention. However, there is an increased risk for ectopic pregnancy, and tubal reocclusion can occur. If pregnancy does not occur following surgery, IVF is recommended, which increases the risks and costs to achieve a pregnancy.

5.2 Proximal Tubal Obstruction

Up to a quarter of tubal disease is due to proximal tubal occlusion [1]. When proximal occlusion is diagnosed on HSG, or no fill is witnessed on chromopertubation at the time of laparoscopy, it can be attributed to transient spasm of the utero-tubal ostia, obstruction from mucus or debris, or a true tubal blockage. True proximal occlusion results most often from salpingitis isthmica nodosa (SIN), PID, or endometriosis and the resulting fibrosis. As noted earlier, a diagnosis of proximal occlusion is due to tubal spasm approximately two-thirds of the time, especially if unilateral. Bilateral proximal occlusion poses a greater concern for real anatomic obstruction.

5.2.1 Tubal Cannulization

Tubal cannulization may be performed under fluoroscopic guidance or hysteroscopically with laparoscopic confirmation. Both methods employ a coaxial catheter system with an outer guide catheter and a flexible inner catheter with a guide wire. While tubal patency rates of over 80% can be achieved with both, the subsequent ongoing pregnancy rates are significantly higher with hysteroscopic cannulation (48.9% vs 15.6%, respectively) [1]. This may be due to the added benefit of being able to simultaneously diagnose and treat other pelvic pathologies at time of laparoscopy or that direct visualization leads to gentler manipulation of the tube. The high patency rates with tubal cannulation are likely achieved by dislodging plugs of mucus and/or debris from the tubal lumen. Histologic evaluation of resected proximal tubal segments in cases where tubal cannulation was unsuccessful revealed true anatomic obliteration of the lumen in 93% of the cases [16].

5.2.1.1 Preoperative Considerations

- If proximal tubal occlusion is diagnosed at initial HSG, it is often appropriate to proceed with laparoscopy to confirm the diagnosis and attempt surgical correction.
- Before attempting surgical treatment of proximal obstruction, as with all tubal disease, patient-specific factors should be considered to ensure that tubal surgery would be the more appropriate route to achieve conception over IVF.
- In addition, older patients with other infertility factors may also be better served bypassing tubal surgery for IVF. Unilateral or bilateral tubal obstruction should also play a role in the treatment decision, as the optimal treatment is currently unknown for unilateral obstruction, which may either be treated primarily as unexplained infertility or including tubal factor as the primary diagnosis.

5.2.1.2 Intraoperative Procedure

- Hysteroscopic tubal cannulation is performed with a Novy cornual cannulation set (Cook Medical), which includes an outer catheter with a removable stylet and an inner catheter with a flexible guide wire (see Video 5.1). A surgical assistant performs laparoscopy concurrently.
  - Procedure
    - Once laparoscopic transcervical chromotubation with indigo carmine or methylene blue confirms proximal tubal occlusion, the operative hysteroscope is inserted using saline for uterine distention. We prefer to use the vaginoscopic technique without a speculum or tenaculum but they can be used if cervical dilation is needed.
    - The outer catheter with stylet is inserted through the operative channel of the hysteroscope. Then the stylet is removed and an end cap is used to seal the Luer hub. The inner catheter with guide wire is the placed through the side arm of the outer catheter (Figure 5.1).
  - The outer catheter is advanced to the tubal ostium (Figure 5.2).
  - The inner catheter and guide wire are gently advanced through the outer catheter while the laparoscopic surgeon straightens the isthmic segment of the tube. The catheter with guide wire can be seen to traverse the intramural tubal segment into the proximal isthmus (Figure 5.3).
  - The guide wire is removed and chromopertubation is performed by injecting dilute indigo carmine or methylene blue through the inner catheter to document complete tubal patency while observing laparoscopically (Figures 5.4 and 5.5).
  - The guide wire may be replaced if the contralateral tube also needs to be cannulated. If the proximal occlusion does not yield to gentle pressure with the inner catheter and guide wire, the procedure should be aborted and true obstruction assumed. In these cases, IVF is discussed with the patient postoperatively.
- Microsurgical resection and anastomosis may be considered for cannulation failure in patients where IVF is not an option. However, unlike reversal of tubal ligation, it involves pathologic tubes and cornual anastomosis, which is technically more difficult and carries a lower success rate.
- Risks associated with tubal cannulization are rare and include
  - risks associated with hysteroscopy (bleeding, pain, fluid overload);
  - potential risk for tubal perforation, which is under 10% and is of no clinical significance [1];
  - risk of ectopic pregnancy in a previously blocked tube.

5.2.1.3 Postoperative Considerations

- Success rates of cannulation are high, with approximately 85% bilateral proximal tubal occlusion

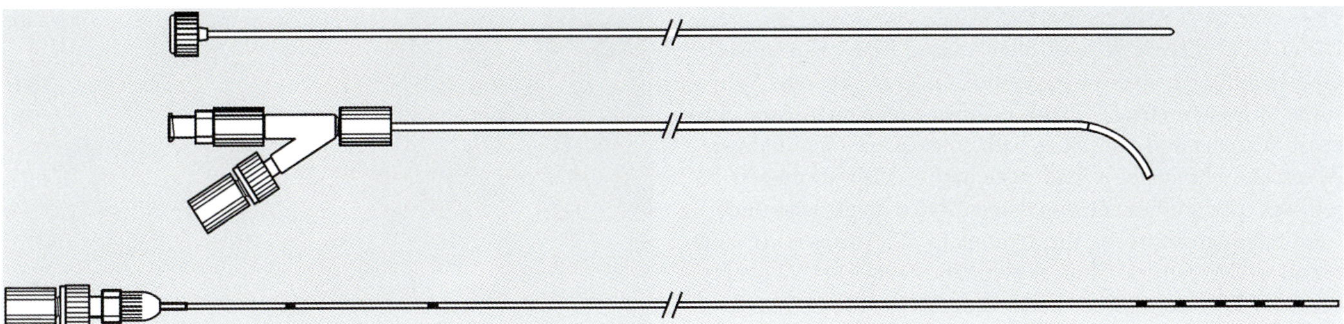

Figure 5.1 The Novy tubal cannulation set consists of a rigid introducer (top), which is inserted into the straight channel of the outer catheter (middle) to facilitate placing the catheter through the operating channel of the hysteroscope. The introducer is removed and the channel capped with a stopper. The guide wire (not shown) is threaded through the inner catheter (bottom), which is then placed through the angled side channel of the outer catheter.

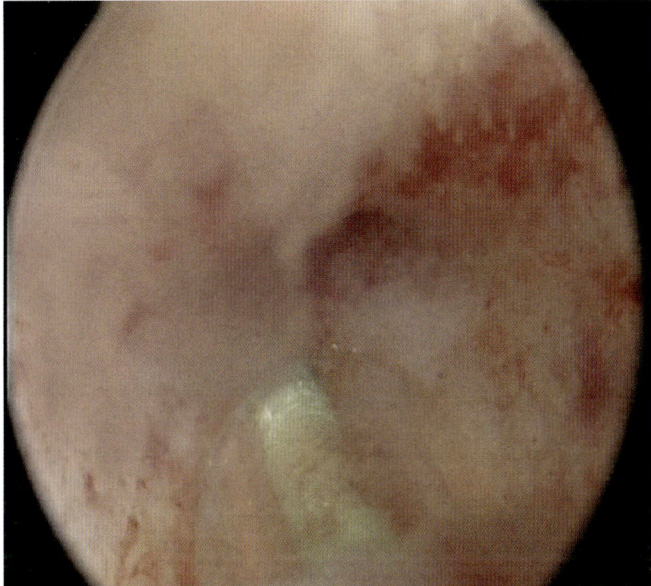

Figure 5.2 The outer catheter is directed to the tubal ostium.

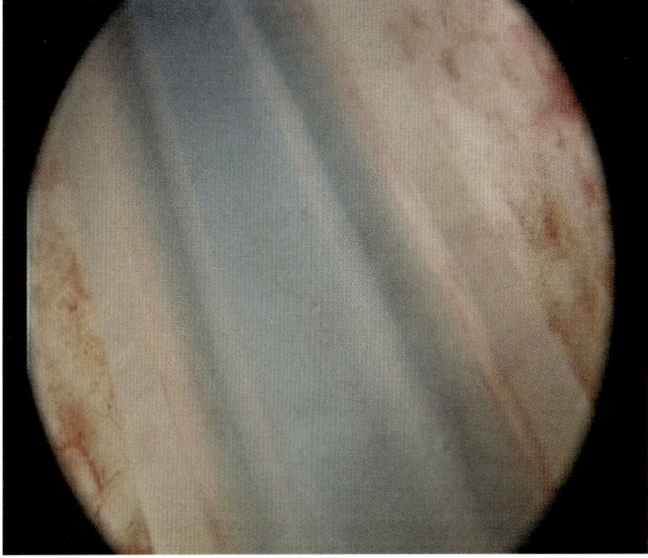

Figure 5.4 The guide wire has been removed and the blue contrast is injected through the inner catheter.

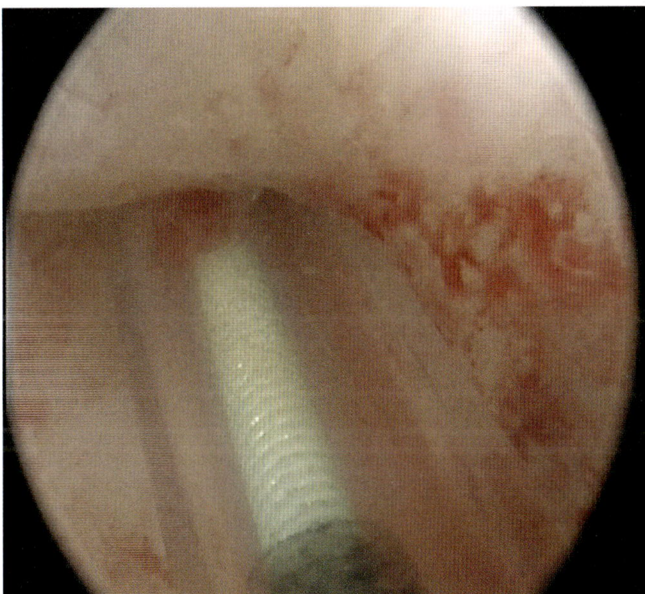

Figure 5.3 The guide wire is cannulating the interstitial segment of the tube and the inner catheter is advanced in the tube over the guide wire.

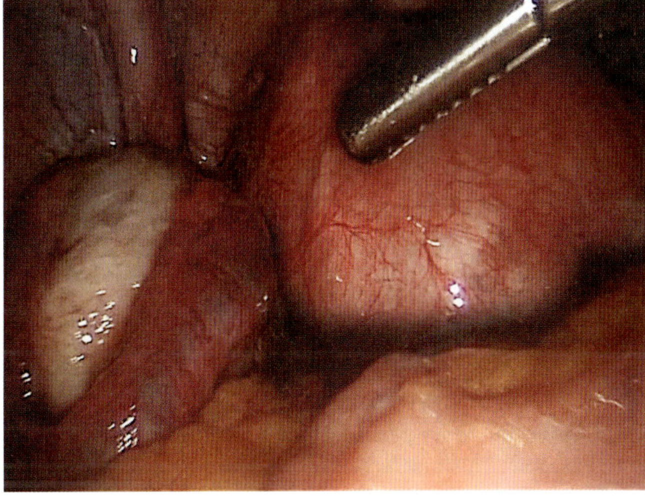

Figure 5.5 Laparoscopy confirms tubal patency.

achieving tubal patency at the end of the procedure. However, up to one-third of cannulizations will subsequently re-occlude [1]. Approximately half of the patients will conceive spontaneously [1,16].

5.3 Distal Tubal Occlusion

Distal tubal disease is most often caused by a prior episode of PID. Other causes of peritonitis such as previous pelvic surgery, endometriosis, and ectopic pregnancy can also cause scarring and adhesions with subsequent tubal damage. A recent meta-analysis and systematic review evaluated 22 retrospective studies encompassing 2,810 patients who underwent salpingostomy in the treatment of hydrosalpinx and found a 27% natural clinical pregnancy rate [12]. However, the included studies were heterogeneous for the exclusion of other infertility factors, surgical technique, surgeon experience, length of follow-up, and especially the degree of tubal damage. Many of the studies did not use a classification system and no stratification was done by extent of disease by those who did. This is very important as only patients with a good prognosis for an intrauterine pregnancy should be considered for neosalpingostomy.

As expected, pregnancy rates are highest in those with mild disease, with rates reported anywhere from 58% to 77% and ectopic pregnancy rates from 2% to 8% [21,22]. Those with severe tubal disease have marginal rates of success (0–22%) and high rates of ectopic pregnancy (0–17%) [21]. Good prognosis features include no more than mild adnexal adhesions, tubal dilation <3 cm, thin pliable tubal walls, and normal-appearing endosalpinx upon opening the tube [18]. If these criteria are not met, the patient would be better served with a salpingectomy.

5.3.1 Neosalpingostomy and Fimbrioplasty

5.3.1.1 Preoperative Considerations

- The decision regarding tubal repair or removal is often made at the time of laparoscopy when the extent of tubal disease can be visualized. Therefore, the patient should be consented for both procedures.
- Preoperative antibiotics should be given to decrease the chance of infection.

5.3.1.2 Intraoperative Procedures

- Historically, tubal repair was performed by laparotomy. However, it should now be performed by minimally invasive endoscopic methods to decrease operative risks, blood loss, postoperative pain, and to hasten recovery time without detrimental effects on success rates [2,19,20]. Laparoscopic neosalpingostomy and fimbrioplasty are the procedures for repairing complete or partial distal tubal occlusion, respectively.
- All procedures are performed using microsurgical technique. This means gentle tissue handling, keeping surfaces moist, avoiding foreign-body contamination from packs and sponges, using fine nonreactive sutures without undue tension, maintaining complete hemostasis through the use of limited and precise electrocoagulation, and taking advantage of the magnification the laparoscope provides.

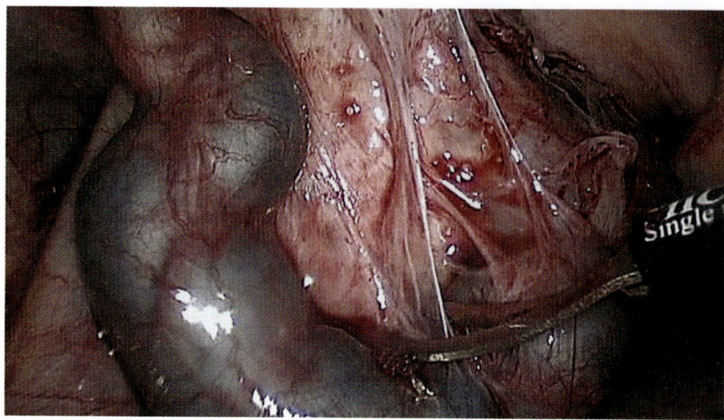

Figure 5.6 Adnexal adhesions are completely excised.

- Since hydrosalpinges are usually the result of a prior pelvic infection, intravenous antibiotics should be administered preoperatively.
- A uterine manipulator is placed for manipulation and chromotubation. An oro-gastric tube and indwelling Foley catheter are placed as for all laparoscopic procedures to reduce the risk of trocar injuries.
- The procedure can be completed with three 5 mm laparoscopic ports, one through the umbilicus and one in each lower quadrant.
- Neosalpingostomy (see Video 5.2):
  - Transcervical chromotubation is performed to confirm that the proximal tube is patent and all adhesions are completely excised (Figure 5.6).
  - Dilute vasopressin (20 units in 100 ml of injectable saline) is injected in the distal mesosalpinx for hemostasis, which limits the need for electrosurgery and potential thermal injury (Figure 5.7).
  - The neosalpingostomy is accomplished by incising the distal end of the hydrosalpinx using a unipolar needle with cutting current. The high power density at the needle tip minimizes thermal spread (Figure 5.8).
  - The incision is opened widely to assess the endosalpinx and evert the edges. If normal tubal mucosa is present, the newly created flaps are everted and sutured to the adjacent tubal serosa with 4-0 Vicryl suture using intracorporeal knot tying. The surgeon and assistant form the knots together. This is easier than the surgeon tying the knots alone and eliminates the need for a third ancillary laparoscopic port (Figures 5.9 and 5.10). The suture end of the SH needle may be straightened using hemostats to form a "ski" to facilitate passing the needle through the 5 mm port.
  - Tubal patency is documented by chromopertubation (Figure 5.11).
  - Interceed is placed over the tube to help prevent postoperative adhesions.
- Fimbrioplasty
  - The steps for performing a fimbrioplasty are exactly the same as for neosalpingostomy described earlier. The only difference is that the existing phimotic distal tubal opening is enlarged with the unipolar needle.

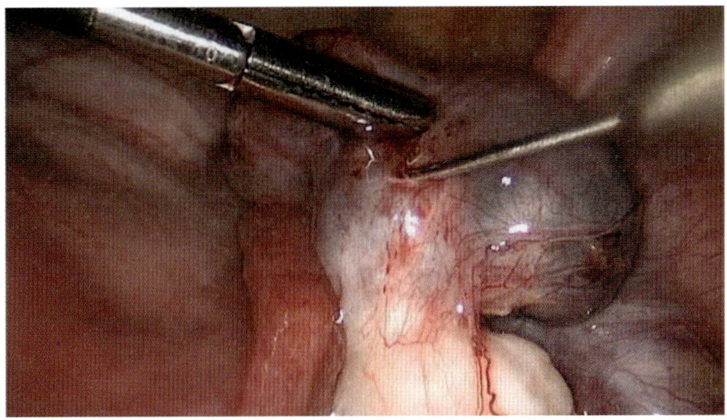

Figure 5.7 Dilute vasopressin is injected in the distal mesosalpinx.

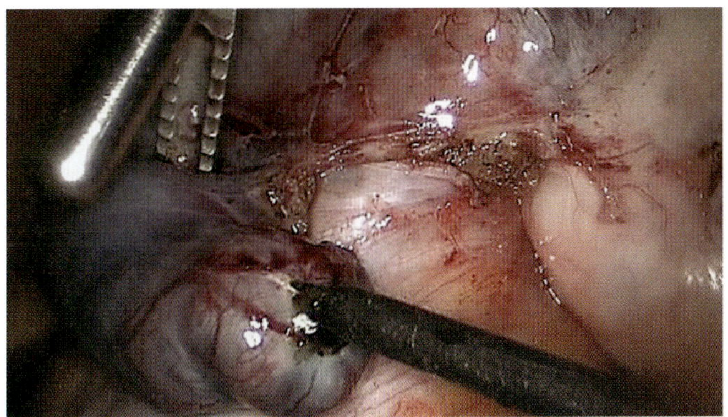

Figure 5.8 The neosapinostomy is created with the monopolar needle with cutting current.

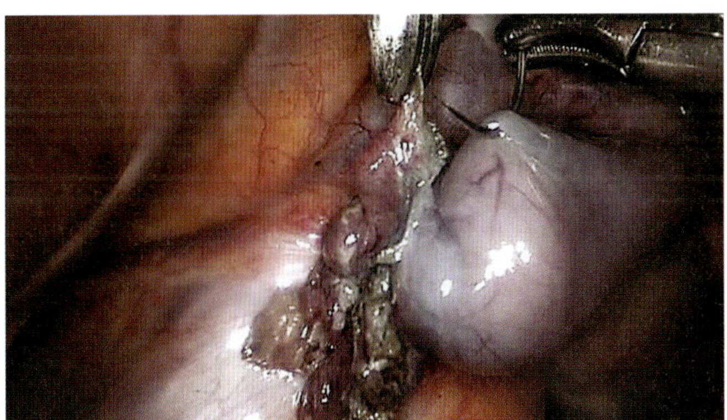

Figure 5.9 The opening is everted with a 4-0 Vicryl suture to the serosa.

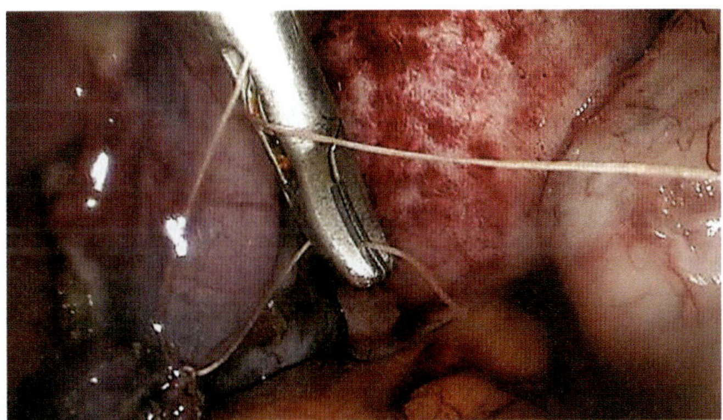

Figure 5.10 The knots are tied intracorporeally.

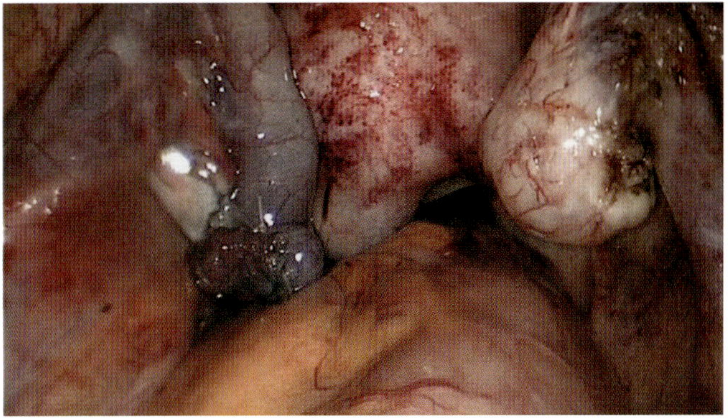

Figure 5.11 Transcervical chromotubation documents tubal patency.

5.3.1.3 Postoperative Considerations

- Patients are instructed to wait two cycles prior to attempting conception and ectopic pregnancy precautions are reviewed.
- Should pregnancy not occur within 6 months of attempting conception after surgical intervention, an HSG should be obtained to ensure continued patency. Salpingectomy prior to IVF would be recommended if re-occlusion occurred.
- Repeat operations for distal occlusion or surgery for patients with both proximal and distal occlusion should be reserved for a very specific subset of patients (where IVF is not an option), as success rates are very low [19].

5.3.2 Salpingectomy

5.3.2.1 Preoperative Considerations

Patients with a poor prognosis for spontaneous conception include those with extensive adhesions, thick-walled massively dilated (>3 cm) tubes, and those with no evidence of normal anatomic luminal mucosa. For these patients, IVF success rates far exceed those of tubal repair with attempted spontaneous conception. However, two meta-analyses have shown that the presence of hydrosalpinges reduce IVF success rates by 50% [23,24]. This may be due to the hydrosalpinx fluid having a direct embryotoxic effect, mechanically flushing the embryos from the uterus or impairing endometrial receptivity [25].

Several studies have demonstrated that salpingectomy prior to IVF restores the success rates back to normal. It is currently unknown whether hydrosalpinges that are not visualized on ultrasonography have the same deleterious effects as those that are dilated enough to been seen by ultrasound, but the current recommendation from a recent Cochrane review endorses either removal or occlusion of a communicating hydrosalpinx prior to IVF [26]. Even a unilateral hydrosalpinx impairs IVF success rates and its removal significantly improves them [27–29].

5.3.2.2 Intraoperative Procedure

- Salpingectomy is best performed laparoscopically with three laparoscopic ports, a 10 mm in the umbilicus and 5 mm in each lower quadrant (see Video 5.3).
  - The procedure can start either proximally or distally. In this figure, the proximal tube was coagulated

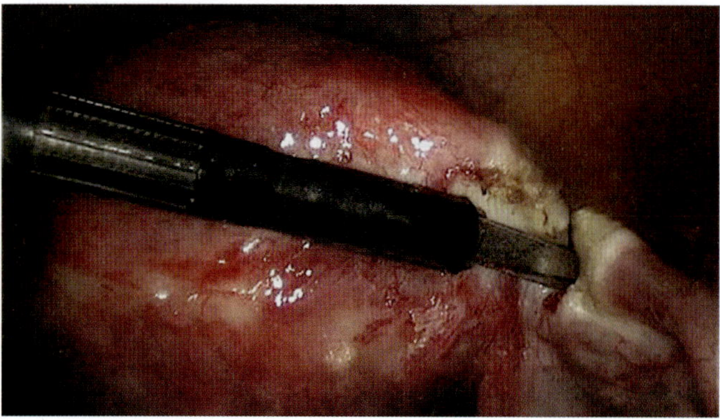

Figure 5.12 The proximal fallopian tube has been cauterized with bipolar graspers and divided with scissors.

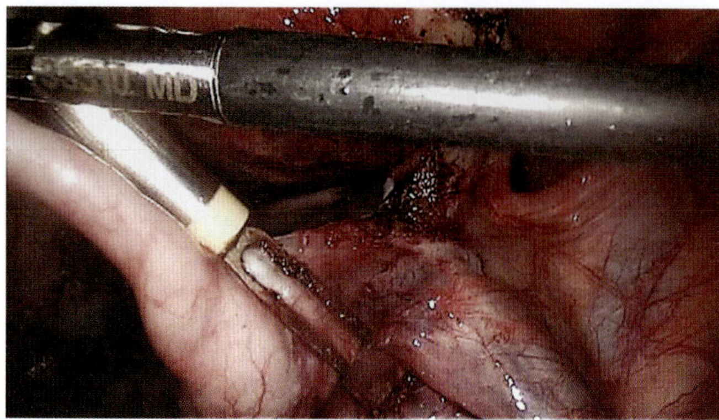

Figure 5.13 The mesosalpinx is being cauterized close to the tube to minimize thermal spread to the ovarian vascular supply.

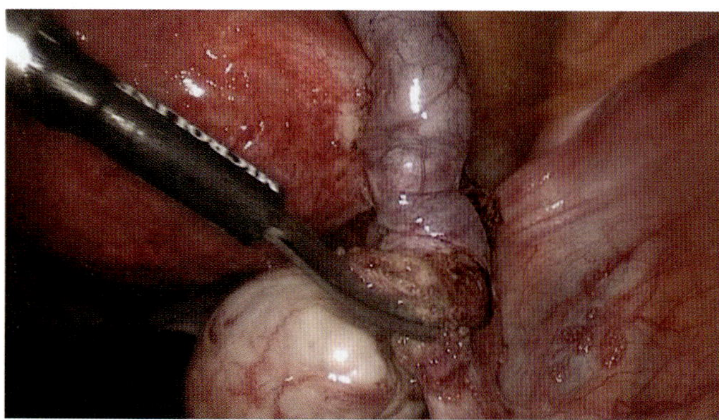

Figure 5.14 The remaining attachment at the distal end is being divided with scissors. The specimen is then removed through the 10 mm umbilical port.

with bipolar grasping forceps and divided with scissors though whatever modality is preferred, i.e., or vessel sealing devices such as LigaSure (Covidien, Minneapolis) or harmonic scalpel may be used (Figure 5.12).

- The mesosalpinx is serially coagulated and divided staying as close to the tube as possible to avoid compromising the ovarian blood supply and potentially leading to diminished ovarian reserve (Figure 5.13).
- The distal end of the tube is divided from the ovary to completely free the tube (Figure 5.14). It is removed through the 10 mm umbilical port while observing through a 5 mm laparoscope in one of the lower-quadrant ports and sent to pathology.
- The abdomen is irrigated and the vascular pedicles are checked for hemostasis while the insufflation pressure is reduced.
- The fascia of the 10 mm umbilical incision should be closed. The pneumoperitoneum is released and the skin incisions are closed.

5.3.2.3 Postoperative Considerations

- Patients may undergo IVF once menses resume.

5.3.3 Tubal Ligation

In cases where extensive pelvic adhesions make performing a salpingectomy difficult or risky, limited data suggests that proximal tubal ligation may provide the same IVF pregnancy outcome benefits as salpingectomy [27]. There is a theoretical concern that proximally occluding a hydrosalpinx may cause further dilation with pain. Therefore, hydrosalpinx should be fenestrated to the fullest extent possible. A few small uncontrolled studies suggested that hysteroscopic proximal tubal occlusion with the Essure device may be an alternative to laparoscopic tubal ligation for treating hydrosalpinges prior to IVF. It may be considered in those patients in whom laparoscopy is not feasible, but there is a hypothetical risk that the trailing coils in the endometrial cavity may have an IUD-like effect.

5.4 Conclusion

Tubal disease accounts for a significant portion of female factor infertility. For relatively young patients with no other significant infertility factors, hysteroscopic tubal cannulation for proximal tubal occlusion and laparoscopic neosalpingostomy for distal tubal disease having a good prognosis should be considered first-line treatments. Salpingectomy, or tubal ligation, should be performed for hydrosalpinges that don't meet the criteria for neosalpingostomy in order to negate their detrimental effects on pregnancy rates with subsequent IVF cycles.

References

1. Honore GM, Holden AE, Schenken RS. Pathophysiology and management of proximal tubal blockage. *Fertil Steril.* 1999;5:785–95.

2. Practice Committee of the American Society of Reproductive Medicine. Optimal evaluation of the infertile female. *Fertil Steril.* 2006;86:S264–7.

3. Evers JL, Land JA, Mol BW. Evidence-based medicine for diagnostic questions. *Semin Reprod Med.* 2003;21:9–15.

4. Dessole S, Meloni GB, Capobianco G, Manzoni MA, Ambrosini G, Canalis GC. A second hysterosalpingography reduces the use of selective technique for treatment of a proximal tubal obstruction. *Fertil Steril.* 2000;73:1037–9.

5. Mol BW, Collins JA, Burrows EA, van der Veen F, Bossuyt PM. Comparison of hysterosalpingography and laparoscopy in predicting fertility outcome. *Hum Reprod.* 1999;14:1237–42.

6. Hamed HO, Shahin AY, Elsamman AM. Hysterosalpingo-constrast sonography versus radiographic hysterosalpingography in the evaluation of tubal patency. *Int J Gynecol Obstet.* 2009;105:215–17.

7.   Ahinko-Hakamaa KM, Huhtala H, Tinkanen H. Confirmation of tubal patency in hysterosalpingo-contrast sonography by transvaginal hydrolaparoscopy. *Acta Obstet Gynecol.* 2009;88:286–90.

8.   Catenacci M, Goldberg JM. Transvaginal hydrolaparoscopy. *Semin Reprod Med.* 2011;29:95–100.

9.   Den Hartog JE, Morre SA, Land JA. Chlamydia trachomatis-associated tubal factor subfertility: immunogenetic aspects and serological screening. *Hum Reprod Update.* 2006;12:719–30.

10. Johnson N, Vanderkerchove P, Lilford R, et al. Tubal flushing for subfertility. *Cochrane Database Syst Rev.* 2009; undefined: pp. CD003718.

11. Society for Assisted Reproductive Technology. Clinic summary report. Available at: www.sartcorsonline.com/rptCSR_PublicMultYear.aspx?ClinicPKID=0. Accessed September 15, 2015.

12. Chu J, Harb HM, Gallos ID, et al. Salpingostomy in the treatment of hydrosalpinx: a systematic review and meta-analysis. *Hum Reprod.* 2015;30:1882–95.

13. Hansen M, Bower C, Milne E, de Klerk N, Kurinczuk J. Assisted reproductive technologies and the risk of birth defects – a systematic review. *Hum Reprod.* 2005;20:328–38.

14. Jackson RA, Gibson KA, Wu YW, Croughan MS. Perinatal outcomes in singletons following in vitro fertilization: a meta-analysis. *Obstet Gynecol.* 2004;103:551–63.

15. El-Chaar D, Yang Q, Gao J, et al. Risk of birth defects increased in pregnancies conceived by assisted human reproduction. *Fertil Steril.* 2009;92:1557–61.

16. Letterie GS, Sakas EL. Histology of proximal tubal obstruction in cases of unsuccessful tubal canalization. *Fertil Steril.* 1991;56:831–5.

17. Pinto AB, Hovsepian DM, Wattanakumtornkul S, Pilgram TK. Pregnancy outcomes after fallopian tube recanalization: oil-based versus water-soluble contrast agents. *J Vasc Interven Radiol.* 2003;14:69–74.

18. Practice Committee of the American Society for Reproductive Medicine. Role of tubal surgery in the era of assisted reproductive technology: a committee opinion. *Fertil Steril.* 2015;103:e37–43.

19. The American Fertility Society classifications of adnexal adhesions, distal tubal occlusion, tubal occlusion secondary to tubal ligation, tubal pregnancies, Mullerian anomalies and intrauterine adhesions. *Fertil Steril.* 1988;9:944–55.

20. Dun EC, Nezhat CH. Tubal factor infertility: diagnosis and management in the era of assisted reproductive technology. *Obstet Gynecol Clin North Am.* 2012;39:551–66.

21. Bontis JN, Theodoridis TD. Laparoscopic management of hydrosalpinx. *Ann NY Acad Sci.* 2006;092:199–210.

22. Nackley AC, Muasher SJ. The significance of hydrosalpinx in in vitro fertilization. *Fertil Steril.* 1998;69:373–84.

23. Milingos SD, Kallipolitis GK, Loutradis DC, et al. Laparoscopic treatment of hydrosalpinx: factors affecting pregnancy rates. *J Am Assoc Gynecol Laparosc.* 2000;7:355–61.

24. Zeyneloglu HB, Arici A, Olive D. Adverse effects of hydrosalpinx on pregnancy rates after in vitro fertilization – embryo transfer. *Fertil Steril.* 1998;70:492–9.

25. Camus E, Poncelet C, Goffinet F, et al. Pregnancy rates after in-vitro fertilization in cases of tubal infertility with and without hydrosalpinx: a meta-analysis of published comparative studies. *Hum Reprod.* 1999;14:1243–9.

26. Practice Committee of the American Society for Reproductive Medicine in collaboration with The Society of Reproductive Surgeons. Salpingectomy for hydrosalpinx prior to in vitro fertilization. *Fertil Steril.* 2008;90:S66–8.

27. Johnson N, van Voorst S, Sowter MC, Strandell A, Mol BW. Surgical treatment for tubal disease in women due to undergo in vitro fertilisation. *Cochrane Database Syst Rev.* 2010;CD002125.

28. Kassabji M, Sims JA, Butlerb L, Muasher SJ. Reduced pregnancy outcome in patients with unilateral or bilateral hydrosalpinx after in vitro fertilization. *Eur J Obstet Gynecol Reprod Biol.* 1994;56:129–32.

29. Murray DL, Sagoskin AW, Widra EA. The adverse effect of hydrosalpinges on in vitro fertilization pregnancy rates and the benefit of surgical correction. *Fertil Steril.* 1998;69:41–5.

30. Shelton KE, Butler L, Toner JP, Oehninger S, Muasher SJ. Salpingectomy improves the pregnancy rate in in-vitro fertilization patients with hydrosalpinx. *Hum Reprod.* 1996;11:523–5.

31. Chan CC, Ng EH, Li CF, Ho PC. Impaired ovarian blood flow and reduced antral follicle count following laparoscopic salpingectomy for ectopic pregnancy. *Hum Reprod.* 2003;18:2175–80.

32. Dar P, Sachs GS, Strassburger D, Bukovsky I, Arieli S. Ovarian function before and after salpingectomy in artificial reproductive technology patients. *Hum Reprod.* 2000;15:142–4.

33. Strandell A, Lindhard A, Waldenstrom U, Thorburn J. Prophylactic salpingectomy does not impair the ovarian response in IVF treatment. *Hum Reprod.* 2001;16:1135–9.

6 Tubal Anastomosis for Reversal of Tubal Ligation

Jeffrey M. Goldberg and Julian A. Gingold

6.1 Background

Surgical sterilization is the most commonly used contraceptive method among couples in the United States [1]. According to the 2002 National Survey of Family Growth, 27% of fertile women relied on female sterilization for birth control, while an additional 9% relied on partner vasectomy [1,2]. While these methods are widely considered safe and effective, regret following female sterilization methods varies widely and has been reported to be as high as 26% [3]. Regret is highest among women who undergo the procedure when less than 30 years old and less than 2 years after the birth of their youngest child [3].

Sterilization procedures are commonly performed laparoscopically using electrocoagulation, Fallope rings, or Hulka or Filshie clips. In addition, partial salpingectomy can be performed at the time of cesarean delivery, transumbically shortly following vaginal delivery, or by interval minilaparotomy using the Parkland or Pomeroy techniques [2,4]. Finally, hysteroscopic insertion of the Essure tubal occlusion device (Bayer, Whippany, NJ) into the tubal ostia has the advantage of being performed as an office procedure.

6.2 Preoperative Considerations

Contraindications to performing tubal anastomosis are final tubal length less than 4 cm, prior ectopic pregnancy or pelvic inflammatory disease, stage 3 or 4 endometriosis, significant adnexal adhesions, and more than a mild male factor [5]. The operative report from the tubal ligation and a semen analysis should be obtained to determine if the patient is a candidate for tubal reversal. Eligible patients are counseled regarding the procedure as well as IVF including the success rates, risks, advantages and disadvantages, and cost.

The advantages of tubal anastomosis are that it is a minimally invasive outpatient procedure, which allows patients to attempt to conceive spontaneously each month, as well as to conceive more than once with no additional intervention (Table 6.1). In most cases, it is less expensive than IVF, especially if more than one cycle is required. The disadvantage is that it carries all of the risks of surgery such as bleeding, infection, organ damage, and reaction to anesthesia as well as postoperative discomfort.

The advantages of IVF are that it is nonsurgical and has high success rates even in patients who are not candidates for tubal anastomosis. Patients may have more than one opportunity to conceive per IVF cycle if extra embryos are available for cryopreservation. The disadvantages of IVF are that it is more labor-intensive with weeks of daily injections, frequent visits for follicle monitoring with pelvic ultrasonography and blood estradiol levels, an outpatient procedure to retrieve the oocytes, and another visit for embryo transfer. Subsequent pregnancy attempts require the thaw and transfer of cryopreserved embryos or additional IVF cycles if no cryopreserved embryos are available. Anecdotally, nearly all eligible patients in our practice opt for tubal anastomosis citing lower cost and that it is more "natural" than IVF as the reasons for their preference. The main risks of IVF are multiple pregnancy, since more than one embryo is often transferred, and ovarian hyperstimulation, which can be potentially life-threatening and require hospitalization. These risks further increase the overall cost of IVF.

6.3 Predictors for Success

Pregnancy rates after tubal anastomosis are stable at 70–90% until they rapidly decrease at age 40 [6–9]. A large population-based study from Australia confirmed the precipitous drop at 40 but the overall pregnancy rates were lower for all groups [10]. This was likely due to multiple surgeons of different skill levels using unspecified techniques. Even including that study, the one-year cumulative pregnancy rates in patients 40 years of age and older is 20–50% [6–10]. These rates are generally better than those achieved with IVF for this age segment. A retrospective cohort of 79 IVF patients and 84 undergoing anastomosis noted a significantly higher cumulative live birth rate with tubal anastomosis versus IVF of 52% for women under 37 years of age, 72% and 52%, respectively $p=0.012$ [11]. For women 37 and older, the anastomosis success rate of 51% was not significantly different from 37% with IVF.

Some studies reported an association between final tubal length and pregnancy rates but others found no difference [7,12]. The sterilization method also significantly impacts success rates, with the best outcomes being achieved following reversal of tubal occlusion by Fallope rings or Filshie or Hulka clips [9].

6.3.1 Financial Considerations

A retrospective cost analysis from Belgium comparing IVF with tubal anastomosis found that the average cost per delivery was double for IVF with a mean of two IVF cycles required [11]. Another cost analysis from the United States confirmed that the cost per pregnancy was double with IVF for women up

Table 6.1 Comparison of Tubal Anastomosis and IVF

	Anastomosis	IVF
Inconvenience	One-time minimally invasive procedure	• Daily injections • Frequent monitoring
Opportunities to conceive	• Can try every month • Can conceive more than once	Limited attempts
Risks	• Surgical risks • Ectopic pregnancy	• Multiple pregnancy • Ovarian hyperstimulation syndrome (OHSS)
Advantages	• More cost-effective • More natural	• Faster time to conception • Preserves fertility • Effective if other infertility factors are present

to age 40. However, the cost for tubal anastomosis was double for women over 40 [13]. An Australian analysis of women between 40 and 47 years reported that the cost per live birth was approximately 10 times more expensive with IVF than with anastomosis [14].

6.4 Surgical Approach

In addition to standard laparotomy with overnight hospitalization, tubal anastomosis may, and should, be performed by minimally invasive outpatient approaches such as minilaparotomy and laparoscopy, with or without robotic assistance. The few studies comparing laparotomy with laparoscopy found no difference in intrauterine or ectopic pregnancy rates. As expected, the operating times were longer with laparoscopy but the hospitalization times were shorter [15]. Since laparoscopic tubal anastomosis is difficult, several shortcuts have been tried such as a one-stitch technique and using clips or glue. The goal of laparoscopic surgery is to duplicate the open procedure. Only the route of access is different. In an effort to overcome the technical difficulties of performing microsurgery through the laparoscope, robotic assistance has been utilized. There are no studies comparing laparoscopic tubal anastomosis with and without robotics. A retrospective study comparing tubal anastomosis with robotics with outpatient minilaparotomy found that robotics added over an hour under anesthesia and $1,450 [16]. Patients returned to work 1 week earlier after robotic anastomosis. The pregnancy rate of 81% with minilaparotomy was not significantly different than the 61% with robotics but that was likely due to the small sample size of 55 patients. Another retrospective study comparing robotic tubal anastomosis with standard laparotomy found no difference in overall pregnancy rates, but the ectopic pregnancy rate was double with robotics [17]. Also, tubal anastomosis with robotics was $2,000 costlier despite the laparotomy patients requiring overnight hospitalization. Regardless of the approach, the steps of performing tubal anastomosis are the same. The author's preferred technique of minilaparotomy is described next.

6.4.1 Operative Technique

The procedure begins by inserting a uterine manipulator for manipulation and chromotubation (see Video 5.3). Diagnostic laparoscopy is performed to assure adequate tubal length and the absence of significant pelvic disease. A 5 cm transverse minilaparotomy is performed approximately 3 cm above the symphysis and carried down to the fascia. The fascia is incised vertically in the midline and the rectus bellies are separated. The peritoneum is then incised vertically and a round wound retractor such as the Mobius (CooperSurgical, Inc., Trumbull, CT) or Alexis (Applied Medical, Rancho Santa Margarita, CA) is placed (Figure 6.1). Dilute vasopressin (20 units in 100 ml of injectable saline) is infiltrated into the mesosalpinx beneath the occluded ends (Figure 6.2). The ends are then mobilized with the unipolar micro-needle with 20 W of cutting current (Figure 6.3). The proximal end is opened with Wescott scissors and patency is confirmed with transcervical chromotubation using dilute indigo carmine or methylene blue dye (Figures 6.4 and 6.5). The distal end is then opened taking care to keep the opening small in order to have similar luminal diameters between the proximal and distal segments (Figure 6.6). Patency of the distal segment is established by retrograde chromotubation by injecting dilute indigo carmine or methylene blue dye transfimbrially with an 18G angiocatheter (Figure 6.7).

The tubal ends are brought together with a 6-0 delayed absorbable suture through the mesosalpinx (Figure 6.8). The actual anastomosis is performed using interrupted 8-0 delayed absorbable suture (though some surgeons prefer Prolene). The first layer is through the muscularis and may include the lumen. The sutures are placed at the 3, 6, 9, and 12 o'clock positions with the 6 o'clock suture placed first. The needle is placed from out to in of one segment and in to out on the other so that the knots are tied extraluminally (Figures 6.9 and 6.10) Transcervical chromotubation is performed to document bilateral tubal patency (Figure 6.11). The serosa is then closed with interrupted 8-0 delayed absorbable suture (Figure 6.12).

6.4.2 Postoperative Considerations

Patients may resume attempts at natural conception with the next menses.

6.5 Essure Reversal

Limited evidence exists to support surgical reversal of Essure device. A retrospective study of 70 patients who underwent bilateral tubouterine implantation and were followed for 1 year

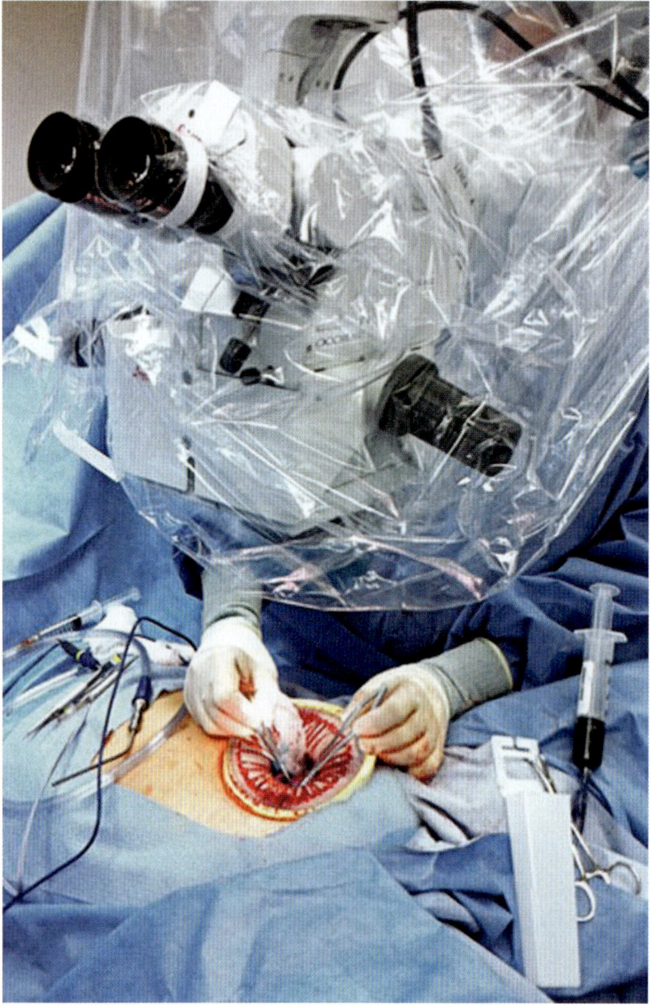

Figure 6.1 Operative setup for microsurgical tubal anastomosis by minilaparotomy with a self-retaining wound retractor.

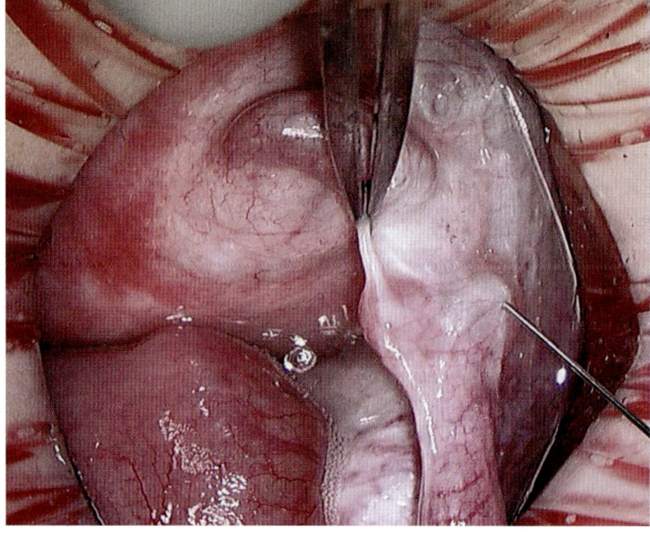

Figure 6.2 Injection of dilute vasopressin into the mesosalpinx.

achieved a 36% pregnancy rate and a 25% live birth rate [18]. There were no ectopic pregnancies. Given the substantially lower success rates with this technique, it should be reserved for patients in whom IVF is not an option.

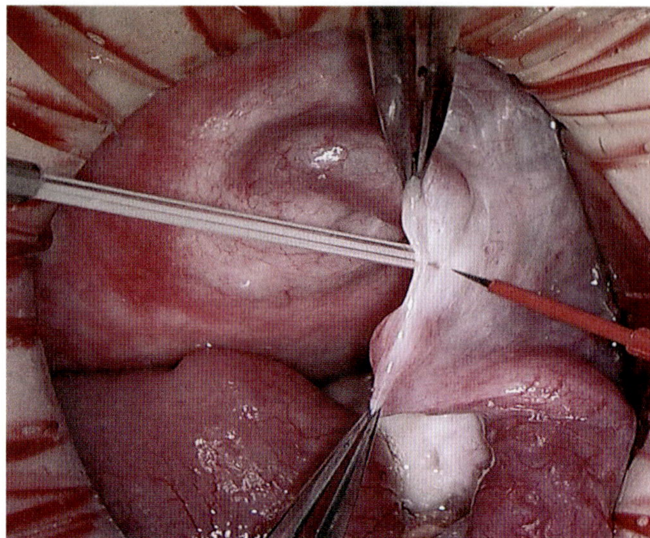

Figure 6.3 Mobilization of the occluded tubal ends with the micro-monopolar needle.

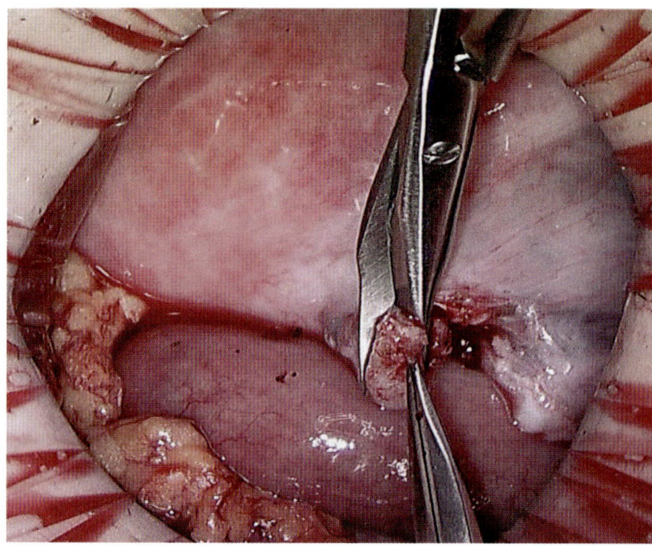

Figure 6.4 Opening the proximal tubal end with Wescott scissors.

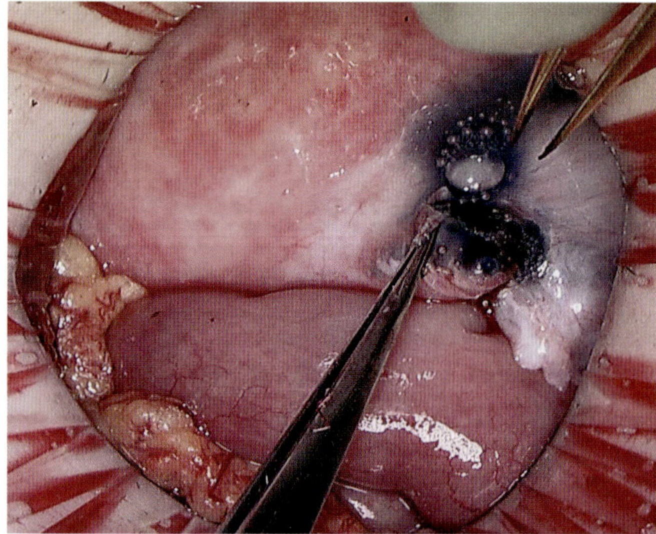

Figure 6.5 Transcervical chromotubation with methylene blue confirming proximal spill.

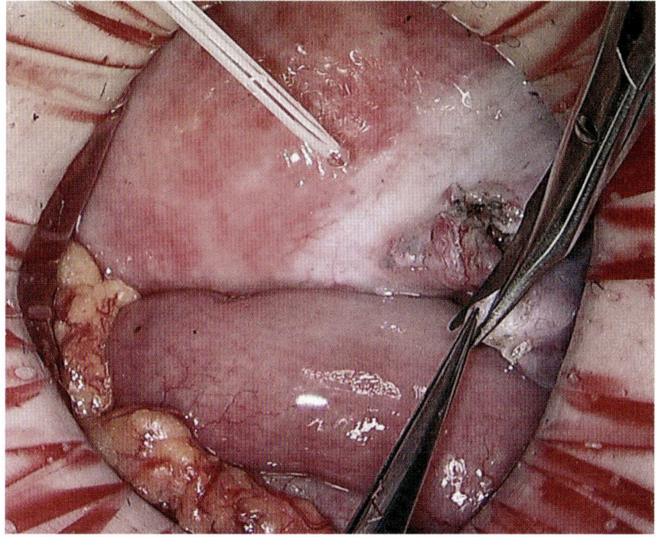

Figure 6.6 Opening the distal tubal end keeping the lumen small.

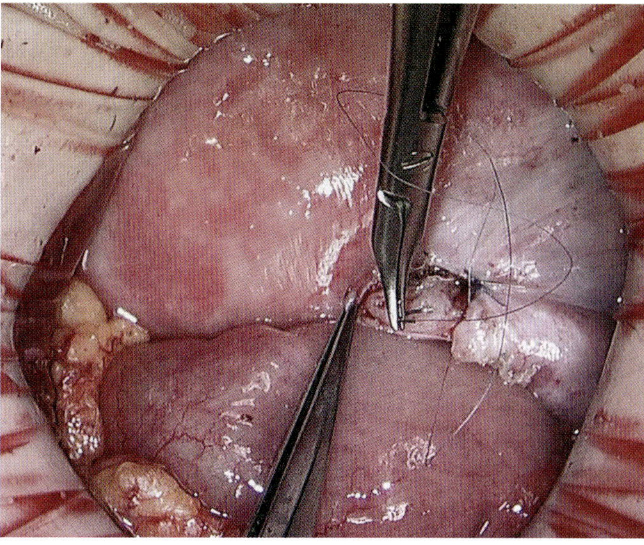

Figure 6.9 The muscularis at the 6 o'clock position is anastomosed with 8-0 suture.

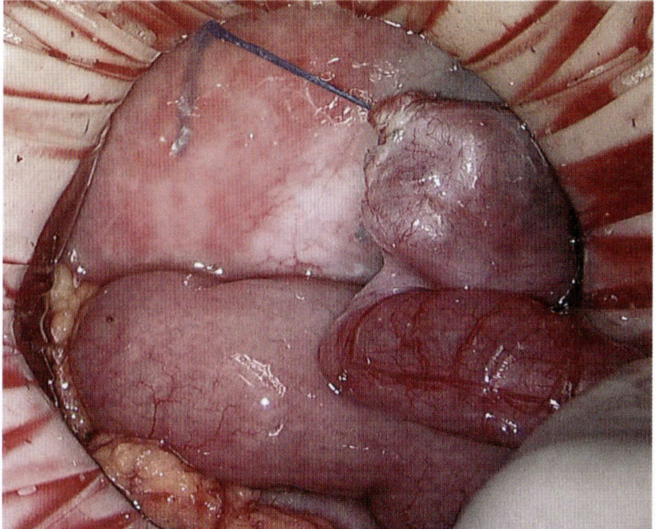

Figure 6.7 Transfimbrial retrograde chromotubation showing patency of the distal tubal segment.

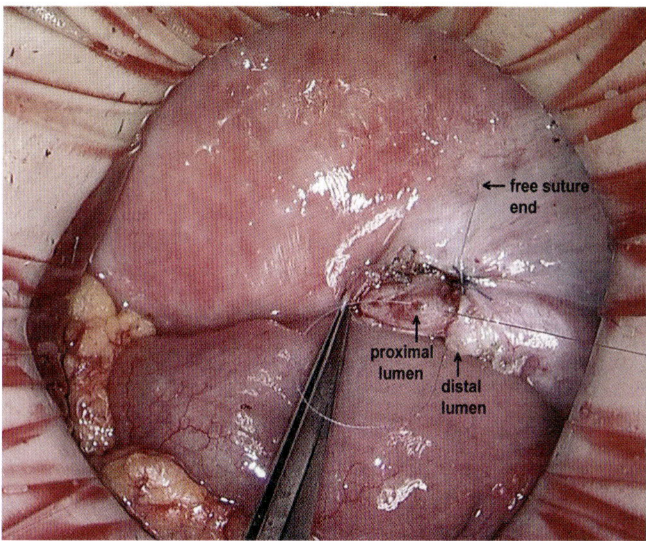

Figure 6.10 The suture is placed from superficial to deep at the distal end and then deep to superficial at the proximal end. The 3, 9, and 12 o'clock sutures are then placed in the same fashion.

6.6 Conclusion

Surgical reversal of tubal sterilization is a highly effective option for restoring fertility, even in older patients. It is often more cost-effective than IVF.

References

1. Mosher WD, Martinez GM, Chandra A, Abma JC, Willson SJ. Use of contraception and use of family planning services in the United States: 1982–2002. *Adv Data*. 2004;1–36.

2. Bartz D, Greenberg JA. Sterilization in the United States. *Rev Obstet Gynecol*. 2008;1:23–32.

3. Hillis SD, Marchbanks PA, Tylor LR, Peterson HB. Poststerilization regret: findings from the United States Collaborative Review of Sterilization. *Obstet Gynecol*. 1999;93:889–95.

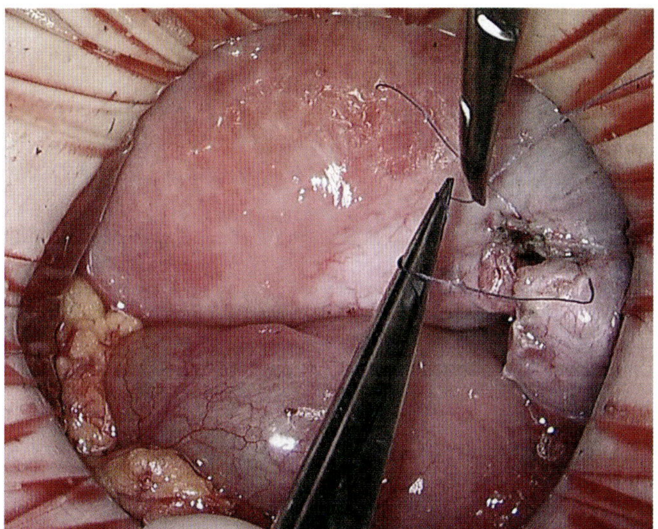

Figure 6.8 The tubal ends are approximated and aligned with a 6-0 suture is placed in the mesosalpinx. All knots are formed with instrument ties.

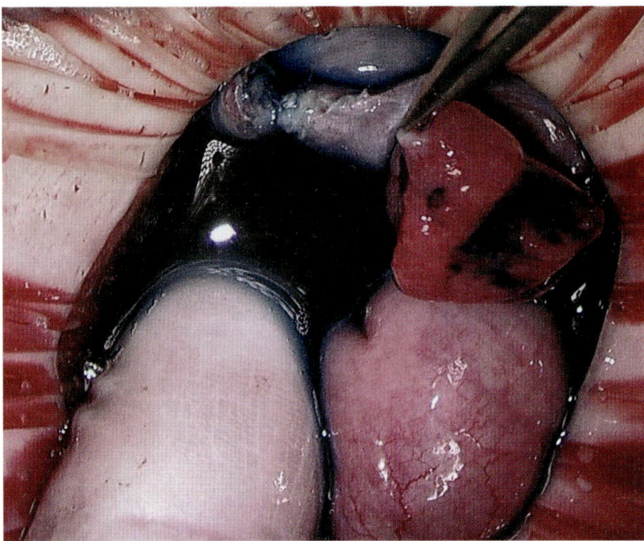

Figure 6.11 Transcervical chromotubation confirming patency of the anastomosis.

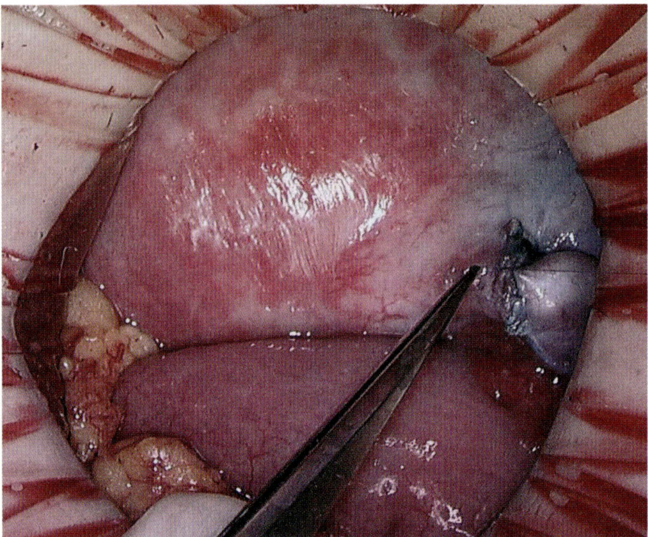

Figure 6.12 Closing the serosa with interrupted 8-0 suture.

4. Peterson HB, Xia Z, Hughes JM, Wilcox LS, Tylor LR, Trussell J. The risk of pregnancy after tubal sterilization: findings from the U.S. Collaborative Review of Sterilization. *Am J Obstet Gynecol.* 1996;174:1161-8-70.

5. Practice Committee of the American Society of Reproductive Medicine. Role of tubal surgery in the era of assisted reproductive technology: a committee opinion. *Fertil Steril.* 2015;103:e37–43.

6. Trimbos-Kemper TC. Reversal of sterilization in women over 40 years of age: a multicenter survey in the Netherlands. *Fertil Steril.* 1990;53:575–7.

7. Kim JD, Kim KS, Doo JK, Rhyeu CH. A report on 387 cases of microsurgical tubal reversals. *Fertil Steril.* 1997;68:875–80.

8. Dubuisson JB, et al. Sterilization reversal: fertility results. *Hum Reprod.* 1995;10:1145–51.

9. Berger GS, Thorp JM, Weaver MA. Effectiveness of bilateral tubotubal anastomosis in a large outpatient population. *Hum Reprod.* 2016;31:1120–5.

10. Malacova E, et al. Live delivery outcome after tubal sterilization reversal: a population-based study. *Fertil Steril.* 2015;104:921–6.

11. Boeckxstaens A, Devroey P, Collins J, Tournaye H. Getting pregnant after tubal sterilization: surgical reversal or IVF? *Hum Reprod.* 2007;22:2660–4.

12. Gomel V. The place of reconstructive tubal surgery in the era of assisted reproductive techniques. *Reprod Biomed Online,* 2015;31:722–31.

13. Messinger LB, et al. Cost and efficacy comparison of in vitro fertilization and tubal anastomosis for women after tubal ligation. *Fertil Steril.* 2015;104:32–38.e4.

14. Petrucco OM, Silber SJ, Chamberlain SL, Warnes GM, Davies M. Live birth following day surgery reversal of female sterilisation in women older than 40 years: a realistic option in Australia? *Med J Aust.* 2007;187:271–3.

15. Cha SH, et al. Fertility outcome after tubal anastomosis by laparoscopy and laparotomy. *J Am Assoc Gynecol Laparosc.* 2001;8:348–52.

16. Rodgers AK, Goldberg JM, Hammel JP, Falcone T. Tubal anastomosis by robotic compared with outpatient minilaparotomy. *Obstet Gynecol.* 2007;109:1375–80.

17. Dharia Patel SP, Steinkampf MP, Whitten SJ, Malizia BA. Robotic tubal anastomosis: surgical technique and cost effectiveness. *Fertil Steril.* 2008;90:1175–9.

18. Monteith CW, Berger GS, Zerden ML. Pregnancy success after hysteroscopic sterilization reversal. *Obstet Gynecol.* 2014;124:1183–9.

Chapter 7

Surgical Management of Ectopic Pregnancy

Bala Bhagavath

7.1 Background

Two percent of all pregnancies occur outside the uterine cavity and the incidence of ectopic pregnancy is higher (5–11%) in patients undergoing infertility management. The rate is as high as 20% in patients who have had prior tubal surgery [1]. This chapter reviews the preoperative considerations, surgical management, and postoperative care of tubal, cornual, cervical, ovarian, and cesarean-section scar ectopic pregnancies as well as extra-pelvic ectopic pregnancies in locations such as the abdomen/peritoneum, omentum, spleen, liver, and the retroperitoneum.

In the United States, the mortality rate due to ectopic pregnancy decreased from 1.15/100,000 deliveries in 1980–1984 to 0.5/100,000 deliveries in 2003–2007. It is projected that the current mortality rate due to ectopic pregnancy is 0.36/100,000 deliveries. Despite this encouraging data, the mortality rate due to ectopic pregnancy was almost seven times higher for African American women and 3.5 times higher for women older than 35 years. Seventy percent of deaths from ectopic pregnancy occurred with tubal pregnancies and 67% were in hospitalized patients [2]. All ethnic groups other than white were more likely to have complications from ectopic pregnancy as one study of low-income-group women had showed [3]. Of greater concern, the incidence of ectopic pregnancy has increased from 19/1,000 pregnancies in 1993 to 26/1,000 pregnancies in 2007 [4]. Infertility treatment increases the risk of ectopic pregnancy and the risk has been tied to the number of oocytes retrieved during controlled ovarian hyperstimulation cycles [5]. The risk of ectopic pregnancy is reduced with transfer of blastocyst-stage embryos and there is no increase in the risk due to ectopic pregnancy with transfer of frozen embryos [6].

7.1.1 Diagnosis

In most fertility clinics, early monitoring of serum hCG results in detection of an ectopic pregnancy prior to the development of any symptoms. The diagnosis is more challenging in the gynecologic clinic or emergency medicine department setting. The hallmark of an ectopic pregnancy is the abnormally slow rise of serum levels of beta subunit of hCG. The original proposal of a 53% rise in levels within a 48-hour period to distinguish abnormal from normal intrauterine pregnancy has now been revised to a minimum level of 35% increase in 48 hours [7]. Abnormally rising hCG levels coupled with an empty uterus on ultrasound raises the suspicion for an ectopic

pregnancy. Using a discriminatory serum hCG level of 3,000 mIU/mL and an empty uterus on transvaginal ultrasound exam, there is still a 0.5% chance of a viable intrauterine pregnancy. Therefore, unless the patient is unstable, it is prudent to check at least one more hCG level in the next few days with repeat of ultrasound before advocating intervention. The sensitivity of ultrasound markers has been analyzed in a recent meta-analysis. Empty uterus, pseudosac, adnexal mass, and fluid in the cul-de-sac have poor sensitivity but reasonably high specificity. As a result, none of these signs can be used to rule out an ectopic pregnancy [8]. A new set of ultrasound criteria was established by the Society of Radiologists in Ultrasound based on the gestational and yolk sacs, crown-rump length and cardiac activity [9]. Novel markers such as interleukin-6 and activin-A have recently been proposed as adjuncts in the diagnosis of tubal pregnancies but no test is of yet 100% sensitive and specific in diagnosing ectopic pregnancy [10,11].

A dedicated multiprofessional team approach to management has shown to increase ultrasound visualization of ectopic pregnancies from 22% to 61% and decrease negative findings at laparoscopy from 13% to 6% [12]. The possible benefits of such a team approach include improvements in communication, education, patient care, and team cohesion [13].

Nontubal pregnancies are often diagnosed late with life-threatening consequences to the affected women [14]. A high index of suspicion has to be maintained at all times to diagnose and treat them expeditiously.

7.1.2 Treatment Considerations

Nonsurgical management of ectopic pregnancy should always be favored where possible, to decrease surgical and anesthetic risks to the patient. Even with ectopic pregnancies occurring in sites other than the fallopian tube, medical management has been shown to be safe and effective [15]. Despite this, surgical management of ectopic pregnancies remains most popular [16,17]. A recent national survey in the UK revealed that 57% of ectopic pregnancies are managed by laparoscopy, 31% medically, 5% by laparotomy, and 6% expectantly [18]. Similar detailed data is not available for the United States. One report from Maryland examined trends from 1999 to 2004. Comparing data for 1994–1999 with 2000–2004, the rate of surgical management of ectopic pregnancy had increased to 88% in hospitalized patients [19]. In another study, use of data from 200 commercial insurance companies from 2002 to 2007 revealed that Methotrexate treatment increased from 11% to 35% whereas laparotomy rate decreased from 40% to 33%. No data was reported on the use of laparoscopic approach. The failure rate for methotrexate treatment was 14% in this study [20]. Surgical management should be reserved for patients who are not eligible for medical or expectant management. When surgical management is chosen, a laparoscopic approach should be taken. A prospective study covering 10 years from 2003 to 2013 showed that after 4 years, they were consistently able to treat all ectopic surgeries, whether hemodynamically stable or not, by laparoscopy [21].

7.2 Tubal Pregnancy (Other Than in the Interstitial Portion)

The most common location (95%) of an ectopic pregnancy is in the fallopian tube [14]. Traditionally, salpingectomy of the affected tube has been the standard of care. In the past two decades, earlier clinical diagnosis has enabled most patients to be treated medically or with salpingostomy to preserve the affected tube. Multiple retrospective studies have shown that the pregnancy rate and recurrent ectopic pregnancy rate after salpingostomy (50–88% and 8%, respectively) are no different compared with salpingectomy (55–68% and 8%, respectively) [22–25]. It may be advantageous to perform a second-look laparoscopy 3 months after salpingostomy in those who have significant adhesions at the time of salpingostomy. In a randomized trial, investigators showed the cumulative pregnancy rate at 36 months was significantly better (60% vs 30%) in women who have significant adhesions at salpingostomy who then had a second-look laparoscopy [26]. Another retrospective study of 334 salpingostomies performed by laparoscopy showed that failure of treatment is more likely with ectopic pregnancies larger than 33.5 mm in diameter. In addition, salpingostomies performed for tubal pregnancies located near the fimbrial end or the cornual end were more likely to fail [27]. The European Surgery in Ectopic Pregnancy study group performed a cost–benefit analysis in a randomized trial. It concluded that the surgical or postoperative follow-up cost is more for the salpingostomy group compared with the salpingectomy group with a higher risk for persistent trophoblast in the salpingostomy group. It was acknowledged that cost of any subsequent IVF cycle was not included in this analysis [28].

Concerns have been raised regarding ovarian reserve being adversely affected after salpingectomy. A prospective study of 131 patients with ectopic pregnancy showed that regardless of whether the patients had methotrexate, methotrexate followed by salpingectomy (15 patients), or salpingectomy, the pre-treatment and post-treatment anti-müllerian hormone levels were not significantly different 3 months after treatment [29].

7.2.1 Diagnosis

The gold standard for the diagnosis of tubal pregnancy is laparoscopy followed by histopathological confirmation after examination of the tissue removed at surgery. Occasionally, a gestational sac with a fetal pole and fetal cardiac activity can be noted outside of the uterine cavity on ultrasound examination.

More frequently, a mass is noticed outside of the uterus and the ovaries with or without the presence of free fluid in the cul-de-sac. Most commonly, the suspicion of tubal pregnancy is entertained with the finding of discriminatory levels of hCG (as discussed under the general diagnosis section earlier) and an empty uterus. Ectopic pregnancy has been documented in the stump of the tube that was previously removed and should be considered if symptoms suggest that possibility [30].

7.2.2 Treatment Considerations

There is no difference in subsequent intrauterine or repeat ectopic pregnancy rates between salpingectomy and salpingostomy (see Video 7.1). The intrauterine pregnancy rate was 56% in salpingectomy vs 61% in salpingostomy and the repeat ectopic pregnancy rate was 5% vs 8%, respectively, neither of which was statistically significant [31]. Concerns have been raised about the effect of salpingectomy on ovarian reserve. A retrospective study of 118 women who underwent IVF after salpingectomy or salpingostomy showed no difference in the number of eggs retrieved [32].

In standard three-port laparoscopic salpingostomy, the uterus is laterally deviated to the contralateral side of the ectopic pregnancy while the distal part of the affected tube is grasped with atraumatic graspers and pulled to the ipsilateral side. Dilute vasopressin (20–30 units in 100 ml of saline) can be injected into the mesosalpinx beneath the ectopic (Figure 7.1). A monopolar needle or scissors is then used to incise the tube on the anti-mesenteric border over the ectopic bulge (Figure 7.2). The products of conception will often spontaneously extrude out. Manual compression on the exterior of the tube beneath the ectopic can facilitate expressing the products of conception through the salpingostomy incision (Figure 7.3). The products may also be flushed out using hydrodissection. In any case, it is important to avoid placing graspers in the incision to extract the tissue as it tends to cause more bleeding, which can be difficult to control, leading to excessive thermal injury from electrocautery or even the need for salpingectomy.

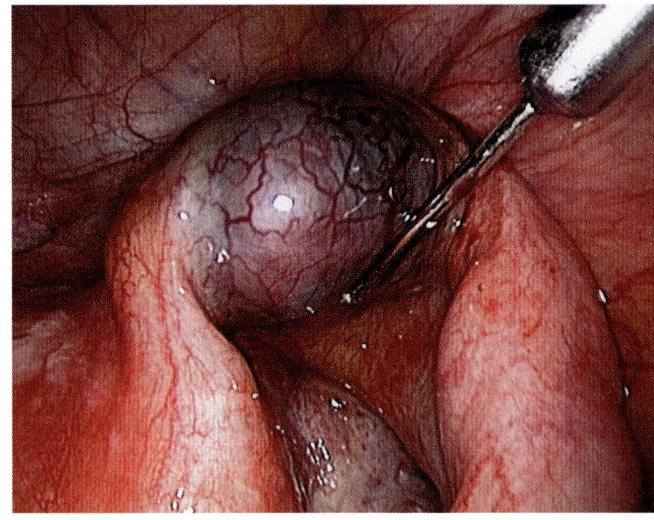

Figure 7.1 Dilute vasopressin is injected in the mesosalpinx beneath an unruptured isthmic ectopic.

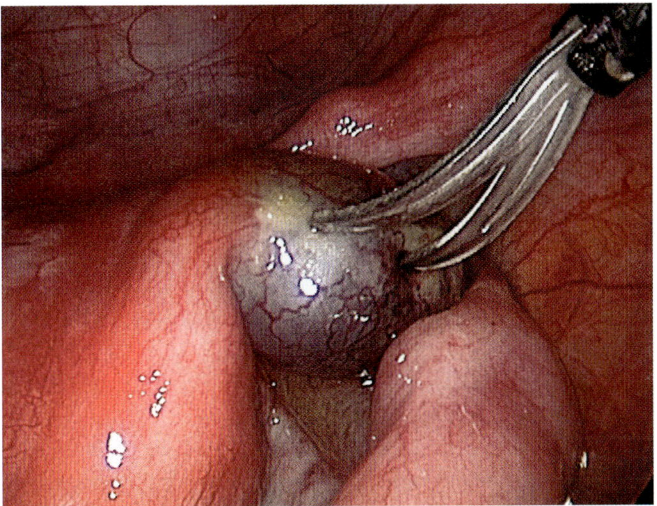

Figure 7.2 The antimesenteric surface of the ectopic bulge is incised with scissors.

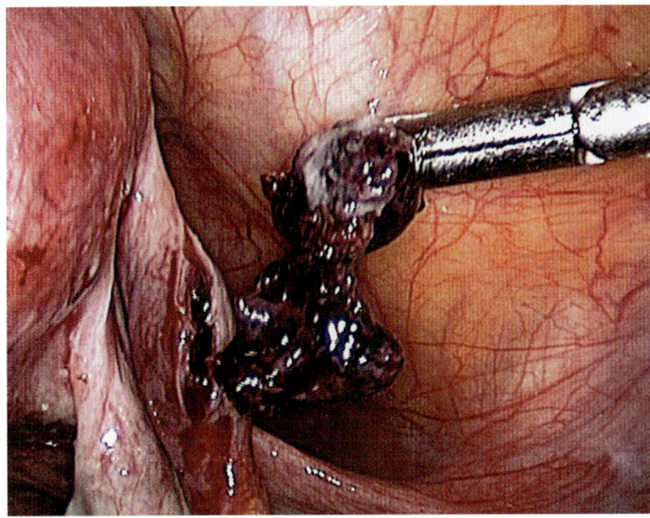

Figure 7.4 The products of conception are removed from the peritoneal cavity.

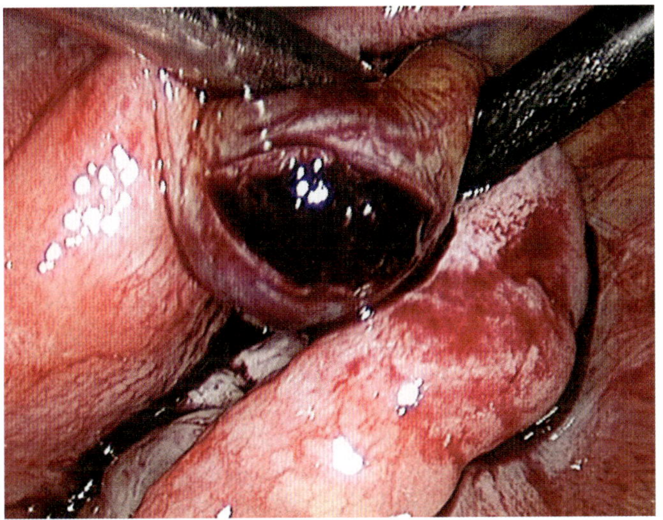

Figure 7.3 External compression is used to express the products of conception through the salpingostomy incision.

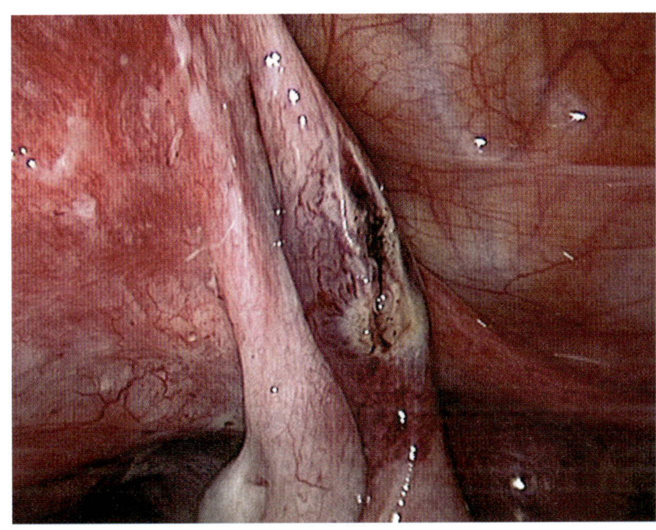

Figure 7.5 Hemostasis is assured and the salpingostomy incision is left open.

The products of conception must be meticulously removed from the pelvis to avoid persistence of the trophoblastic tissue (Figure 7.4). Salpingostomy is left open to heal by secondary intention (Figure 7.5).

Salpingectomy can be started at the cornual or fimbriated end. The mesosalpinx, as well as the proximal tube, are coagulated with bipolar cautery then divided with scissors (Figures 7.6–7.9). Care must be taken to stay as close to the mesenteric border of the fallopian tube as possible to prevent possible compromise of the blood supply to the ovary. Advanced sealing devices can be used instead of the bipolar graspers and scissors. A single-port approach can also be used for both salpingostomy as well as salpingectomy and the principles are similar to multiport approach [33,34]. Regardless of the approach, the products of conception should be carefully removed, preferably after placing them in a tissue removal bag.

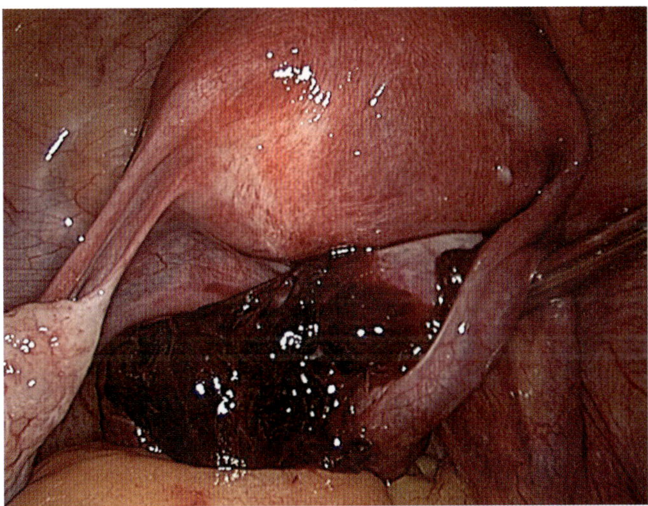

Figure 7.6 This is a ruptured ampullary ectopic pregnancy.

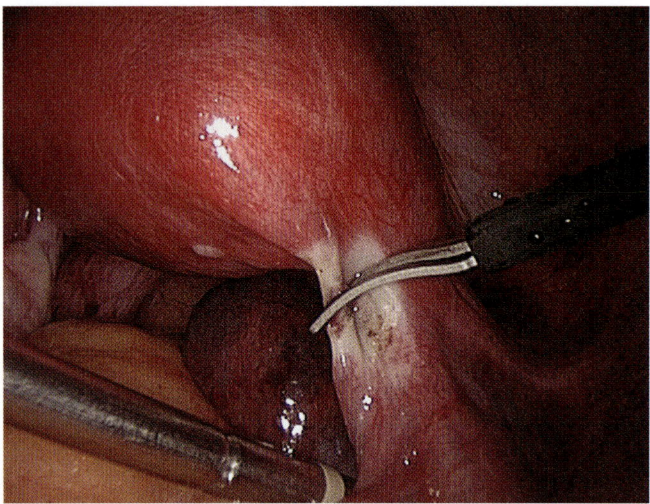

Figure 7.7 The proximal tube is coagulated and divided.

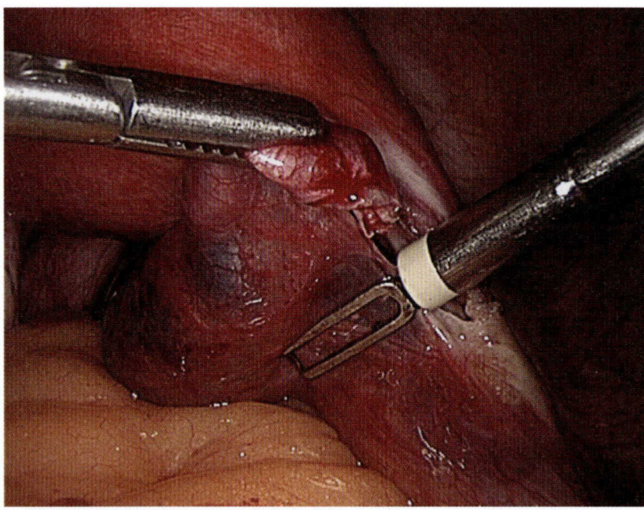

Figure 7.8 The mesosalpinx is coagulated close to the tube to avoid compromising the ovarian vascular supply.

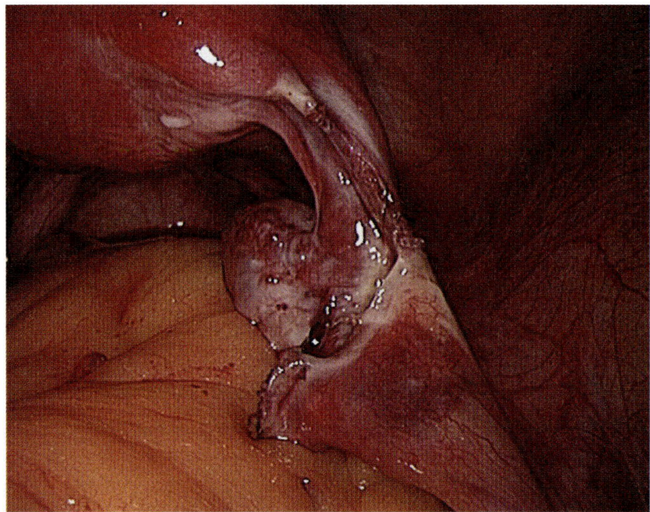

Figure 7.9 The tube has been removed through the 10 mm umbilical port, taking care not to leave any products of conception behind.

7.3 Cornual or Interstitial Pregnancy

Although some authors make the distinction that interstitial pregnancy occurs in the interstitial portion of the fallopian tube and cornual pregnancy occurs in a rudimentary uterine horn of a unicornuate uterus, in this chapter, cornual pregnancy is used to mean a pregnancy in the interstitial portion of the fallopian tube. The risk factors for cornual pregnancy are no different than for other tubal pregnancies, but in one series 71% of patients had previous bilateral salpingectomies [35]. Therefore, a high index of suspicion has to be entertained in order to diagnose this condition.

In one case series of 17 patients, the majority of patients (68%) underwent laparoscopic management of the cornual pregnancy as opposed to medical treatment. In patients who desired another pregnancy, 58% were successful regardless of the type of treatment [36]. Another recent series of patients reported a pregnancy rate of 39% after surgery [35].

7.3.1 Diagnosis

A triad of ultrasound signs was proposed by Timor-Titsch including an empty uterine cavity, an eccentrically placed gestational sac, and a thin myometrium surrounding the gestational sac that is < 5 mm. Ackerman added a fourth sign of a bright echogenic line extending from the uterine cavity to the cornua running to one side of the gestational sac called the "interstitial line." Use of all four criteria results in 80% sensitivity and 98% specificity for the diagnosis of ectopic pregnancy [37].

7.3.2 Treatment Considerations

Compared with laparotomy, laparoscopic management of the cornual pregnancy has the advantages of faster recovery and decreased morbidity. However, effective hemostasis is a prime concern and surgeons must possess the requisite laparoscopic suturing skills. As a result, many patients undergo laparotomy with resection of the affected cornua. Others have advocated a hysteroscopic approach with either resection, use of urologic stone retriever forceps, or injection of methotrexate to treat the gestational sac [38,39]. Most surgeons favor a laparoscopic approach and in experienced hands, the outcome is as good as with other tubal pregnancies managed by laparoscopy [40].

Techniques described for hemostasis can be broadly classified into chemical vasoconstrictive agents (dilute vasopressin), securing of the ascending branch of the uterine artery using suture (endoloop, encircling suture around the base of the ectopic, square suture that is carried through and through the anterior and posterior walls of the uterus), automatic stapler, electro-cautery, fibrin glue, and uterine artery ligation [41].

A standard, three-port laparotomy approach is sufficient to manage the condition. A single-port approach has also been reported. If the ascending branch of the uterine artery is to be suture ligated, the double-impact devascularization technique can be used [41]. A 0-Proline or similar suture can be used to take a first bite along the medial border of the cornual ectopic after infiltrating with dilute vasopressin solution (20–30 units of vasopressin in 100 ml of normal saline) traversing from the superior to the inferior margin of the ectopic. The needle should then be reversed and the bite taken in the posterior to the anterior direction underneath the ectopic, through the mesosalpinx. The knot is then tied over the fundus, thus constricting the ectopic as well as the ascending branch of the uterine artery. More than two bites can be employed to achieve a good purse-string effect. An alternative method is to use an endoloop device to encircle the base of the ectopic gestation. This does not quite secure the ascending branch of the uterine artery but does not require any suturing skills [42].

The cornual ectopic may be treated by cornuostomy or wedge resection. Monopolar cautery or harmonic scalpel can be used to create a linear cornuostomy to allow evacuation of the contents with laparoscopic suction irrigator and/or graspers. Once the contents have been evacuated, the defect should be closed in one or two layers using interrupted or running sutures. If bidirectional barbed suture is available, all the above steps requiring suture can be achieved without any knot-tying skills. It has been reported that removal of the contents of the gestational sac alone is sufficient and it is not necessary to remove the sac. This reportedly decreases the risk of excessive bleeding and does not increase the risk of persistent ectopic tissue after the surgery [43,44].

Wedge resection of the cornua is the classic treatment for the condition. This is more likely to result in higher blood loss. After injection of dilute vasopressin, a monopolar needle or harmonic scalpel is used to resect the cornual ectopic before closing the defect using standard or bidirectional barbed suture. Reports of rupture and dehiscence in subsequent pregnancies have been published for patients with wedge resection but the safety of cornuostomy remains to be established [45].

7.4 Rudimentary Horn Pregnancy

Pregnancies in the rudimentary uterine horn of a unicornuate uterus can be mistaken for a pregnancy in a bicornuate uterus, cornual pregnancy, or abdominal pregnancy. Tsafrir proposed the following criteria to diagnose a pregnancy in the uterine horn: (1) asymmetric bicornuate uterine pattern; (2) absence of a visual continuity between the cervical canal and the uterine cavity containing the pregnancy; and (3) presence of myometrial tissue surrounding the gestational sac [46]. Rudimentary horn pregnancies may progress into the second trimester, leading to late rupture with severe intraperitoneal hemorrhage. They are best managed by laparoscopic excision of the rudimentary horn.

7.5 Cervical Pregnancy

Cervical pregnancies are relatively rare and comprise about 1% of all ectopic pregnancies [47].

7.5.1 Diagnosis

The classic sign of cervical pregnancy on ultrasound is an hourglass uterus. The uterus appears narrow with an enlarged cervix narrowing at the internal os. The differential diagnosis is a pregnancy in the process of miscarrying. Fetal cardiac activity may be present and Doppler ultrasonography may reveal increased vascularity surrounding a true ectopic pregnancy [48]. Both of these features will be absent with an aborting pregnancy.

7.5.2 Treatment Considerations

Due to its rarity and variable presentation, a standard treatment for cervical pregnancy has not been established. Options include medical treatment with methotrexate, systemically or by ultrasound-guided local instillation [49]. Surgical treatment with curettage may be performed followed by Foley balloon tamponade to limit bleeding from the placental bed [50]. Alternatively, or in addition, uterine artery embolization may be performed prior to curettage [48].

7.6 Cesarean Scar Pregnancy

There is some debate as to whether these are true ectopic pregnancies as they occur within the uterus, although in the lower uterine segment. Although conservative management of cesarean scar pregnancy has been reported to result in live birth, the vast majority of pregnancies are terminated secondary to the risk of rupture, bleeding, and placenta accreta [51].

7.6.1 Diagnosis

The cesarean scar pregnancy can be mistaken for a cervical pregnancy, pregnancy implanted in the lower uterine segment, or a miscarriage in progress. On ultrasound examination, these pregnancies will be located within the anterior myometrium with little or no myometrium between the gestational sac and the bladder [48].

7.6.2 Treatment Considerations

Treatment options include local injection of methotrexate, suction evacuation of the gestational sac, hysterotomy, and hysterectomy [52,53].

Suction curettage, with the additional use of a Foley balloon for tamponade in case of profuse bleeding, was shown to be safe and effective in a series of 19 patients, of whom 16 were successfully treated [53].

7.7 Ovarian Pregnancy

Ovarian ectopic pregnancy is diagnosed intraoperatively by the presence of Spiegelberg's criteria.

1. The gestational sac is in the region of the ovary.
2. The fallopian tube is intact on the side of the ectopic.
3. The ectopic pregnancy is attached to the uterus by the ovarian ligament.
4. Histological examination confirms presence of ovarian tissue in the wall of the gestational sac.

Although this set of criteria holds true today, it is possible to diagnose these using ultrasound. The etiology is not known but associated risk factors include fertility treatment and use of intrauterine device [54]. Ovarian pregnancies frequently present with rupture and severe blood loss compared with tubal pregnancies [55].

7.7.1 Diagnosis

Preoperative diagnosis by ultrasonography has reasonable accuracy [56]. However, distal tubal pregnancies, ruptured ovarian pregnancies with absence of yolk sac or fetal pole and normal corpus luteum, make the diagnosis challenging [47].

7.7.2 Treatment Considerations

Laparoscopic excision of the ectopic gestation with sparing of the ovarian tissue is the treatment of choice although laparoscopic approach is reported to be less likely to be used by surgeons compared to tubal pregnancies [54]. Monopolar cautery or harmonic scalpel can be used to perform the wedge resection of the ovary, taking care to remove as little of healthy ovarian tissue as possible. If the ovary cannot be saved, a salpingo-oophorectomy should be considered. Management with methotrexate as first line of treatment is not recommended for fear of rupture and uncontrolled bleeding.

7.8 Heterotopic Pregnancy

In a recent analysis of assisted reproductive technology (ART) pregnancies, 5% of all ectopic pregnancies were heterotopic – pregnancies in two different locations, one usually in the uterine cavity and the other in any of the ectopic pregnancy locations detailed earlier and later than this section [57]. The higher risk is attributed to ART and quite specifically to more than one embryo being transferred.

7.8.1 Diagnosis

Diagnosis is extremely difficult as visualization of the normal intrauterine pregnancy gives a false sense of security to care providers. A high index of suspicion must be entertained in any patient with a history of assisted reproductive technologies.

7.8.2 Treatment Considerations

Specific treatment of the ectopic pregnancy depends on the location of the ectopic, the hemodynamic stability of the patient, and her desire to continue the intrauterine pregnancy. Local injection of methotrexate, KCl, and hyperosmolar glucose have been reported with subsequent delivery of a normal, healthy baby, though methotrexate is a concern if the intrauterine pregnancy is desired [58]. Laparoscopic salpingostomy or salpingectomy may also be performed with continuation of the intrauterine pregnancy.

7.9 Abdominal Pregnancy

Abdominal pregnancies occur when the oocyte is fertilized in the peritoneal cavity or the preimplantation embryo is expelled from the fimbriated end of the fallopian tube. They have been documented in the peritoneum, omentum, bowel, spleen, liver, and retroperitoneum [59]. The most common location is on the serosal surface of the uterus and the peritoneum covering the adnexa, which constituted 48% of cases in one case series of 31 patients. The next common location was bowel (30%). There were three fetal deaths among 27 fetuses in 22 patients and 7 maternal deaths among 26 patients, making this a condition with very high maternal and fetal mortality rates [60].

7.9.1 Diagnosis

The diagnosis can be confirmed by ultrasound examination with additional magnetic resonance imaging or computerized tomography if indicated. The diagnostic findings include an empty uterus, gestational sac with a fetus that is not surrounded by myometrium, unusual lie of the fetus if advanced gestational age with low amniotic fluid volume, and poor visualization of the placenta. More unusual locations such as spleen and liver are typically diagnosed usually after a negative laparoscopy leads to MR or CT imaging [48].

7.9.2 Treatment Considerations

The management of abdominal pregnancies depends on the hemodynamic stability of the mother, the gestational age, and the condition of the fetus and poses two therapeutic dilemmas. The first is whether to allow a previable pregnancy to continue at the expense of putting the mother at risk if she were to start bleeding profusely. The second is the management of the placenta at delivery. Removal of placenta almost always results in severe bleeding and can damage the organ(s) of attachment.

Leaving the placenta in can lead to potentially life-threatening consequences such as hemorrhage, sepsis, disseminated intravascular coagulation, fistula formation, and bowel obstruction. If the decision is made to leave the placenta in, methotrexate may be administered to the patient prior to the surgery or immediately postsurgery. Use of methotrexate before or after surgery is not universally accepted and the benefits are unclear [61].

If a decision is made to remove placenta at the time of surgery, selective embolization of the bleeding placental bed can be undertaken intraoperatively. Abdominal packing of the placental bed, followed by removal after a few days has also been reported [61].

Pregnancies in other locations such as spleen and liver have been treated conservatively with a combination of intramuscular methotrexate and percutaneous ultrasound-guided local injection of methotrexate into the gestational sac. Surgical treatment should be reserved as a last resort [62].

References

1. Strandell A, Thorburn J, Hamberger L. Risk factors for ectopic pregnancy in assisted reproduction. *Fertil Steril.* 1999;71(2):282–6.

2. Creanga AA, Shapiro-Mendoza CK, Bish CL, Zane S, Berg CJ, Callaghan WM. Trends in ectopic pregnancy mortality in the United States: 1980–2007. *Obstet Gynecol.* 2011;117(4):837–43.

3. Stulberg DB, Cain L, Dahlquist IH, Lauderdale DS. Ectopic pregnancy morbidity and mortality in low-income women, 2004–2008. *Hum Reprod.* 2016;31(3):666–71.

4. Trabert B, Schwartz SM, Peters U, et al. Genetic variation in the sex hormone metabolic pathway and endometriosis risk: an evaluation of candidate genes. *Fertil Steril.* 2011;96(6):1401–6.e3.

5. Acharya KS, Acharya CR, Provost MP, et al. Ectopic pregnancy rate increases with the number of retrieved oocytes in autologous in vitro fertilization with non-tubal infertility but

not donor/recipient cycles: an analysis of 109,140 clinical pregnancies from the Society for Assisted Reproductive Technology registry. *Fertil Steril.* 2015;104(4):873–8.

6. Santos-Ribeiro S, Tournaye H, Polyzos NP. Trends in ectopic pregnancy rates following assisted reproductive technologies in the UK: a 12-year nationwide analysis including 160,000 pregnancies. *Hum Reprod.* 2016;31(2):393–402.

7. Morse CB, Sammel MD, Shaunik A, et al. Performance of human chorionic gonadotropin curves in women at risk for ectopic pregnancy: exceptions to the rules. *Fertil Steril.* 2012;97(1):101,6.e2.

8. Richardson A, Gallos I, Dobson S, Campbell BK, Coomarasamy A, Raine-Fenning N. Accuracy of first-trimester ultrasound in diagnosis of tubal ectopic pregnancy in the absence of an obvious extrauterine embryo: systematic review and meta-analysis. *Ultrasound Obstet Gynecol.* 2016;47(1):28–37.

9. Doubilet PM, Benson CB, Bourne T, Blaivas M, Society of Radiologists in Ultrasound Multispecialty Panel on Early First Trimester Diagnosis of Miscarriage and Exclusion of a Viable Intrauterine Pregnancy, Barnhart KT, et al. Diagnostic criteria for nonviable pregnancy early in the first trimester. *N Engl J Med.* 2013;369(15):1443–51.

10. Rajendiran S, Senthil Kumar GP, Nimesh A, Dhiman P, Shivaraman K, Soundararaghavan S. Diagnostic significance of IL-6 and IL-8 in tubal ectopic pregnancy. *J Obstet Gynaecol.* 2016:1–3.

11. Barnhart KT. Novel diagnostic tests of ectopic pregnancy, if at first you don't succeed. *Am J Obstet Gynecol.* 2015;212(1):4–6.

12. Berry J, Davey M, Hon MS, Behrens R. Optimising the diagnosis of ectopic pregnancy. *J Obstet Gynaecol.* 2016;36(4):437–9.

13. Bharathan R, Farag M, Hayes K. The value of multidisciplinary team meetings within an early pregnancy assessment unit. *J Obstet Gynaecol.* 2016;3:1–5.

14. Parker VL, Srinivas M. Non-tubal ectopic pregnancy. *Arch Gynecol Obstet.* 2016;294(1):19–27.

15. Hunt SP, Talmor A, Vollenhoven B. Management of non-tubal ectopic pregnancies at a large tertiary hospital. *Reprod Biomed Online.* 2016;33(1):79–84.

16. Berry J, Davey M, Hon MS, Behrens R. A 5-year experience of the changing management of ectopic pregnancy. *J Obstet Gynaecol.* 2016;36(5):631–4.

17. Berretta R, Dall'Asta A, Merisio C, et al. Tubal ectopic pregnancy: our experience from 2000 to 2013. *Acta Biomed.* 2015 14;86(2):176–80.

18. Taheri M, Bharathan R, Subramaniam A, Kelly T. A United Kingdom national survey of trends in ectopic pregnancy management. *J Obstet Gynaecol.* 2014;34(6):508–11.

19. Sewell CA, Anderson JR. Update on trends for inpatient surgical management of tubal ectopic pregnancy in Maryland. *South Med J.* 2011;104(7):488–94.

20. Hoover KW, Tao G, Kent CK. Trends in the diagnosis and treatment of ectopic pregnancy in the United States. *Obstet Gynecol.* 2010;115(3):495–502.

21. Odejinmi F, Rizzuto I, Oliver R, Alalade A, Agarwal N, Olowu O. Beyond guidelines: effectiveness of a programme in achieving operative laparoscopy for all women requiring surgical management of ectopic pregnancy. *Gynecol Obstet Invest.* 2015;80(1):46–53.

22. Jamard A, Turck M, Pham AD, Dreyfus M, Benoist G. Fertility and risk of recurrence after surgical treatment of an ectopic pregnancy (EP): salpingostomy versus salpingectomy. *J Gynecol Obstet Biol Reprod (Paris).* 2016;45(2):129–38.

23. Li J, Jiang K, Zhao F. Fertility outcome analysis after surgical management of tubal ectopic pregnancy: a retrospective cohort study. *BMJ Open.* 2015;5(9):e007339.

24. Cheng X, Tian X, Yan Z, et al. Comparison of the fertility outcome of salpingotomy and salpingectomy in women with tubal pregnancy: a systematic review and meta-analysis. *PLoS One.* 2016;11(3):e0152343.

25. Demirdag E, Guler I, Abay S, Oguz Y, Erdem M, Erdem A. The impact of expectant management, systemic methotrexate and surgery on subsequent pregnancy outcomes in tubal ectopic pregnancy. *Ir J Med Sci.* 2017;186(2):387–92.

26. Li Z, Liu J, Min W, Zhang D, Yang X, Sun Y. Effect of second-look laparoscopy on subsequent fertility outcome after laparoscopic salpingostomy for tubal pregnancy: a randomized controlled study. *J Minim Invasive Gynecol.* 2015;22(4):612–8.

27. Kayatas S, Demirci O, Kumru P, Mahmutoglu D, Saribrahim B, Arinkan SA. Predictive factors for failure of salpingostomy in ectopic pregnancy. *J Obstet Gynaecol Res.* 2014;40(2):453–8.

28. Mol F, van Mello NM, Strandell A, et al. Cost-effectiveness of salpingotomy and salpingectomy in women with tubal pregnancy (a randomized controlled trial). *Hum Reprod.* 2015;30(9):2038–47.

29. Sahin Y, Kelestimur F. Medical treatment regimens of hirsutism. *Reprod Biomed Online.* 2004;8(5):538–46.

30. Karadeniz RS, Tasci Y, Altay M, Akkus M, Akkurt O, Gelisen O. Tubal rupture in ectopic pregnancy: is it predictable? *Minerva Ginecol.* 2015;67(1):13–9.

31. Mol F, van Mello NM, Strandell A, et al. Salpingotomy versus salpingectomy in women with tubal pregnancy (ESEP study): an open-label, multicentre, randomised controlled trial. *Lancet.* 2014;383(9927):1483–9.

32. Odesjo E, Bergh C, Strandell A. Surgical methods for tubal pregnancy – effects on ovarian response to controlled stimulation during IVF. *Acta Obstet Gynecol Scand.* 2015;94(12):1322–6.

33. Carbonnel M, Revaux A, Frydman R, Yazigi A, Ayoubi JM. Single-port approach to benign gynecologic pathology. A review. *Minerva Ginecol.* 2015;67(3):239–47.

34. Nicollerat JA. Elevated plasma glucose levels increase risk for complications. *Diabetes Educ.* 2000;26 Suppl:11–3.

35. Wang J, Huang D, Lin X, et al. Incidence of interstitial pregnancy after in vitro fertilization/embryo transfer and the outcome of a consecutive series of 38 cases managed by laparoscopic cornuostomy or cornual repair. *J Minim Invasive Gynecol.* 2016;23(5):739–47.

36. Nikodijevic K, Bricou A, Benbara A, et al. Cornual pregnancy: management and subsequent fertility. *Gynecol Obstet Fertil.* 2016;44(1):11–16.

37. Moawad NS, Mahajan ST, Moniz MH, Taylor SE, Hurd WW. Current diagnosis and treatment of interstitial pregnancy. *Am J Obstet Gynecol.* 2010;202(1):15–29.

38. Grindler NM, Ng J, Tocce K, Alvero R. Considerations for management of interstitial ectopic pregnancies: two case reports. *J Med Case Rep.* 2016;10(1):106.

39. Leggieri C, Guasina F, Casadio P, Arena A, Pilu G, Seracchioli R. Hysteroscopic methotrexate injection under ultrasonographic guidance for interstitial pregnancy. *J Minim Invasive Gynecol.* 2016;23(7):1195–9.

40. Nirgianakis K, Papadia A, Grandi G, McKinnon B, Bolla D, Mueller MD. Laparoscopic management of ectopic pregnancies: a comparison between interstitial and "more distal" tubal pregnancies. *Arch Gynecol Obstet.* 2017;295(1):95–101.

41. Afifi Y, Mahmud A, Fatma A. Hemostatic techniques for laparoscopic management of cornual pregnancy: double-impact devascularization technique. *J Minim Invasive Gynecol.* 2016;23(2):274–80.

42. Faioli R, Berretta R, Dall'Asta A, et al. Endoloop technique for laparoscopic cornuectomy: a safe and effective approach for the treatment of interstitial pregnancy. *J Obstet Gynaecol Res.* 2016;42(8):1034–7.

43. Soriano D, Vicus D, Mashiach R, Schiff E, Seidman D, Goldenberg M. Laparoscopic treatment of cornual pregnancy: a series of 20 consecutive cases. *Fertil Steril.* 2008;90(3):839–43.

44. Ross R, Lindheim SR, Olive DL, Pritts EA. Cornual gestation: a systematic literature review and two case reports of a novel treatment regimen. *J Minim Invasive Gynecol.* 2006;13(1):74–8.

45. Liao CY, Tse J, Sung SY, Chen SH, Tsui WH. Cornual wedge resection for interstitial pregnancy and postoperative outcome. *Aust N Z J Obstet Gynaecol.* 2017;57(3):342–5.

46. Tsafrir A, Rojansky N, Sela HY, Gomori JM, Nadjari M. Rudimentary horn pregnancy: first-trimester prerupture sonographic diagnosis and confirmation by magnetic resonance imaging. *J Ultrasound Med.* 2005;24(2):219–23.

47. Hosni MM, Herath RP, Mumtaz R. Diagnostic and therapeutic dilemmas of cervical ectopic pregnancy. *Obstet Gynecol Surv.* 2014;69(5):261–76.

48. Dibble EH, Lourenco AP. Imaging unusual pregnancy implantations: rare ectopic pregnancies and more. *AJR Am J Roentgenol.* 2016:1–13.

49. Goldberg JM, Widrich T. Successful management of a viable cervical pregnancy by single-dose methotrexate. *J Womens Health Gend Based Med.* 2000;9(1):43–5.

50. Frishman GN, Melzer KE, Bhagavath B. Ectopic pregnancy in a cesarean-section scar: the patient >6 weeks into an ectopic pregnancy, underwent local treatment. *Am J Obstet Gynecol.* 2012;207(3):238.e1–238.e2.

51. Abraham RJ, Weston MJ. Expectant management of a caesarean scar pregnancy. *J Obstet Gynaecol.* 2012;32(7):695–6.

52. Liu S, Durai S. Management of a case of caesarean scar pregnancy and all its complications. *BMJ Case Rep.* 2016 May 17;2016. DOI: 10.1136/bcr,2016–215111.

53. Polat I, Ekiz A, Acar DK, et al. Suction curettage as first line treatment in cases with cesarean scar pregnancy: feasibility and effectiveness in early pregnancy. *J Matern Fetal Neonatal Med.* 2016;29(7):1066–71.

54. Joseph RJ, Irvine LM. Ovarian ectopic pregnancy: aetiology, diagnosis, and challenges in surgical management. *J Obstet Gynaecol.* 2012;32(5):472–4.

55. Melcer Y, Smorgick N, Vaknin Z, Mendlovic S, Raziel A, Maymon R. Primary ovarian pregnancy: 43 years experience in a single institute and still a medical challenge. *Isr Med Assoc J.* 2015;17(11):687–90.

56. Plotti F, Di Giovanni A, Oliva C, Battaglia F, Plotti G. Bilateral ovarian pregnancy after intrauterine insemination and controlled ovarian stimulation. *Fertil Steril.* 2008;90(5):2015.e3–e5.

57. Perkins KM, Boulet SL, Kissin DM, Jamieson DJ, National ART Surveillance (NASS) Group. Risk of ectopic pregnancy associated with assisted reproductive technology in the United States, 2001–2011. *Obstet Gynecol.* 2015;125(1):70–8.

58. Tsakos E, Tsagias N, Dafopoulos K. Suggested method for the management of heterotopic cervical pregnancy leading to term delivery of the intrauterine pregnancy: case report and literature review. *J Minim Invasive Gynecol.* 2015;22(5):896–901.

59. Patel C, Feldman J, Ogedegbe C. Complicated abdominal pregnancy with placenta feeding off sacral plexus and subsequent multiple ectopic pregnancies during a 4-year follow-up: a case report. *J Med Case Rep.* 2016;10:37.

60. Hymel JA, Hughes DS, Gehlot A, Ramseyer AM, Magann EF. Late abdominal pregnancies (>/=20 weeks gestation): a review from 1965 to 2012. *Gynecol Obstet Invest.* 2015;80(4):253–8.

61. Kunwar S, Khan T, Srivastava K. Abdominal pregnancy: methods of hemorrhage control. *Intractable Rare Dis Res.* 2015;4(2):105–7.

62. Python JL, Wakefield BW, Kondo KL, Bang TJ, Stamm ER, Hurt KJ. Ultrasound-guided percutaneous management of splenic ectopic pregnancy. *J Minim Invasive Gynecol.* 2016;23(6):997–1002.

Surgical Management of Uterine Myomas

John C. Petrozza

In women of reproductive age, fibroids are known to cause menorrhagia [1], infertility [2], adverse obstetrical outcomes, dyspareunia [3], and, if the fibroids are large, bladder and bowel symptoms, back pain, pelvic pressure or pain, and ureteral compression along with hydronephrosis [4]. The goal of the reproductive surgeon, in regard to symptomatic uterine fibroids, is quite simple: make the uterus normal. By doing this, you alleviate the patients of their symptoms, reduce the risk for fibroid recurrence, and provide an opportunity for the woman to carry a pregnancy to term. The goal of this chapter is to help you determine when to offer a myomectomy, how to prepare for the surgery, and the surgical techniques needed to be successful.

8.1 Diagnosis

Imaging is the cornerstone of helping to characterize the nature of the uterus, determine if any masses are present, and helping to guide any additional tests. Typically, a pelvic ultrasound is arranged as the first-line test, as it is 95–100% sensitive in detecting fibroids and is quite cost-effective, especially when the fibroids are small and the size of the uterus is less than 10 weeks [5]. However, when the fibroids are large or the uterus starts to expand beyond the pelvic brim, the ability to ascertain the number and location of the fibroids becomes more difficult. In addition, the presence of an ovarian cyst should be factored into surgical planning. Of course, if the size of the uterus and fibroids dictates that an abdominal approach is the best option to remove the fibroids, or a hysterectomy is chosen, then there is probably no need for further imaging, except when there is a question of adenomyosis versus fibroids, whereby magnetic resonance imaging (MRI) may help differentiate these a little better.

A sonohysterogram or saline infusion sonohysterography helps in determining whether the fibroid is abutting or encroaching into the endometrial cavity and is more superior to just an ultrasound or hysteroscopy in determining the amount of fibroid intracavitary versus intramural (Figure 8.1). Compared to hysteroscopy, a sonohysterogram allows you to actually measure the size of the fibroids.

MRI, while more costly than an ultrasound or sonohysterogram, is really the best tool to accurately determine the size and location of all uterine fibroids (Figure 8.2).

By looking at the sagittal and coronal images, you can develop a map of the fibroids and determine the best surgical approach to normalize the uterus, especially if you are contemplating a laparoscopic approach [6]. Just as important, MRI images are much easier to interpret than ultrasound images, especially for the patient, which ultimately helps involve the patient in the decision-making process. In addition to mapping the fibroids, MRI images can be used to assess whether the fibroid is degenerating or calcified, and can help raise concern for a sarcoma if the fibroid edges are irregular, lymphadenopathy is present, peritoneal excrescences are seen, or if diffusion studies suggest hypercellularity within the fibroids [7].

8.2 Preoperative Evaluation

In addition to a thorough medical history, especially one that looks for a family history of bleeding disorders or diseases that may predispose the patient to a higher risk for sarcoma or endometrial cancer, medications that may predispose to intraoperative bleeding, or other comorbidities that may impact the safety of the surgery or prolong the recovery, thorough pelvic and abdominal exams are mandatory. A bimanual, even if the uterus is large, can help you gauge the presence of any lower-uterine-segment fibroids. During the bimanual exam, it is important to determine if there will be enough lateral space to place your ports. This is the time when you start to think about port placement, if you are considering a laparoscopic approach.

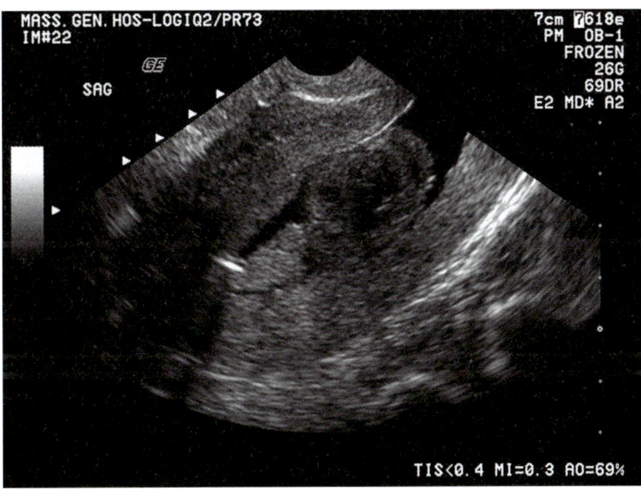

Figure 8.1 Sonohysterogram of type 0 submucosal fibroid and endometrial polyp.

(A)

(B)

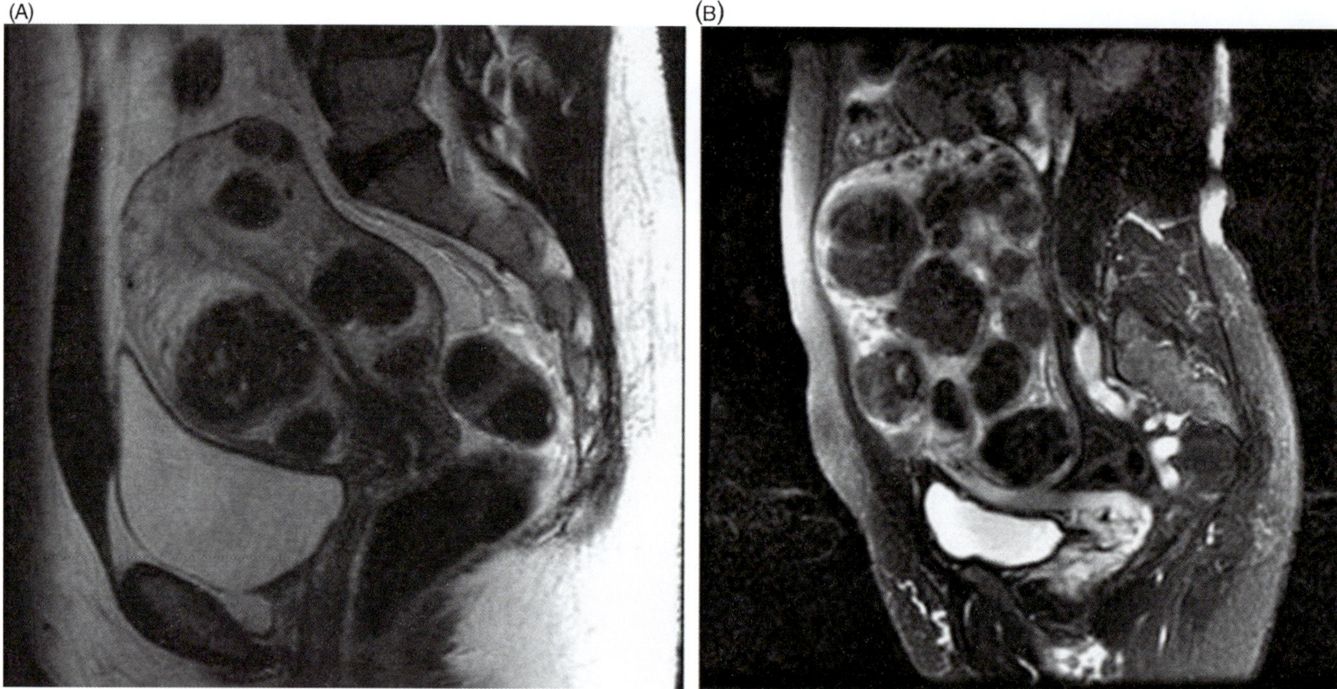

Figure 8.2 MRI (sagittal) views of fibroid uterus. Uterus A is amenable to laparoscopy. Uterus B is more appropriate for an abdominal approach.

An assessment of complete blood count (CBC) and thyroid-stimulating hormone (TSH) level should have been done at the initial visit and addressed if abnormal. For women older than the age of 35 who have risk factors for endometrial cancer (unopposed estrogen, polycystic ovarian syndrome, obesity, Lynch syndrome, Cowden syndrome, Tamoxifen therapy) it is not unwise to consider an endometrial biopsy for reassurance [8]. All women older than the age of 45 with abnormal bleeding and fibroids should also have an endometrial sampling done [9].

Perhaps the most important thing to do prior to the surgery is review the imaging studies. If there are multiple fibroids and an MRI was done, review the images with your surgical team. Create an expectation of how many fibroids you are expecting to remove and where you might have some difficulties during the case. Like an athlete "visualizes" before their race or game, the surgeon should have a mental picture of what they expect to see and what they will do if they encounter certain situations.

If the patient is anemic due to blood loss, reducing blood with a GnRH agonist, oral contraceptives, or tranexamic acid may be helpful [10]. In addition, oral or intravenous iron supplements may be of benefit. In some case, and after consultation with a hematologist, erythropoietin-stimulating agents may be indicated or even blood transfusion. Consider having intraoperative blood salvage if you expect extensive blood loss or if the patient refuses any possibility of blood product use [11].

Shrinking the fibroids prior to a myomectomy or hysterectomy is sometimes helpful, especially for abdominal cases where you can potentially increase the chances of elevating the uterus through a Pfannensteil incision and avoid the need for a vertical one, or in hysterectomy cases where you can potentially decrease the uterine size to one that is manageable laparoscopically or perhaps increase the odds of extracting the uterus and fibroids vaginally. GnRH agonists will decrease fibroid volume up to 40% over a three-month period, as will aromatase inhibitors, progesterone receptor modulators, and GnRH antagonists [12]. None are Food and Drug Administration (FDA) approved for this purpose.

8.3 Surgical Approach for Myomectomy

There are many variables that must be considered when determining the best approach for a myomectomy.

1. Size of the uterus.
2. Number of fibroids.
3. Location of fibroids.
4. Surgeon skill.
5. Prior pelvic and abdominal surgeries.
6. Patient preference.
7. Patient's body habitus.

Ultimately, the approach should offer the best opportunity to remove all fibroids and ensure a healthy, normal uterus. For women who are trying or hope to conceive in the future, I have yet to have a patient who successfully conceived after an open myomectomy complain that we did not perform her surgery laparoscopically. Alternatively, I see many patients in my fibroid clinic for second opinions who present with a recurrence of fibroids, when in reality, after reviewing prior imaging and operative notes, their "recurrence" is actually fibroids that were never removed in the first place. Indeed, 27–62% of women will have myomas seen on ultrasound 5–10 years after their initial surgery and 10–25% will require a second surgery [13,14]. Typically, the larger the uterus and the more numerous the fibroids, the greater the risk.

For a laparoscopic myomectomy to be efficient, there needs to be enough room to place your ports, apply traction and torque to your instruments, and enough distance between your camera and the fibroids. Once a uterus gets above 16 weeks' size, the case becomes more difficult. Pedunculated fibroids are easy to tackle, as are most subserosal fibroids. Anterior fibroids are generally more approachable than posterior fibroids, except when they start to encroach near the bladder. The more fibroids there are, the longer it will take to remove them, suture, and extract the tissue. There are few data to help us determine what size or number of fibroids should be used to decide one approach over the other. Fibroids that were associated with major complications included myomas greater than 5.0 cm, greater than three myomas removed, broad ligament fibroids, and intramural fibroids [15]. As technology has become better (flexible laparoscopes, high-definition cameras and monitors, barbed suture, etc.) and surgeons better trained, these parameters have changed. In our practice we feel comfortable approaching cases with fibroids greater than 10 cm or more than seven fibroids.

Perhaps the biggest limiting factor, at least in our hands, for a laparoscopic approach are cases where there are significant submucosal involvement either from one large fibroid or multiple smaller ones. Also, cases where there are multiple intramural fibroids that will not be easily seen or felt during the laparoscopy usually forces me to recommend an abdominal approach.

Robotic-assisted laparoscopic myomectomy or hysterectomy is much more time-consuming and expensive compared to traditional laparoscopy, with no clear improvement in outcomes, based on very limited studies [16]. However, its true advantage lies in its ability to make laparoscopy easier for the general gynecologist, hopefully allowing for more appropriate laparoscopic procedures to be done.

Overall, laparoscopy allows for a shorter recovery and lower overall risk for complications compared to abdominal myomectomy and should always be considered. But never hesitate to do an open procedure if it will ensure an efficient procedure and the best opportunity to remove all fibroids and normalize the uterus.

8.4 Techniques

Although the entry approach is different for a laparoscopic versus an open approach, once the surgeon begins removing the fibroids, the basic principles remain:

1. Employ techniques to minimize blood loss.
2. Minimize tissue injury.
3. Identify the fibroids pseudocapsule.
4. Use countertraction on the fibroid and sharp dissection to help you stay within the pseudocapsule as you isolate the fibroid.
5. Close all dead space in the remaining defect, suturing in layers if needed.
6. Achieve hemostasis.
7. Close the serosa using the least reactive method and suture possible to minimize adhesion formation.

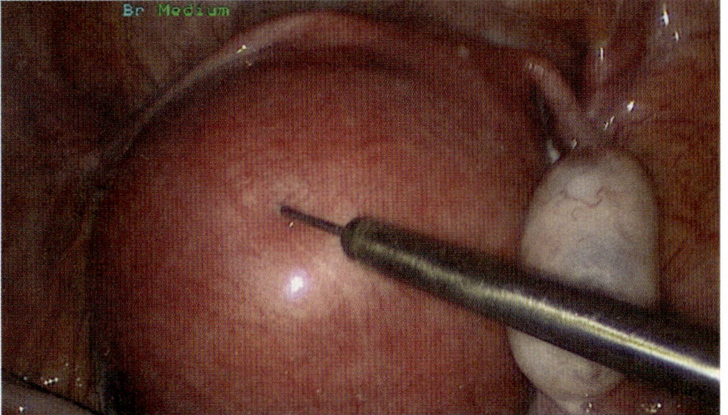

Figure 8.3 Injecting vasopressin under serosa.

8. Use some form of adhesion barrier over the myomectomy sites.
9. Extract the tissue from the body using an efficient technique that minimizes tissue dispersion.

Minimizing blood loss during incision into the fibroid is important, yet none of the pharmacologic or mechanical techniques alone have been shown to reduce the rate of blood transfusion. Likewise, there are few data looking at combinations of pharmacologic and mechanical devices. Vasopressin is the most commonly used pharmacologic agent and randomized studies have shown that blood loss is less when compared to placebo and comparable or less when compared to a uterine artery tourniquet [17,18]. Of course, it is easy to inject vasopressin via laparoscopy or an open procedure, but it is technically difficult to place a uterine artery tourniquet laparoscopically, and thus it is rarely used with this approach. Vasopressin comes in 20-unit vials and is often diluted, typically 20 units in 100 ml of saline. The half-life of an intramuscular injection is 10–20 minutes and the duration of action is 2–8 hours. The maximum safe dose is not known, but some studies suggest no more than six units should be used [19]. It is contraindicated in women with cardiovascular, vascular, and renal disease. We try to avoid injecting directly into the myometrium, but rather inject just under the serosa, allowing the superficial venous system to take the medicine into the deeper layers. This also helps avoid an intravascular injection. Vasopressin should be injected before each uterine incision. Instead of injecting into multiple sites, injecting into one site near your anticipated incision line should be adequate (Figure 8.3). If more vasopressin is needed, keep your needle in place and just switch out your syringe.

A uterine artery tourniquet is more suited for an open myomectomy. Make a small 1.0 cm incision in the broad ligament just above the uterocervical junction. Take care to find a clear area away from the uterus. Use a ¾-inch Penrose drain or similar catheter and pass behind the uterus and through the incisions, tightening and securing the ends anteriorly with a Kelly clamp. Avoid applying too much tension, as you may tear the broad ligament and uterine artery or vein. The goal is to compress the vessels and reduce blood flow [20].

Occlusion of the ovarian arteries is best accomplished by placing an atraumatic clamp, such as a bulldog clamp, bilaterally across the uterine ovarian ligament. There are laparoscopic bulldog clamps that can be detached from the end of their laparoscopic introducer and retrieved very easily with the same device.

Intraoperative blood salvage is a great ancillary tool to use, especially if you are anticipating blood losses that would warrant a transfusion based on the patients starting blood count. The goal is to avoid a blood transfusion. Utilizing the machine because you anticipate a 500 cc blood loss in a patient with a hematocrit of 42% is not cost effective or clinically meaningful. However, having it available for a patient with a hematocrit of 30% where you anticipate a blood loss greater than 500 cc may be more realistic. Blood loss is generally more pronounced when many fibroids are removed, especially those that are intramural and deeply penetrating the myometrium, as well as the length of the surgery [21].

In cases where extensive bleeding is encountered, in a last-ditch effort to save the uterus, uterine artery ligation or uterine artery embolization may be employed. Uterine artery embolization is best done in these cases with an absorbable media such as Gelfoam˚, as the impact of using more permanent occlusive particles on fertility and pregnancy are not well known [22].

Gentle tissue handling is just as important in laparoscopic surgery as it is in an open case, perhaps even more so. Due to the cooling and drying effect of the CO_2 gas insufflation, the tissue may be more prone to desiccation and more traumatized by pressure and pulling than what it is exposed to in open gases. Every attempt should be made to avoid grasping and pulling on the serosal surface (Figure 8.4) and the use of warm, humidified CO_2 gas has been advocated to avoid tissue damage and reduce post-operative pain.

Minimizing tissue damage also means using thermal energy that has the least amount of dispersion. Most often this is a monopolar device with a needle tip, an ultrasonic device, or a CO_2 laser. In open cases, you can even use a scalpel, although we favor a monopolar needle tip on a cutting mode for open cases and an ultrasonic device for laparoscopic cases (Figure 8.5).

The ultimate key to a myomectomy, the one step that will help minimize blood loss, is to find the myoma's pseudocapsule. The pseudocapsule is a compressed layer of myometrium that is relatively avascular. Just above this plane, however, is a very vascular myometrial layer that bleeds quite easily. While this seems quite intuitive, in practice there are times where it is difficult to discern the perfect plane. Prior use of GnRH agonists, prior uterine myomectomies, the presence of coexisting adenomyosis, and degenerating fibroids can all distort the pseudocapsule [23]. More importantly, a malignancy can also do this. If you have difficulty finding the pseudocapsule and there is no other reason to explain a distorted tissue plane, send off a sample of the mass for a frozen section analysis. Although a frozen section is not definitive, any ambiguous or positive result warrants an open procedure. It is better to cut deep into the fibroid and work back to find the pseudocapsule rather than cutting too shallow and digging through myometrium to find the right plane (Figure 8.6).

Once you identify the plane, make sure your incision is large enough to remove the fibroid. If the incision is not large

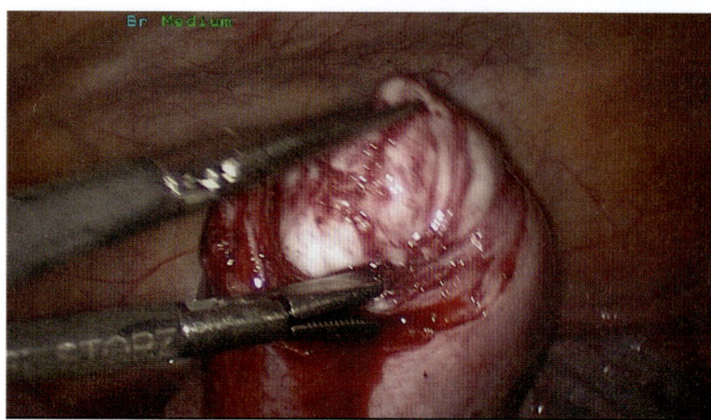

Figure 8.4 Avoid excessive serosal damage. Note that Allis grasper is holding myometrium and not serosa.

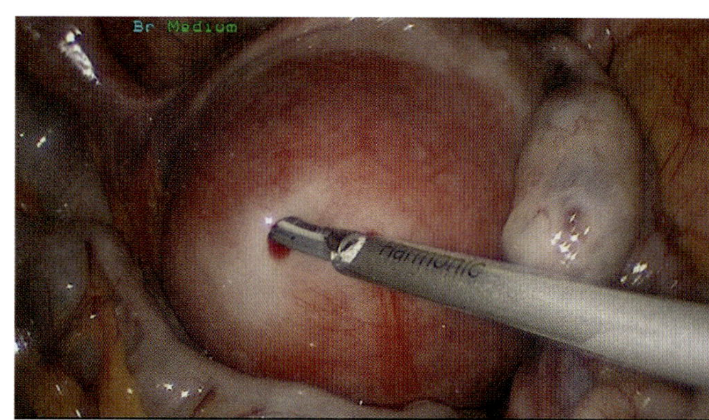

Figure 8.5 Minimize thermal damage. An ultrasonic device is used to make uterine incision.

enough, it will be easy to drift from the appropriate tissue plane and you will be applying too much force on the myometrium and serosa as you try to create better exposure. You know you have made the appropriate incision when you start to see the fibroid deliver itself as you dissect it out (Figure 8.7).

A myoma screw, single-tooth tenaculum, sharp towel clamp, or triple hook clamp should be used to grab the fibroid and provide countertraction (Figure 8.8).

This facilitates identifying the fibers of the pseudocapsule that cling to the fibroid. Sharp dissection will facilitate cutting these fibers. When dissecting, stay above the developing groove and focus on loosening the loose fibers. Some clinicians advocate using the end of a scalpel of insert their fingers or a sponge stick to help pull down these fibers. I discourage this as it tends to traumatize the myometrium more and distorts your planes. As the dissection gets further into the tissue plane, pull the serosa back and grab the knuckle of tissue that forms above the dissection area with an Allis clamp (Figure 8.9). This will keep you from tearing the serosa and provide better exposure.

Fibroids that are just below an enucleated fibroid should be removed through the same incision. However, it can be argued that fibroids that are more lateral and less accessible should be removed through a separate incision. This may prevent causing more damage to the myometrium and reduce the risk of an inadvertent entry into the uterine cavity.

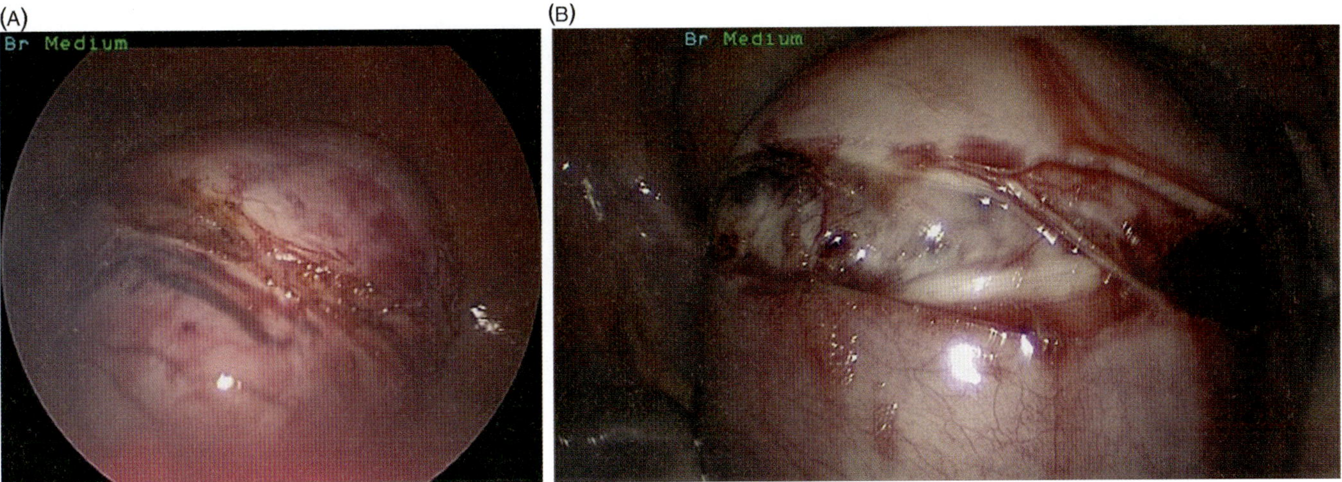

Figure 8.6 Uterus A incision is not deep enough. Uterus B incision has reached myoma and pseudocapsule is exposed.

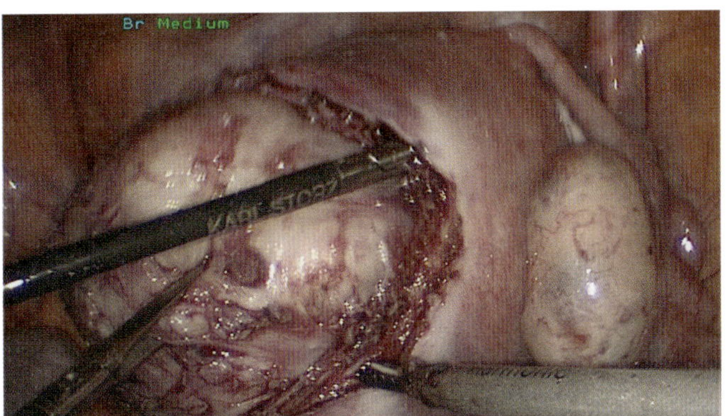

Figure 8.7 Incision is large enough that myoma starts to extrude itself with minimal countertraction.

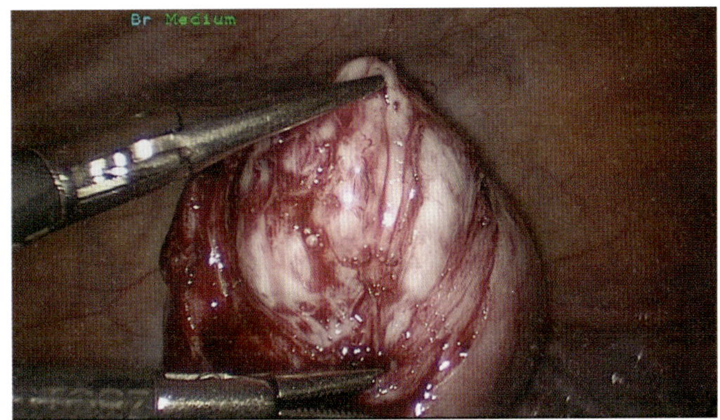

Figure 8.9 Allis clamp holds on to knuckle of pseudocapsule and myometrium to help define tissue plane.

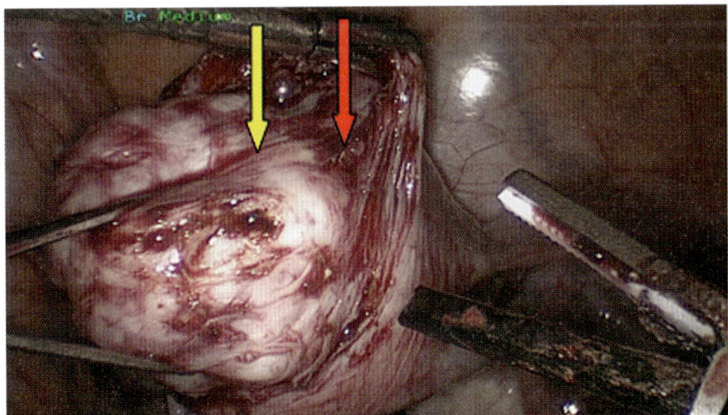

Figure 8.8 Countertraction with tenaculum helps define fibers that need to be released. The yellow arrow shows the fibers that need to be released. Avoid cutting too far down (red arrow) as you'll get into myometrium and bleeding.

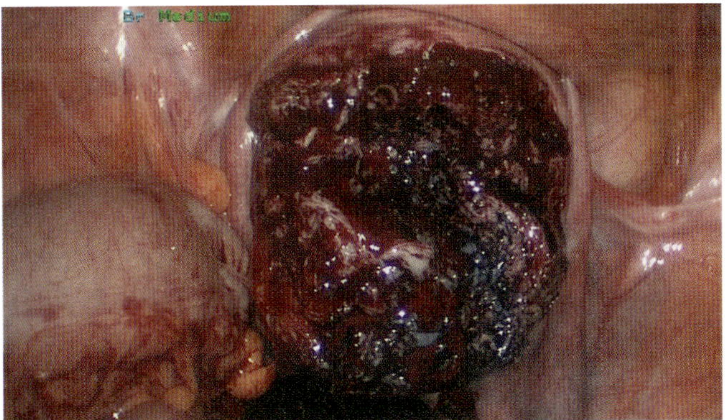

Figure 8.10 Methylene blue dye indicates cavity has been entered.

If there is concern that you may enter the cavity, instilling some methylene blue dye into the cavity at the start of the case will aid in identifying the cavity and facilitate a proper repair. If the cavity is entered, there is no need to identify the endometrium and reapproximate it with suture (Figure 8.10).

The inadvertent suture in the uterine cavity will predispose for adhesions. Instead, reapproximate the myometrium above the endometrium, which will bring the endometrium together with less risk of placing an inadvertent stitch into the uterine cavity. It is best to close each defect once the fibroid(s) from that incision is removed. This will help minimize blood loss. Following the general principles of surgery, you want to completely close the dead space within the uterine defect. Typically a braided polyglactin (Vicryl®) suture is used or a barbed suture is employed. The benefit of the barbed suture is that it applies an even tension along the suture line and keeps the tissue

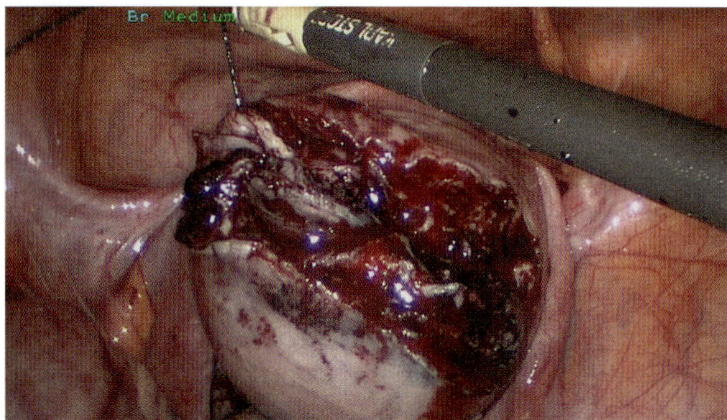

Figure 8.11 Closing defect in layers using barbed suture.

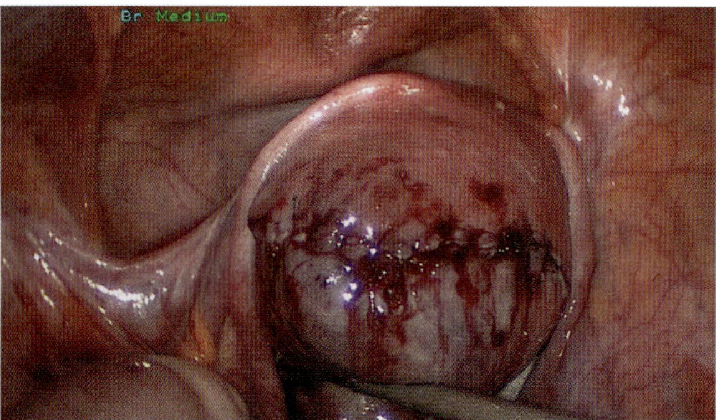

Figure 8.12 Serosal closure.

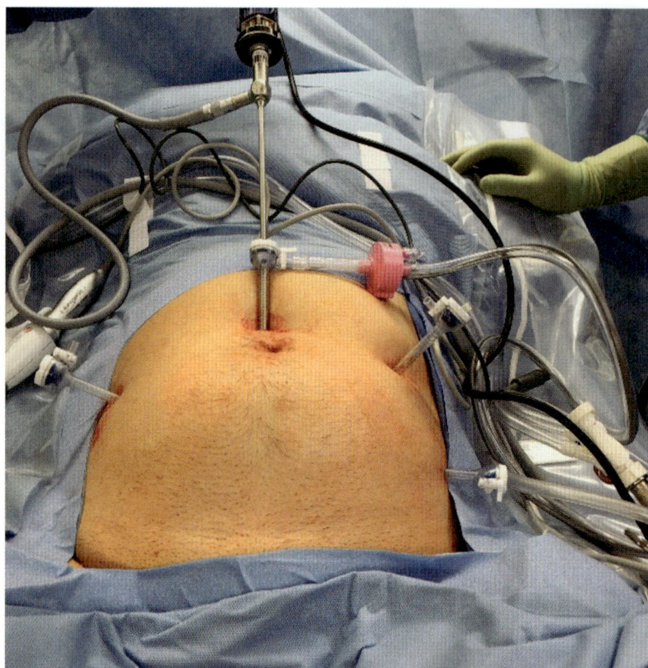

Figure 8.13 Laparoscopic port placement.

well-approximated. It also does not require tying a knot, which is helpful when suturing laparoscopically. The sutures can be placed interrupted, figure-of-eights, or running. Avoid locking your suture line, as this may cause tissue necrosis and promote poor healing. Use as many layers as you need to close the dead space and to reduce any tension for your serosal closure (Figure 8.11).

The serosa is typically closed with a monofilament suture, such as 3-0 or 4-0 PDS. There are no data showing that a baseball stitch prevents adhesion formation any better than a simple running stitch, but intuitively, it makes more sense that hiding as much suture below the serosa exposes less foreign material and perhaps results in less adhesion formation (Figure 8.12). Following that principle, closing the serosa in a manner similar to a subcuticular stitch may be more appealing.

If there is oozing that cannot be controlled, the use of a fibrin-promoting product can be used, although there is very little data that they are any better than just placing another suture layer or figure-of-eight stitch. Most times, serosal bleeding can be controlled with a cautery device.

As reproductive surgeons, it is paramount that we try to minimize the risk of postoperative adhesion formation. The most important step is meticulous technique and gentle tissue handling. For open myomectomies, hyaluronic acid sheets (Seprafilm®), which are quite brittle, can be placed over the uterine incisions. Likewise, oxidized regenerated cellulose sheets (Interceed®) can also be used. For the latter, the area must be dry and hemostatic to be effective. For laparoscopic cases,

oxidized cellulose sheets or an icodextrin solution (Adept®) can be used. Both sheet barriers have been shown effective in reducing adhesion formation but data on icodextrin are less encouraging based on only a few small studies [24–26].

8.5 Laparoscopic Myomectomy

The benefits of a laparoscopic approach are quite clear, but it requires a surgeon who feels comfortable and is skilled in laparoscopic suturing (see video; this video demonstrates the enucleation of a 4.0 cm intramural fibroid, multilayered suturing of the myometrium, and closure of the serosal layer in a baseball stitch fashion). It will also require careful, contained removal of the fibroids through an exit point, either abdominally or vaginally.

The success of a laparoscopic approach hinges on correct port placement. The camera port should be placed well above most superior fibroid or the fundus of the uterus. You must take into account the pulling and twisting of the fibroid as it is enucleated and starts to creep up higher toward your camera. You can never have too much space between your camera and pathology. Depending on which side you like to suture, this is where you should place your suturing ports. The upper port should be high enough to allow you to tug on fibroids during the dissection process, while the lower one should be far enough from the upper port to keep your instruments from crossing each other too much. Typically, this should be at least 9.0 cm. The lower port should be in the same vertical plane, or slightly more lateral than the upper port. Typically, these are lateral to the inferior epigastric artery. On the opposite side, another port should be placed to help with grasping and dissection. Avoid putting this too low, or it will be less effective. We use 5 mm ports for all our sites, including the camera (Figure 8.13). Some

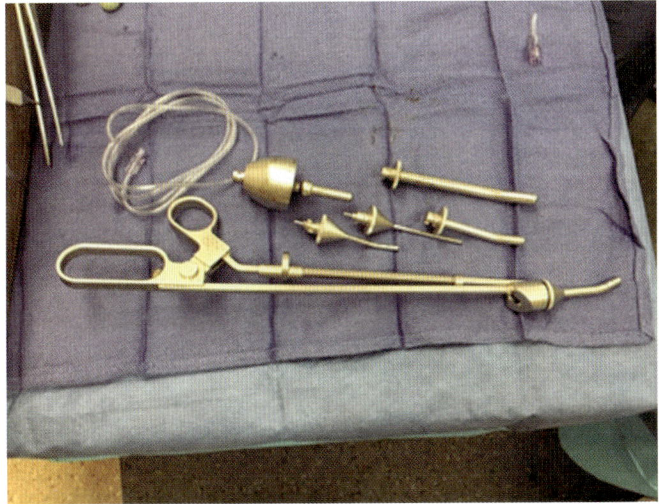

Figure 8.14 Pelosi uterine manipulator.

surgeons prefer to have a lateral 10 or 12mm port to help facilitate suture and needle entry. If using a 5 mm port, you can pass your suture and needle by removing the trocar and passing directly through the incision, then replacing your trocar once the suture is in the abdominal cavity.

Uterine incisions should be horizontal rather than vertical, which allows for easier suturing. With robot-assisted laparoscopy, this is not the case, as vertical incisions are just as easy to close as transverse ones due to the articulation capabilities of the instruments. For uterine manipulation, we prefer to use a reusable device, such as the Pelosi (Figure 8.14). This device is strong, durable, articulates at the tip, and offers excellent exposure.

8.6 Abdominal Myomectomy

The benefits of an open myomectomy is the ability to utilize your tactile sense to find fibroids that are not clearly seen and would have been missed with a laparoscopic approach. It also allows for meticulous closure and the opportunity to remove fibroids that have a significant submucosal component. Most fibroids can be approached through a Pfannestiel incision. The incision can be extended laterally and the fascia taken off the rectus up the level of the umbilical ring to aid in exposure. A Maylard incision can be used to create even more exposure, and compared to a vertical incision, has less postoperative pain and better cosmesis. The uterus is typically brought up through the incision, which gives excellent exposure and avoids the need to pack the bowel and minimizes spillage of blood and debris into the abdominal cavity (Figure 8.15).

8.7 Hysterectomy versus Myomectomy

It is important to take into account the patient's wishes when it comes to choosing a procedure to treat symptomatic fibroids. There are no guidelines that state that a hysterectomy must be done if the patient has completed her childbearing. Nor is there any strong evidence showing that myomectomies are associated clinically with more morbidity than a hysterectomy.

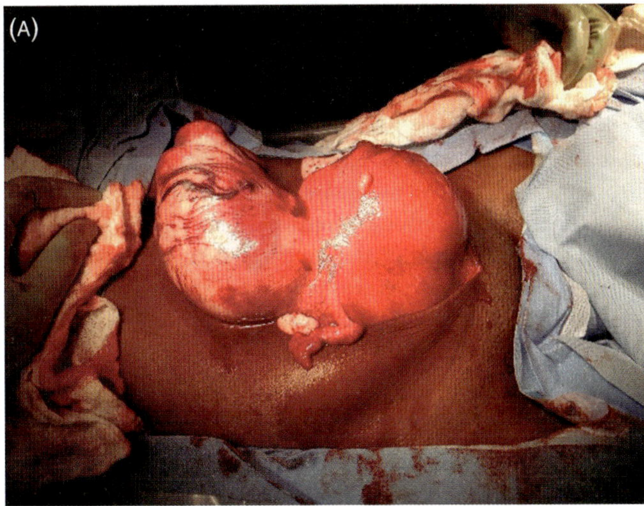

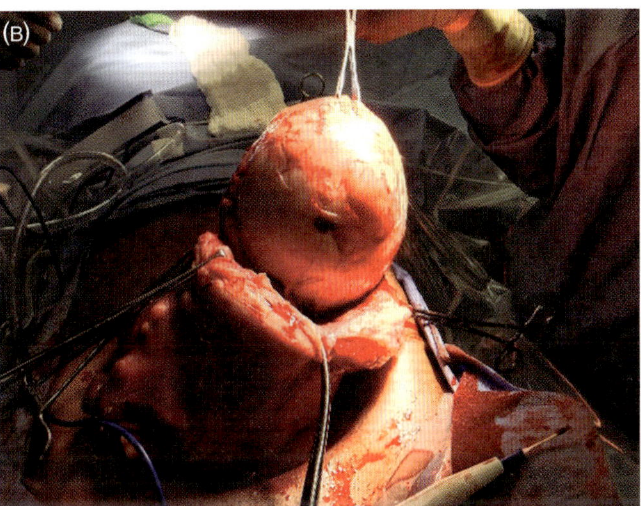

Figure 8.15 Exteriorizing the uterus and dissecting out myoma.

In general, it is typically easier to do a laparoscopic hysterectomy than a laparoscopic myomectomy, and this should be discussed with the patient, but ultimately it is a decision that the patient should be involved with.

8.8 Laparoscopic Myolysis

Thermal or freezing destruction of a myoma, without extracting the destroyed tissue, is the basis for myolysis. Radiofrequency is the newer modality and is considered to be the easiest to master. A metal device is inserted laparoscopically into the myoma, and a bipolar current is then directed in a spherical manner, destroying the tissue. It is done with ultrasound guidance to prevent excessive thermal spread. It does not require uterine incisions or suturing and appears to be well tolerated with adequate symptom relief [27]; however, the studies are limited and more data is needed before it becomes universally accepted.

8.9 Hysteroscopic Myomectomy

The European Society of Hysteroscopy classified submucosal fibroids in the following manner [28]:

Type 0 – entirely within the uterine cavity

Type I – less than 50% in the myometrium

Type II – more than 50% in the myometrium

A recent classification called size, topography, extension of the base, penetration into the myometrium, and lateral wall involvement (STEP-W) uses more information, such as myoma size, topography, length of myoma base, myometrial penetration, and location within the cavity to determine whether a hysteroscopic approach is feasible [29]. The higher the score, the less likely a hysteroscopic approach will work. In general, type II fibroids and fibroids larger than 3.0 cm are more difficult and may require a second hysteroscopy to remove.

The use of a GnRH agonist to decrease fibroid size may be helpful and prevent a two-stage procedure, but clinical data on this approach are limited. Dilute vasopressin (20 units in 100 cc saline) injected intracervically at the start of the procedure has been shown in some small studies to facilitate cervical dilation and minimize hysteroscopic fluid absorption. Likewise, vaginal misoprostol administered at least 4–5 hours prior to the procedure has shown the same benefit.

Small type 0 fibroids, generally less than 0.5–1.0 cm, can sometimes be removed with a simple operative hysteroscope and scissors. A hysteroscopic single-tooth tenaculum can then be used to retrieve the fibroid through a dilated cervix. In general, a resectoscope using a wire loop technique or a hysteroscopic morcellator will be utilized. The resectoscope historically was a monopolar device that required the use of hypotonic distention media. If the fluid deficit was excessive, greater than 1000 cc, there was the concern of severe hyperammonia, hyponatremia, and hypokalemia and associated cardiac and neurologic disturbances [30]. Recent advancements in bipolar design have forged the popularity of newer resectoscopes that can utilize physiologic solution, larger fluid deficits, and greater safety for the patient [31]. The ability to operate longer due to acceptable higher fluid deficits can potentially reduce the number of two-step procedures. Since higher fluid deficits are allowed, it is even more imperative that communication between the surgeon and anesthesiologist is robust. A long case with a 2-liter deficit, along with 1–2 liters of intravenous fluid given by the anesthesiologist could lead to fluid overload and flash pulmonary edema. If fluid deficits are creeping up during the case, it is not unreasonable for the anesthesiologist to decrease the IV flow rate or stop it all together.

Another interesting phenomenon with the bipolar resectoscopes, especially the smaller diameters scopes with 5.0 mm loops, is that the bipolar energy will start to weaken and thin the loop over time. Thus, if you are using the loop to elevate and separate the myoma, cutting the tissue, and doing this several times, these smaller loops can break. It may be more prudent to use a larger resectoscope for these cases.

The wire loop technique utilizes some of the same principles as described above for open or laparoscopic myomectomies:

1. Minimize thermal energy.
2. Handle the tissue gently.
3. Identify the pseudocapsule for type I and II fibroids and use this plane to elevate and separate the myoma from the underlying myometrium.
4. Safely remove the tissue and minimize dispersal of the tissue.

Using the loop electrode, tissue plane between the myometrium and fibroid can be identified. This technique works well for all submucosal fibroid types. Typically, the plane will be identified closest to you, and as you elevate the tissue with the inactive electrode, you will start to see some of the lateral plane develop. Cut the elevated fibroid with the activated electrode (70–100 W in cutting mode) and you will then start to see the posterior part of the tissue plane come into view. At some point, you will have to extract the fibroid chips, which can be done under direct visualization using the loop or blindly using a small polyp forceps or even a suction using a D&C catheter. The deflation of the uterine cavity during this process will cause the myometrium to start to push the remaining fibroid into the uterine cavity. When you replace the resectoscope, continue to dissect out the fibroid in a similar manner. Make sure all fibroid pieces are extracted at the end of the case.

The hysteroscopic morcellator (tissue extraction device) works best for type 0 and some type I fibroids. In general, softer tissue is quite easy to remove with this device, which is why it works wells for endometrial polyps and retained products of conception. Studies have indicated that procedure time is significantly less with the morcellator devices versus the resectoscope [32]. Very dense or calcified fibroids are more difficult to remove. Preoperative imaging can help you determine if the tissue is more likely to be soft, degenerating, calcified, or dense, which can then help you determine which instrument is best to use. These devices also use physiologic distention media such as saline or lactated ringers and the same rules apply as described for the bipolar resectoscope. The cutting window for the device is at the distal tip and laterally positioned. Cutting is started by bringing the aperture to the tissue to be cut and applying pressure against the fibroid. The cut tissue is removed through the suction tubing and into a bag in the fluid collection canister. There may be instances where you may have to change the resecting blade, especially in long cases involving dense fibroids. Sometimes, increasing the rotation speed of the blade will help cut through the fibroid. In general, fibroids larger than 3.0 cm are best handled with a resectoscope. It is also wise to have resectoscope on standby for your hysteroscopic morcellator cases. Newer hysteroscopic morcellators have started to employ radiofrequency technology to cut tissue and secure any bleeding areas.

8.10 Laparoscopic Tissue Extraction

There has been recent concern that power morcellation may increase the risk for dissemination of malignant tissue, specifically sarcomas. The actual prevalence of sarcomas has been intensely reviewed, with the best evidence suggesting that it is approximately 1:352 to 1:1000 cases [33]. There is also the concern that even-spreading benign tissue will create parasitic

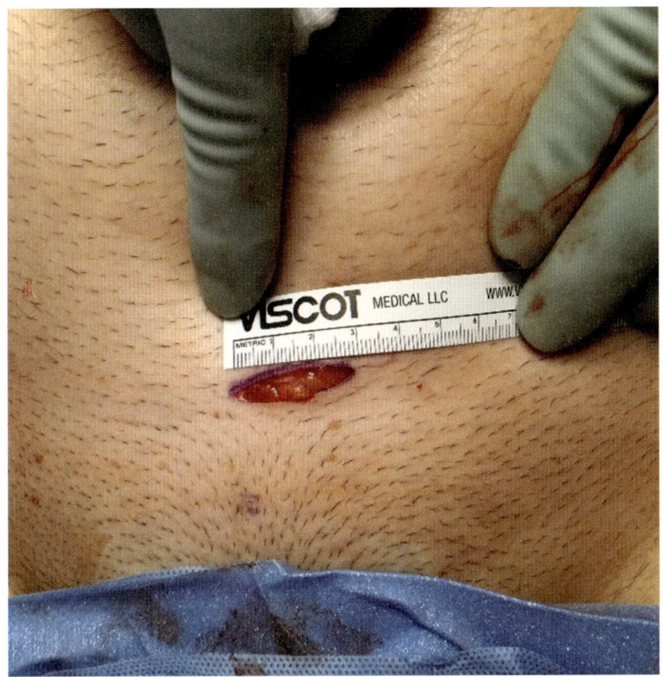

Figure 8.16 Suprapubic incision for tissue extraction site.

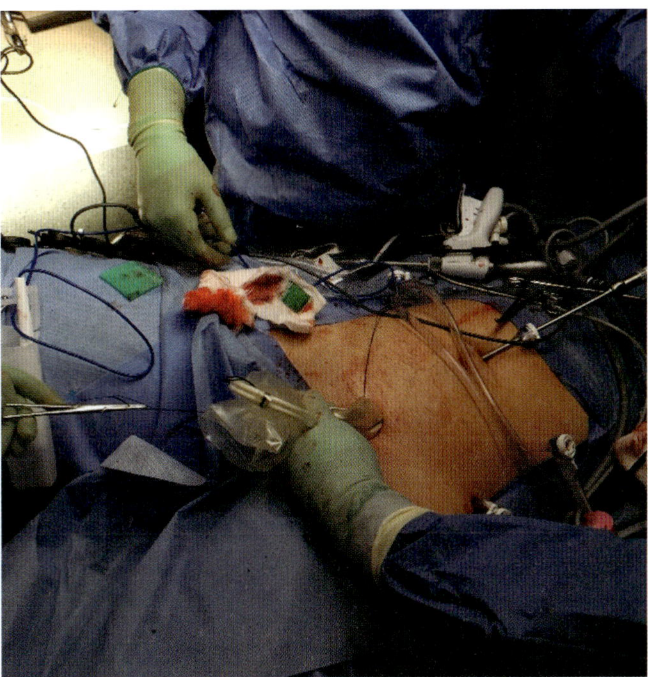

Figure 8.17 Tissue extraction bag introduced through suprapubic incision.

fibroid formation, which clearly has been reported more frequently over the last 10 years. Morcellation of a sarcoma is associated with a worsened prognosis [34]. Any serious concern for a possible sarcoma warrants an abdominal approach to surgery or at the very least, no use of power morcellation. Risk factors include [35]:

1. postmenopausal women;
2. history of tamoxifen therapy for over 2 years;
3. history of pelvic irradiation;
4. history of childhood retinoblastoma;
5. personal history of hereditary leiomyomatosis and renal cell carcinoma; and
6. black race.

The FDA issued an advisory statement regarding the use of power morcellators and the reflex reaction by many surgeons and societies was to incorporate contained power or hand morcellation, despite the lack of any evidence that it was safer [36]. What is clear is that the use of containment systems has increased surgical time and cost and forced many surgeons to perform abdominal procedures. The increase in abdominal procedures has also increased perioperative morbidity.

The technique for contained hand morcellation involves either extending a preexisting port site to 3.0 cm, creating an Omega incision at the umbilicus, or making a suprapubic incision (Figure 8.16). It is best to discuss with the patient what she prefers.

A containment bag is dropped through the incision into the abdominal cavity (Figure 8.17).

A large trocar with a balloon sleeve can be then inserted into the incision to help maintain pneumoperitoneum (Figure 8.18). Some surgeons will also use a gel port, one that is typically used in single-site laparoscopic procedures.

The bag is then opened in the pelvis and the fibroid(s) grasped and dropped into it. The bag opening is then brought up through the incision and opened (Figure 8.19).

The bag is pulled taunt to help elevate the tissue and the myoma is grasped with a Kocher clamp or triple-hook clamp. Using a #10 blade, the tissue is cut using c-incisions into the tissue while gently pulling the tissue (Figure 8.20). Rocking the tissue back and forth will also help elevate it through the incision.

Dense fibroids will take longer to extract, while soft tissue will be removed quite efficiently (Figure 8.21).

Once the tissue is removed, the trocar should be replaced, and the pelvis and abdomen inspected for any injuries or tissue remnants. The pelvis and abdomen should then be irrigated liberally.

References

1. Fraser IS, Critchley HO, Munro MG, Broder M. Writing Group for this Menstrual Agreement Process. A process designed to lead to international agreement on terminologies and definitions used to describe abnormalities of menstrual bleeding. *Fertil Steril.* 2007;87(3):466.

2. Pritts EA, Parker WH, Olive DL. Fibroids and infertility: an updated systematic review of the evidence. *Fertil Steril.* 2009;91(4):1215.

3. Lippman SA, Warner M, Samuels S, Olive D, Vercellini P, Eskenazi B. Uterine fibroids and gynecologic pain symptoms in a population-based study. *Fertil Steril.* 2003;80(6):1488.

4. Bansal T, Mehrotra P, Jayasena D, Okolo S, Yoong W, Govind A. Obstructive nephropathy and chronic kidney disease secondary to uterine leiomyomas. *Arch Gynecol Obstet.* 2009;279(6):785.

5. Dueholm M, Lundorf E, Hansen ES, Ledertoug S, Olesen F. Accuracy of magnetic resonance imaging and transvaginal

(A)

(B)

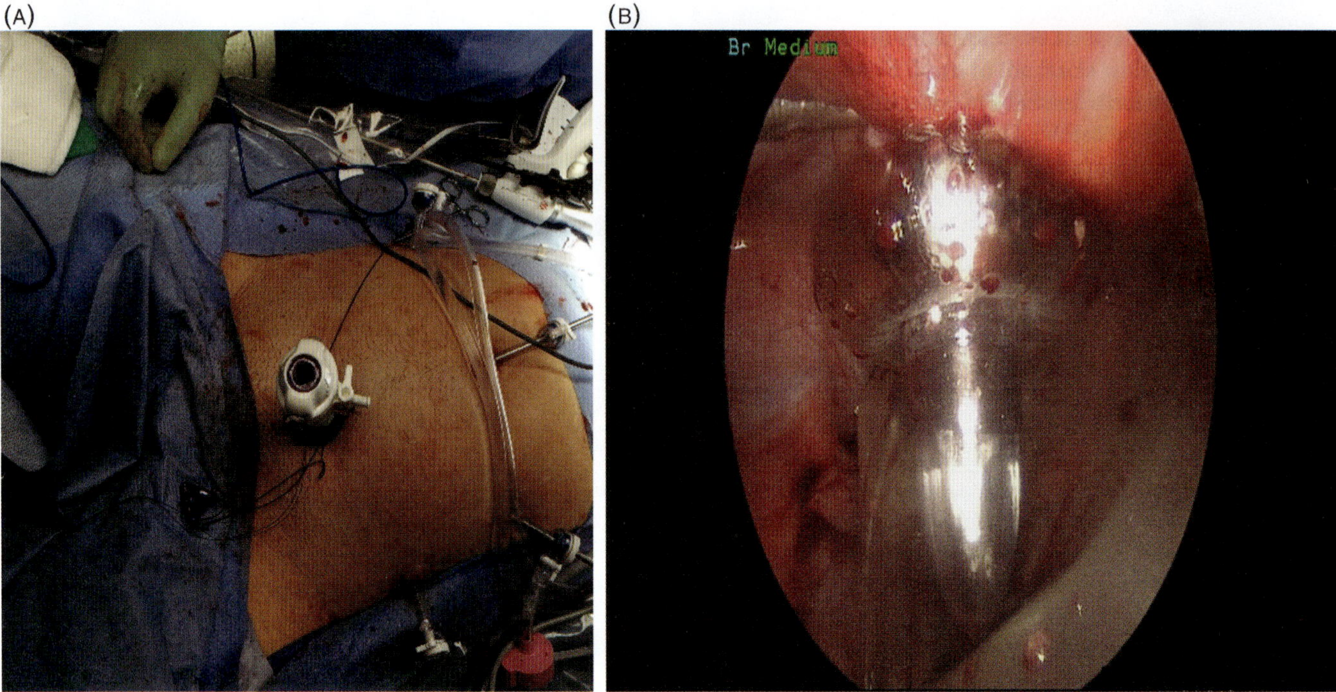

Figure 8.18 After bag is inserted, a balloon trocar helps maintain pneumoperitoneum and offers another access point into the abdominal cavity.

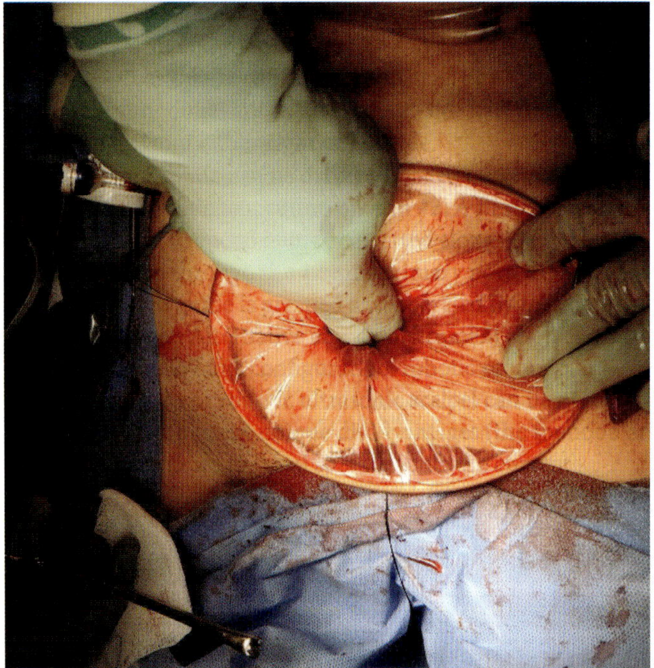

Figure 8.19 Tissue extraction bag brought out through suprapubic incision.

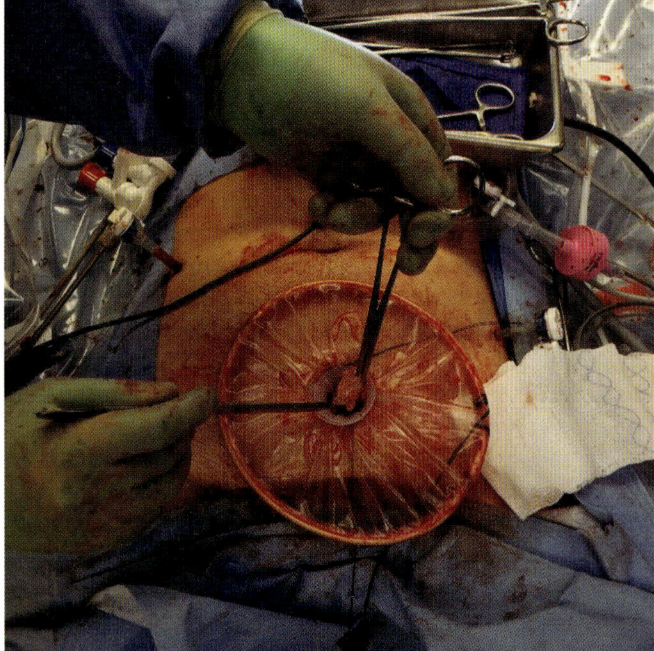

Figure 8.20 Extracting myoma using c-incision technique.

ultrasonography in the diagnosis, mapping, and measurement of uterine myomas. *Am J Obstet Gynecol.* 2002;186(3):409.

6. Omary RA, Vasireddy S, Chrisman HB, et al. The effect of pelvic MR imaging on the diagnosis and treatment of women with presumed symptomatic uterine fibroids. *J Vasc Interv Radiol.* 2002;13(11):1149.

7. Lin G, Yang LY, Huang YT, et al. Comparison of the diagnostic accuracy of contrast-enhanced MRI and diffusion-weighted MRI in the differentiation between uterine leiomyosarcoma/smooth muscle tuor with uncertain potential and benign leiomyoma. *J Magn Reson Imaging.* 2016;43(2):333.

8. Smith RA, von Eschenbach AC, Wender R, et al. American Cancer Society guidelines for the early detection of cancer: update of early detection guidelines for prostate, colorectal, and endometrial cancers. *CA Cancer J Clin.* 2001;51:38.

9. Committee on Practice Bulletins – Gynecology. Diagnosis of abnormal uterine bleeding in reproductive-aged women. Practice Bulletin No. 128. *Obstet Gynecol.* 2012;120:197.

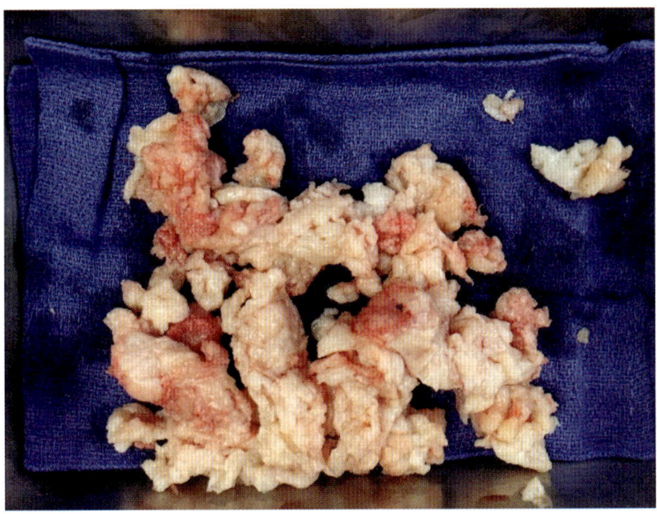

Figure 8.21 Extracted myoma.

10. Lethaby A, Vollenhoven B, Sowter M. Pre-operative GnRH analogue therapy before hysterectomy or myomectomy for uterine fibroids. *Cochrane Database Syst Rev.* 2001;(2):CD000547.

11. West S, Ruiz R, Parker WH. Abdominal myomectomy in women with very large uterine size. *Fertil Steril.* 2006;85(1):36.

12. Broekmans FJ. GnRH agonists and uterine leiomyomas. *Hum Reprod.* 1996;11 Suppl 3:3.

13. Fedele L, Parazzini F, Luchini L, Mezzopane R, Tozzi L, Villa L. Recurrence of fibroids after myomectomy: a transvaginal ultrasonographic study. *Hum Reprod.* 1995;10(7):1795.

14. Thompson LB, Reed SD, McCrummen BK, Warolin AK, Newton KM. Leiomyoma characteristics and risk of subsequent surgery after myomectomy. *Int J Gynaecol Obstet.* 2006;95(2):138.

15. Sizzi O, Rossetti A, Malzoni M, et al. Italian multicenter study on complications of laparoscopic myomectomy. *J Minim Invasive Gynecol.* 2007;14(4):453.

16. Barakat EE, Bedaiwy MA, Zimberg S, Nutter B, Nosseir M, Falcone T. Robotic-assisted, laparoscopic, and abdominal myomectomy: a comparison of surgical outcomes. *Obstet Gynecol.* 2011;117(2 Pt 1):256.

17. Kongnyuy EJ, Wiysonge CS. Interventions to reduce haemorrhage during myomectomy for fibroids. *Cochrane Database Syst Rev.* 2011;(11):CD005355.

18. Fletcher H, Frederick J, Hardie M, Simeon D. A randomized comparison of vasopressin and tourniquet as hemostatic agents during myomectomy. *Obstet Gynecol.* 1996;87(6):1014.

19. Frishman G. Vasopressin: if some is good, is more better? *Obstet Gynecol.* 2009;113(2 Pt 2):476.

20. Taylor A, Sharma M, Tsirkas P, Di Spiezio Sardo A, Setchell M, Magos A. Reducing blood loss at open myomectomy using triple tourniquets: a randomised controlled trial. *BJOG.* 2005;112(3):340.

21. Ginsburg ES, Benson CB, Garfield JM, Gleason RE, Friedman AJ. The effect of operative technique and uterine size on blood loss during myomectomy: a prospective randomized study. *Fertil Steril.* 1993;60(6):956.

22. Helal AS, Abdel-Hady el-S, Refaie E, El Shamy M, El Fattah RA, Mashaly Ael M. Preliminary uterine artery ligation versus pericervical mechanical tourniquet in reducing hemorrhage during abdominal myomectomy. *Int J Gynaecol Obstet.* 2010;108(3):233.

23. Deligdisch L, Hirschmann S, Altchek A. Pathologic changes in gonadotropin releasing hormone agonist analogue treated uterine leiomyomata. *Fertil Steril.* 1997;67(5):837.

24. Diamond MP. Seprafilm Adhesion Study Group. Reduction of adhesions after uterine myomectomy by Seprafilm membrane (HAL-F): a blinded, prospective, randomized, multicenter clinical study. *Fertil Steril.* 1996;66(6):904.

25. Mais V, Ajossa S, Piras B, Guerriero S, Marongiu D, Melis GB. Prevention of de-novo adhesion formation after laparoscopic myomectomy: a randomized trial to evaluate the effectiveness of an oxidized regenerated cellulose absorbable barrier. *Hum Reprod.* 1995;10(12):3133.

26. Broek RP, Stommel MW, Strik C, van Laarhoven CJ, Keus F, van Goor H. Benefits and harms of adhesion barriers for abdominal surgery: a systematic review and meta-analysis. *Lancet.* 2014;383(9911):48–59. Epub 2013 Sep 27.

27. Chudnoff SG, Berman JM, Levine DJ, Harris M, Guido RS, Banks E. Outpatient procedure for the treatment and relief of symptomatic uterine myomas. *Obstet Gynecol.* 2013;121(5):1075–82.

28. Wamsteker K, Emanuel MH, de Kruif JH. Transcervical hysteroscopic resection of submucous fibroids for abnormal uterine bleeding: results regarding the degree of intramural extension. *Obstet Gynecol.* 1993;82(5):736.

29. Lasmar RB, Xinmei Z, Indman PD, Celeste RK, Di Spiezio Sardo A. Feasibility of a new system of classification of submucous myomas: a multicenter study. *Fertil Steril.* 2011;95(6):2073–7.

30. Istre O, Jellum E, Skajaa K, Forman A. Changes in amino acids, ammonium, and coagulation factors after transcervical resection of the endometrium with a glycine solution used for uterine irrigation. *Am J Obstet Gynecol.* 1995;172(3):939.

31. Dyrbye BA, Overdijk LE, van Kesteren PJ, et al. Gas embolism during hysteroscopic surgery using bipolar or monopolar diathermia: a randomized controlled trial. *Am J Obstet Gynecol.* 2012 Oct;207(4):271.e1–6.

32. Pampalona JR, Bastos MD, Moreno GM, et al. A comparison of hysteroscopic mechanical tissue removal with bipolar electrical resection for the management of endometrial polyps in an ambulatory care setting: preliminary results. *J Minim Invasive Gynecol.* 2015;22(3):439–45.

33. Mahnert N, Morgan D, Campbell D, Johnston C, As-Sanie S. Unexpected gynecologic malignancy diagnosed after hysterectomy performed for benign indications. *Obstet Gynecol.* 2015;125(2):397–405.

34. Park JY, Park SK, Kim DY, et al. The impact of tumor morcellation during surgery on the prognosis of patients with apparently early uterine leiomyosarcoma. *Gynecol Oncol.* 2011;122(2):255–9. Epub 2011 May 12.

35. Tropé CG, Abeler VM, Kristensen GB. Diagnosis and treatment of sarcoma of the uterus. A review. *Acta Oncol.* 2012;51(6):694–705.

36. US Food and Drug Administration (FDA), Obstetrics and Gynecology Devices Advisory Committee. FDA executive summary: Laparoscopic power morcellation during uterine surgery for fibroids, Washington, DC, 2014. www.fda.gov/advisorycommittees/calendar/ucm400221.htm.

Chapter 9

Laparoscopic Surgery for the Management of Endometriosis

Vadim Morozov, Nisha Lakhi, and Ceana H. Nezhat

9.1 Introduction

Endometriosis affects women worldwide. One study demonstrated the prevalence and incidence rates of endometriosis respectively to be 8.1 and 3.5 per 1000 women [1]. Although much has been studied and discovered about this disease in the last few decades, its etiology and clinical manifestations remain an enigma for many professionals involved in the treatment and care of women with endometriosis [2]. The symptoms are variable and may not be related to the extension of the disease. These symptoms include dysmenorrhea, deep dyspareunia, chronic pelvic pain, intestinal and/or urinary cyclical symptoms, and infertility [3].

There are three distinct types of endometriosis: superficial endometriosis, ovarian endometriomas, and deeply infiltrating endometriosis (DIE). This differentiation is important in the therapeutic management of the disease. In 1996, the American Society for Reproductive Medicine (ASRM) revised an established surgical classification categorizing the disease in four different stages defined by a point system according to the surgical findings [4]. The pathophysiology of endometriosis, its effects on local surrounding organs and tissues, and the mechanisms by which it causes pain and possibly infertility has been studied extensively [5].

Surgical management of endometriosis is directed toward alleviating the symptoms of the disease, preserving organ function, and, in cases of compromised fertility, reestablishing the reproductive potential of the affected patient. Surgical diagnosis and eradication of endometriosis, combined with medical suppression, can provide the most favorable long-term results. Conservative and medical management of endometriosis exists, yet the discussion of those approaches is outside the scope of this chapter.

9.2 Preoperative Evaluation and Diagnosis

Although the diagnosis of endometriosis can be suspected from clinical examination as well as the patient's history and narrative description, it is widely accepted that the gold standard for diagnosis is either direct visualization of endometriotic lesions and implants or pathologically confirmed biopsy of the lesion. Currently, video-laparoscopic diagnosis and treatment of endometriosis is preferential to laparotomy. Both have shown similar results as far as treatment and outcomes are concerned. A detailed vaginal and rectovaginal digital examination supplanted with transvaginal ultrasonography (TVUS) and at times transrectal ultrasonography (TRUS) are noninvasive methods used to help with the diagnosis of endometriosis and to strategize multidisciplinary treatment plans if needed [6].

Treatment depends on the age of the patient, the location of the disease, the severity of symptoms, and the desire for future fertility. Surgical intervention is usually indicated for pain, infertility, or impaired function of the involved organ, such as the bladder, ureter, or bowel.

9.3 Surgical Treatment of Pelvic Endometriosis

Video-laparoscopic surgery for the diagnosis and potential treatment of endometriosis begins with a careful examination of abdominal and pelvic anatomy. Broadly speaking, endometriosis can be divided into four categories:

1. Superficial peritoneal endometriosis.
2. Ovarian endometrioma.
3. Deep infiltrating endometriosis (>5 mm implants).
4. Extragenital endometriosis (e.g., diaphragmatic, pulmonary, etc.).

Visual inspection of the uterus, fallopian tubes, ovaries, bladder reflection, and cul-de-sac with utero-sacral ligaments are routinely performed. Para-ovarain fossae are examined bilaterally with the retraction of the adnexum away from the underlying peritoneum. Even though typical powder-burn and cherry-red spot lesions are easily identified (Figure 9.1), the surgeon should look for atypical presentation of endometriosis, such as white and clear lesions vesicular lesions (Figure 9.2), and peritoneal retractions.

Examination of the intestines, omentum, curvature of the stomach, the gallbladder, and both lobes of the liver is carried out. Visualization of the spleen, if possible, is done as well. Inspection of both hemidiaphragms is performed for signs of diaphragmatic endometriosis (Figure 9.3). Mossy endometriosis secondary to ascites has also been described (Figure 9.4) [7]. The surgical management of the extragenital endometriosis including endometriosis of the thoracic cavity and diaphragm is outside of the scope of this discussion.

As demonstrated by Sutton in 1994 and confirmed by Abbott 10 years later [4,8], both laparoscopic excision of endometriosis and laparoscopic ablation have produced significant reduction in pelvic pain. The greatest reduction in pain scores after treatment was observed in stages II and III (ASRM

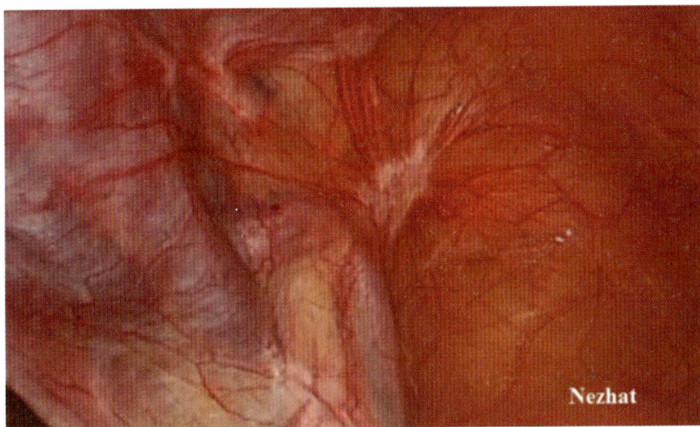

Figure 9.1 Atypical endometriosis lesion.

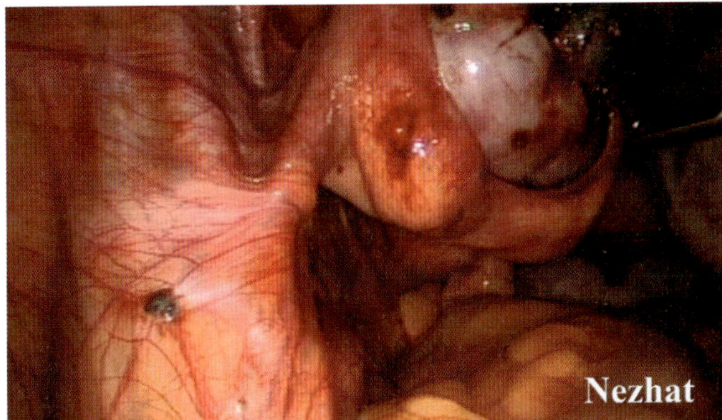

Figure 9.2 Typical blue endometriosis lesion.

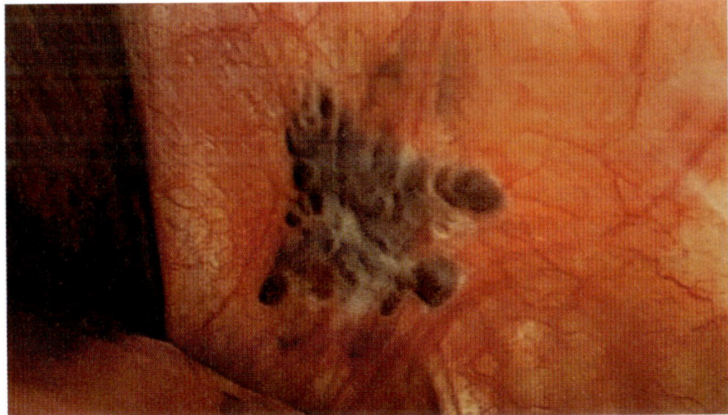

Figure 9.3 Endometriosis of the diaphragm behind the liver.

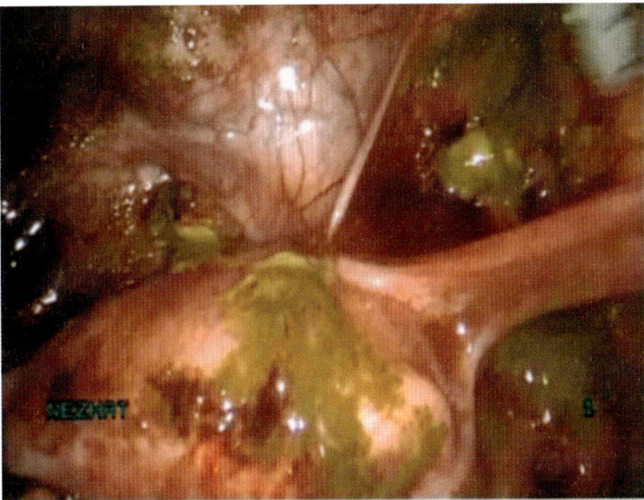

Figure 9.4 Mossy endometriosis secondary to ascites *(video)*.
Video Link: www.fertstert.org/article/S0015-0282(16)62663–8/ abstract [7].

classification), while stage I showed moderate improvement in pain scores [4]. Nevertheless, in a randomized, placebo-controlled trial, laparoscopic excision of endometriosis resulted in significantly more symptomatic relief than laparoscopy alone (80% vs. 32%) [7].

9.4 Management of Superficial Peritoneal Endometriosis

Once the endometriosis lesions are identified, the important nearby anatomic structures are visualized and identified. Very often, the visible endometriosis lesion represents "the tip of the iceberg," with underlying retroperitoneal disease being larger than the visible lesion. The laparoscopic hydro dissection technique is utilized successfully and with good results [9]. In instances where superficial endometriosis implants are positioned away from underlying structures (e.g., ureter or the bowel), simple excision of the peritoneal implant is carried out:

1. Peritoneum with identified lesion is tented up utilizing grasping forceps (Figure 9.5).

2. Small 4–5 mm incisional window is made next to the peritoneal implant with either laser, laparoscopic scissors, or electrosurgical instrument (Figure 9.6).

3. Hydro dissection is utilized to create a "cushion" and help with interface separation. The fluid entering the retroperitoneal space moves the lesion slightly away and medial from vital underlying structures and provides a "heat sink" for thermal spread during further use of electrosurgery. The tip of the laparoscopic suction-irrigator is then inserted into the incision and the high-pressure irrigation with either normal saline or lactated Ringer's solution is performed (Figure 9.7).

4. Peritoneal implant is removed utilizing traction-counter traction technique and either sharp dissection or preferred energy device (CO_2 laser vs. monopolar current vs. ultrasonic energy) (Figure 9.8).

5. Meticulous homeostasis is achieved with superficial bipolar fulguration, if anatomy allows, utilizing bipolar forceps (Figure 9.9).

6. The removed specimen is sent to pathology for final examination.

7. Use of adhesion-prevention agents is controversial but could be applied laparoscopically if warranted.

Vaporization and ablation of superficial peritoneal implants is also performed with the help of various energy devices, although in our practice vaporization and excision remains the

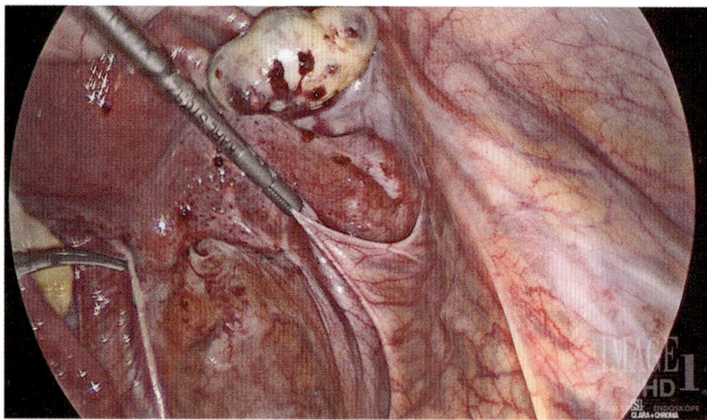

Figure 9.5 Step 1: Grab peritoneum away from sidewall and ureter.

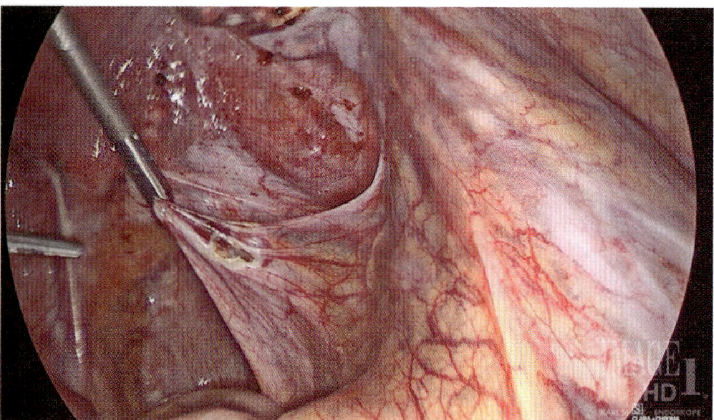

Figure 9.6 Step 2: Make incision and allow pneumo dissection.

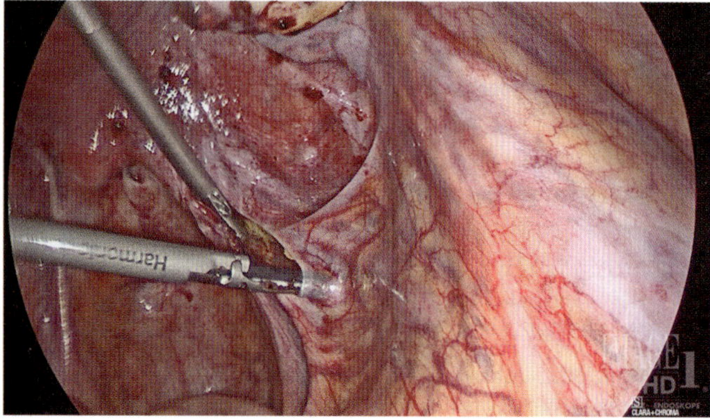

Figure 9.7 Step 3: Extend peritoneum incision parallel to retroperitoneal structure.

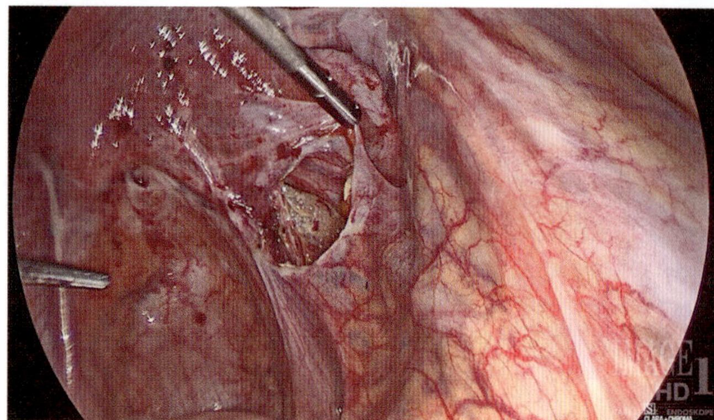

Figure 9.8 Step 4: Separate lesion from ureter.

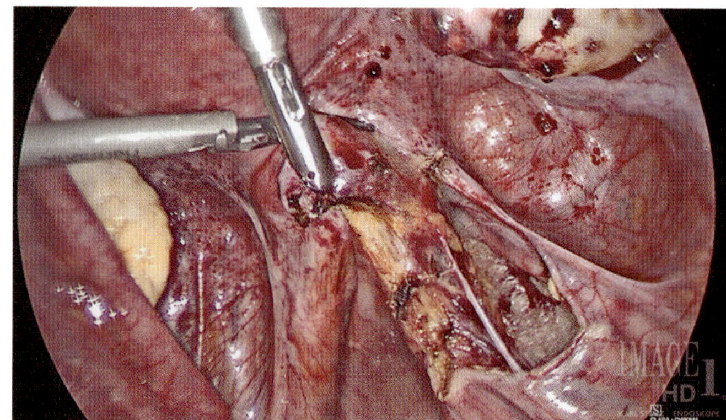

Figure 9.9 Step 5: Excise the endometriotic lesion.

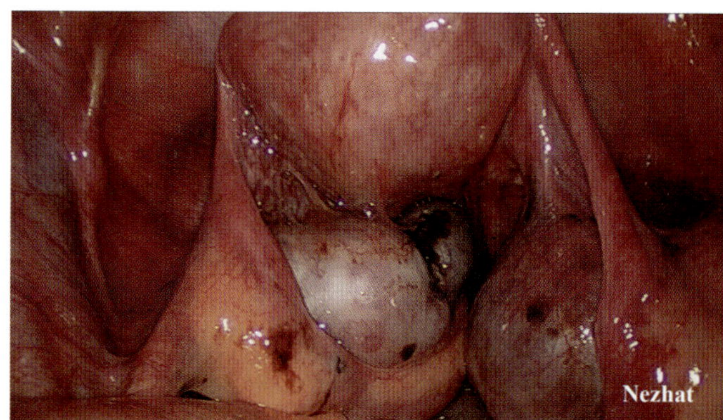

Figure 9.10 Bilateral ovarian endometriomas (left: type I endometrioma, right: type II endometrioma).

most favorable option depending on the location and depth of penetration of the lesions.

9.5 Management of Ovarian Endometriomas

The European Society of Human Reproduction and Embryology recommends surgical and histology evaluation of cysts > 3 cm in diameter and with characteristics of ovarian endometriomas (Figure 9.10).

Ovarian endometriomas should be distinguished from superficial endometriosis of the ovary (Figures 9.11 and 9.12).

Surgical excision of endometriomas via a stripping technique has been demonstrated to be superior to cyst drainage and ablation, while the effect of endometriosis treatment on overall fertility remains unknown. Excisional surgery has shown to improve spontaneous pregnancy rates 9–12 months after surgery compared to ablative surgery [10].

The typical surgical procedure can be described as follows:

If the ovary with the endometrioma is adherent to the pelvic sidewall, peritoneal dissection with ureterolysis is performed to free the ovary from its attachments.

1. Adhesions between the affected ovary and the uterus and/ or broad ligaments are lysed sharply or with the help of preferred energy sources.

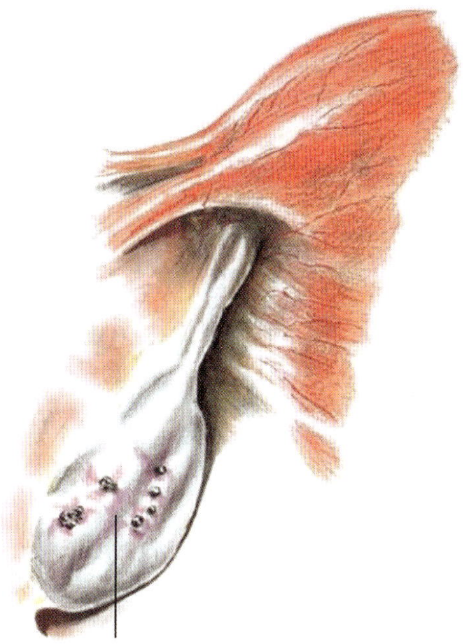

Figure 9.11 Superficial endometriosis involving the surface of the ovary.

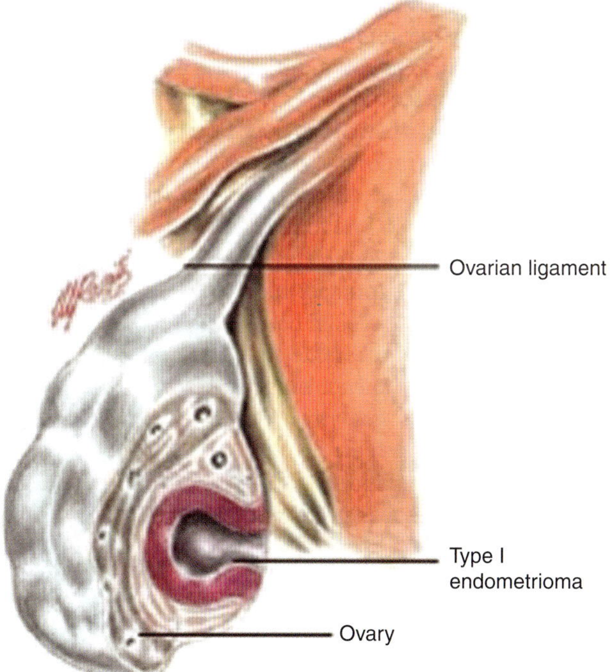

Figure 9.12 Ovarian endometrioma.

2. Utilizing traction-counter traction techniques, the capsule of the cyst is removed by striping technique: chocolate fluid that sometimes leaks during cystectomy is suctioned and copiously irrigated for complete evacuation (Figure 9.13).

3. Electrosurgery is reserved for cases where superficial fulguration is required; suturing of the ovary has potential for adhesion formation and future fertility compromise.

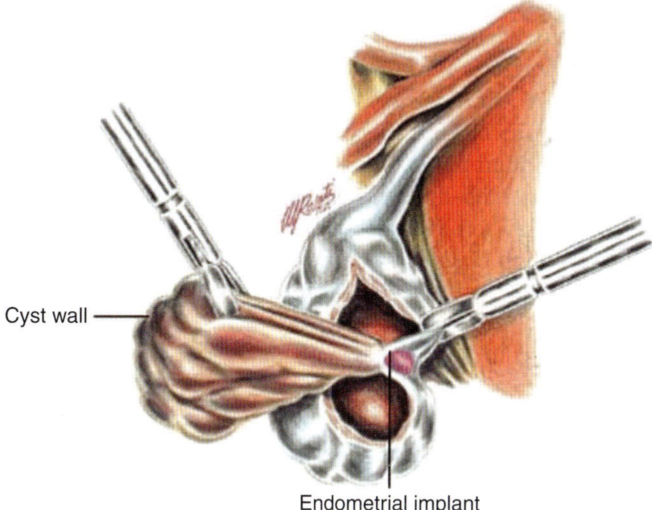

Figure 9.13 Traction-counter traction technique for excision of ovarian endometrium. Note that the entire cyst wall is excised.

However, at times selective intracortical suturing with fine monofilament absorbable sutures such as 4-0 Polydixanone for approximation of ovarian edges is necessary.

4. Use of adhesion-prevention agents is controversial but can be accomplished laparoscopically based on surgeon's preference. Wrapping of the fallopian tubes in adhesion barriers have been reported to cause adhesions and must be avoided.

9.6 Management of Deeply Infiltrating Endometriosis

Deeply infiltrating endometriosis (DIE) is characterized by endometriotic implants that penetrate more than 5 mm into the affected tissue and is responsible for painful symptoms whose severity is strongly correlated with the depth of the DIE lesions. DIE may involve sites such as the uterosacral ligaments (USL), the rectovaginal septum (RVS), the posterior vaginal wall, the bowel, and the urinary tract. We will discuss the surgical management of colorectal and urinary tract DIE.

9.6.1 Rectovaginal and Pararectal Endometriosis

Resection of pararectal and rectovaginal (RV) lesions start with developing the pararectal space and/or relaxing excision:

1. Rectovaginal digital examination is performed prior to initiation of surgical intervention to gauge the position and the involvement of the disease process.

2. Relaxing excision is made between the ipsilateral ureter and the uterosacral ligament, allowing the mobilization of the uterosacral ligament with the potential lesion medially.

3. Pararectal space, classically defined as a triangle between the hypogastric artery, uterine artery, and the ureter, can be approached either from the opening of the broad ligament above, also known as "the superior approach," or from the peritoneal dissection with ureterolysis.

4. Once pararectal space is developed and noticed to be free of endometriosis, the rectum is retracted to the contralateral side. Use of rectal probes or end-to-end anastomosis (EEA) sizer can facilitate exposure, since it allows for the manipulation of the rectum and aids in pararectal dissection.

5. Uterine manipulator can aid displacing the uterus anteriorly and to the contralateral side.

6. Traction-counter traction is utilized while tenting the lesion with the laparoscopic grasper. The lesion is excised utilizing a variety of laparoscopic instruments, ideally avoiding middle rectal vessels and intramesenteric nerve bundles.

7. The resection of the RV lesion is carried into the vaginal fornices and the lesion is removed with excision of the associated vaginal wall.

8. Vaginal defect is closed and reapproximated with the variety of available absorbable suture material.

Not uncommonly, the lesion will be in very close proximity to the rectal wall and extend all the way to the muscles of the pelvic floor. Routine intraoperative procto-sigmoidoscpy can be performed and the rectum examined "under water" to demonstrate the integrity of the rectal wall and absence of microscopic perforations, particularly if the electrosurgical instruments were used [11].

9.6.2 Endometriosis of Gastrointestinal Tract

The bowel is involved in approximately 10% of endometriosis cases. The most commonly affected sites are the rectum and sigmoid 76%, the appendix 18%, and the cecum 5%. Other segments less frequently involved include the ileum, jejunum, or other parts of small intestine in 3% of the cases [11,12]. The surgery is necessary when the small intestine is affected due to the risk of obstruction and in symptomatic rectosigmoid disease, because medical therapy is either temporarily effective or ineffective. In less than 1%, it invades intestinal lumen, thus detection with colonoscopy is rare.

Treatment of intestinal endometriosis depends on the location of the lesion, single- or multifocal lesions(s), size of the lesion, depth of penetration, skill, and experience of the surgeon and availability of proper instrumentation. Techniques used for excision of gastrointestinal DIE lesions include rectal shaving, disc excision, and segmental resection [11–14]. Shaving of lesions involving bowel mesentery, serosa, or less than 2–3 mm superficial muscularis has been performed with CO_2 lasers since the early 1990s with good long-term results and less morbidity [15]. Trans-abdominal or trans-rectal discoid excision is performed for single infiltrative lesions with more than 5 mm depth of penetration as long as it does not invade more than one-third of the bowel wall [13,14]. Segmental resection with EEA is performed for lesions larger than 3 cm, multifocal lesions, or in cases of narrowing of the lumen [13,14]. The necessity of each particular technique and the surgical outcomes have been debated for decades, with all approaches showing good results when done at high-volume centers and with proper surgical technique.

9.6.3 Shaving Technique

Shaving of bowel endometriosis can be used for more superficial lesions that are not circumferential and do not constrict the lumen of the bowel. The technique is as follows:

1. The lesion involving the bowel wall is identified, palpated using the tip of suction-irrigator, and elevated by grasping forceps. A proctosigmoidoscopy or rectal probe can be used for exposure and to facilitate identification of the lesion if necessary.

2. The ureters are identified and the pararectal spaces are developed bilaterally.

3. The lesion is placed on traction using grasping forceps and full-thickness "shaving" technique is carried out from proximal to distal end using variety of laparoscopic instruments (*video*; Nezhat C, Nezhat F, Nezhat CH. Nezhat's Video-Assisted and Robotic-Assisted Laparoscopy and Hysteroscopy with DVD. 4th edition. New York: Cambridge University Press, 2013).

4. The surgeon should follow the contour of the bowel around the endometriotic nodule. The goal is to free the nodule completely from the bowel wall and to identify the healthy tissue surrounding the nodule (Figure 9.14).

5. After procedure, air is injected into the rectum, which is submerged in the irrigation fluid, and the bowel is compressed above the site of dissection to ensure that there is no leakage. A dilute solution of methylene blue is introduced into the rectum to assess for the thickness integrity of the wall [16].

If the bowel lumen is entered, the defect is repaired by placing several through-and-through single interrupted delayed absorbable sutures (Figure 9.15).

Alternatively, stay sutures are placed in the corners of the opening to the bowel and either trans-abdominal or transanal Endo Stapler is applied for repair.

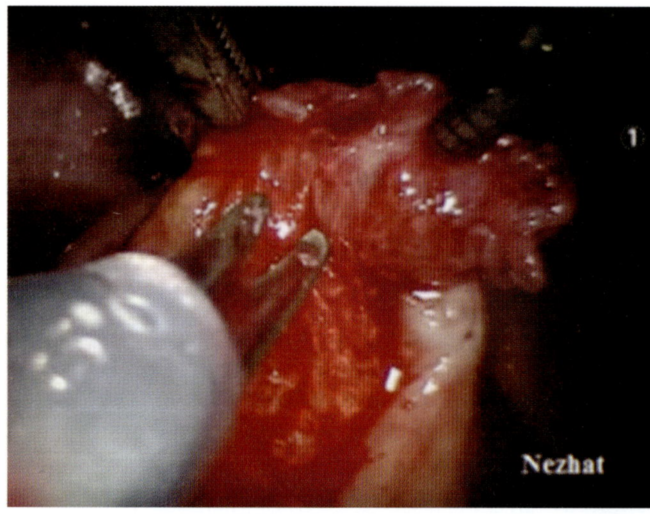

Figure 9.14 Endometriosis nodule being excised from surface of bowel using the rectal shaving technique.

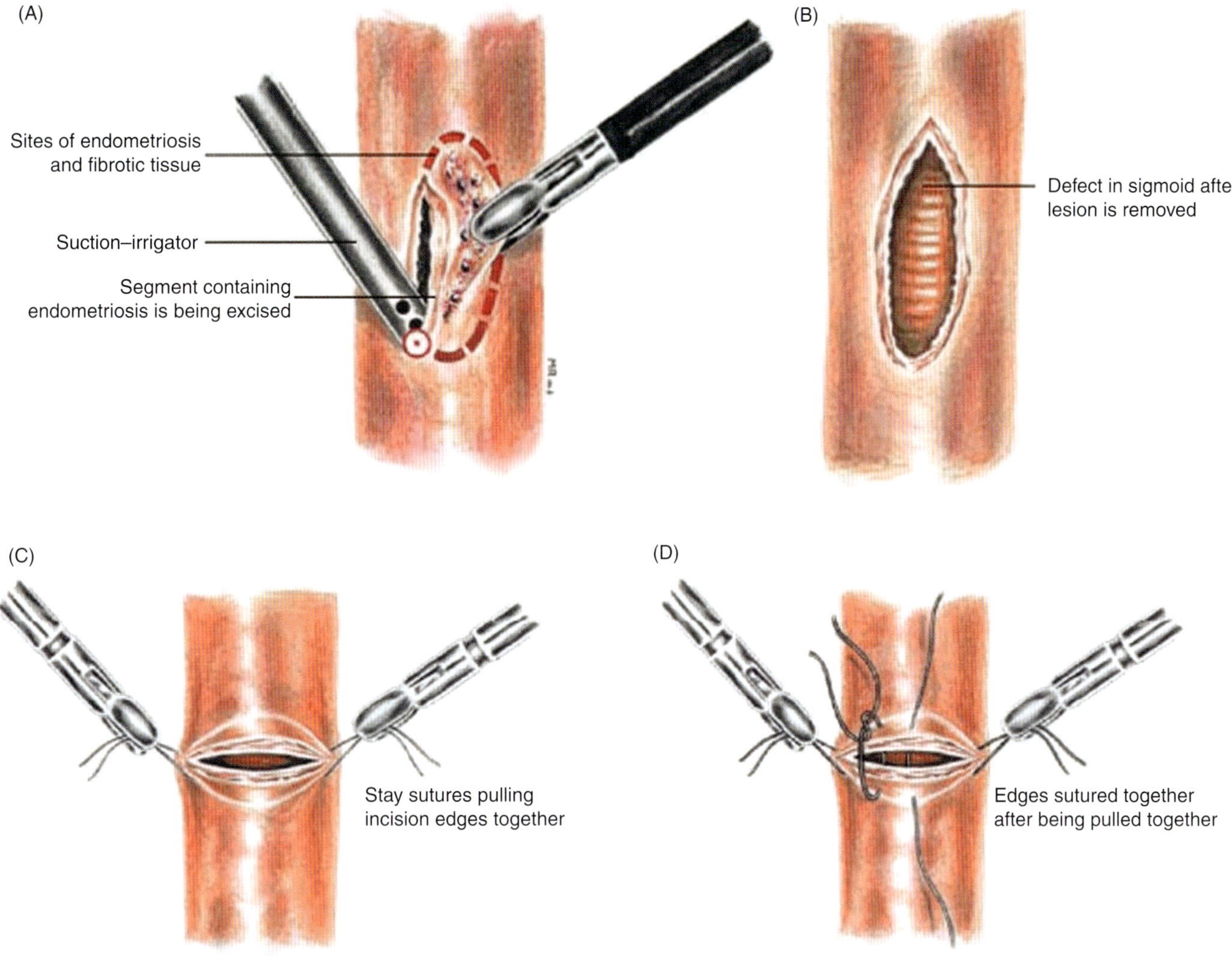

Figure 9.15 Repair of bowel using a single interrupted layer of delayed absorbable suture.

If complete bowel resection is required, this can be achieved by laparoscopically assisted anterior resection and anastomosis (Figure 9.16).

1. The rectum is mobilized entirely with the development of pararectal and presacral spaces.
2. Ureters are identified bilaterally, sometimes with prior stent placement.
3. Hemostasis is achieved using electrosurgical techniques on branches of inferior mesenteric vessels.
4. The rectum is transected proximally to the lesion and the proximal end is prolapsed either transanally, transvaginally, or transabdominally though minilaparotomy (< 4 cm incision).
5. The anvil of a circular stapler is placed into the proximal end and secured with purse-string absorbable suture.
6. The distal end of the rectum and the endometriosis lesion is prolapsed either transanally, transvaginally, or through mini-laparotomy incision and the liner stapler is used to separate and remove the lesion.
7. The rectal stump is brought back into the pelvis, the anvil is attached to the shaft of the circular stapler,

and stapler is fired under laparoscopic guidance completing EEA.

The bowel is examined for possible stricture and leaks by proctosigmoidoscopy with examination "under water" technique described previously [16].

9.6.4 Discoid Resection

Discoid resection entails wedge resection of the anterior wall of the rectum. Two techniques have been described in the literature: (1) resection of the endometrial nodule followed by suture repair or (2) resection of the endometrial nodule using either linear stapler trans-abdominally (Figure 9.17) or circular stapler trans-anally [15,17,18].

1. After adhesiolysis, ureterolysis and dissection of retrocervical region are performed as described earlier.
2. The lateral and anterior wall of the bowel are dissected in order to surround the lesion.
3. A cut through the lesion is performed in order to free it from the posterior aspect of the uterus and/or the vagina. Sometimes, residual lesions are left and can be removed separately.

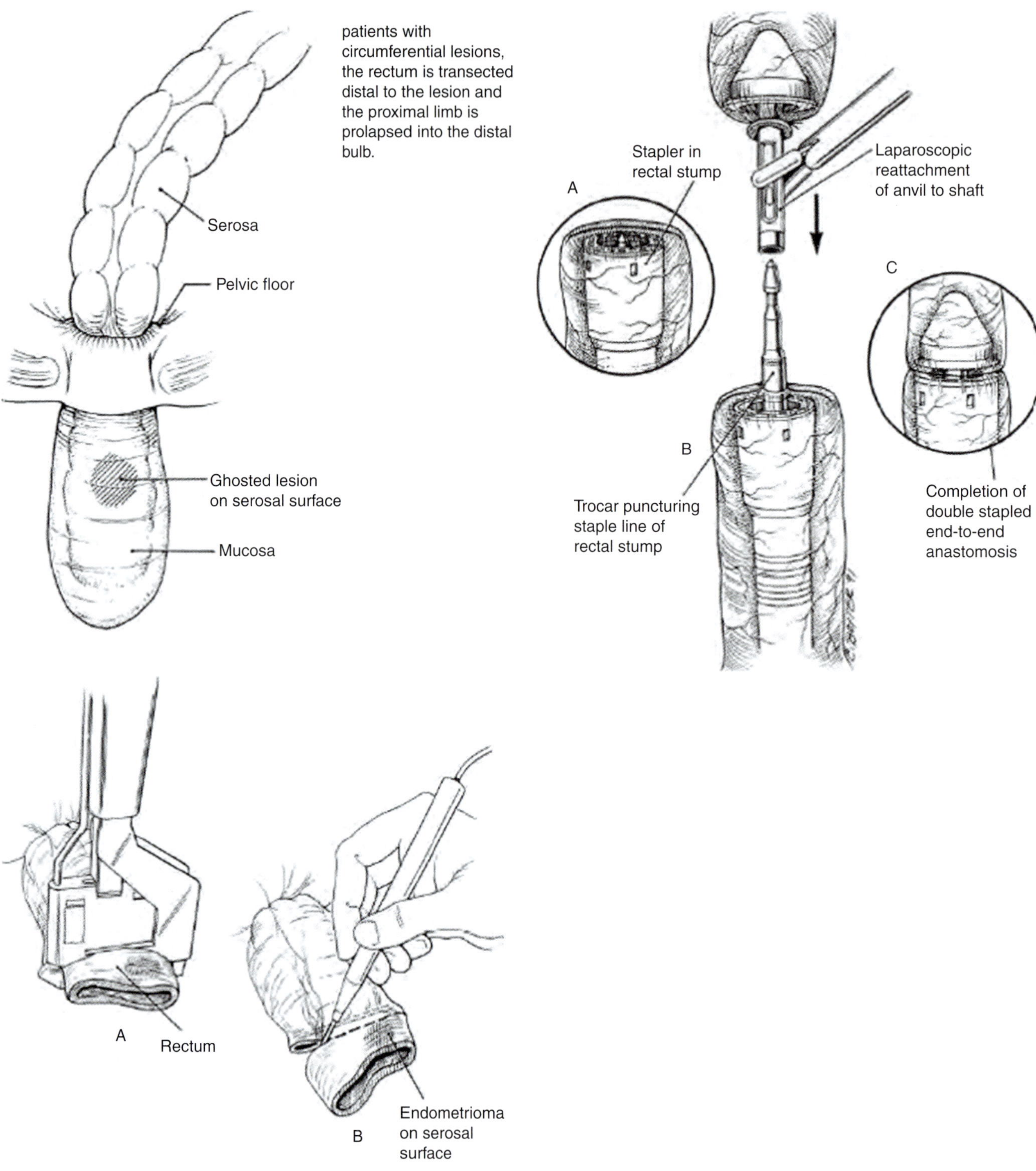

Figure 9.16 Laparoscopic technique of low anterior resection.

4. Stay sutures are placed lateral to the endometriotic lesion, identifying the areas to be excised.
5. The stapler is inserted and opened, positioning the lesion in the gap between the ogiva (tip) and its shoulder.
6. Using two instruments, each thread of the suture is held, providing a downward traction on the bowel, helping imbricate the affected area into the hollow, while the stapling device is being closed.
7. The stapler is activated.
8. The excised area is inspected and should contain the endometriotic lesion as well as the suture.
9. Examination with air insufflation and under-fluid emersion and blue dye test are performed as described above.

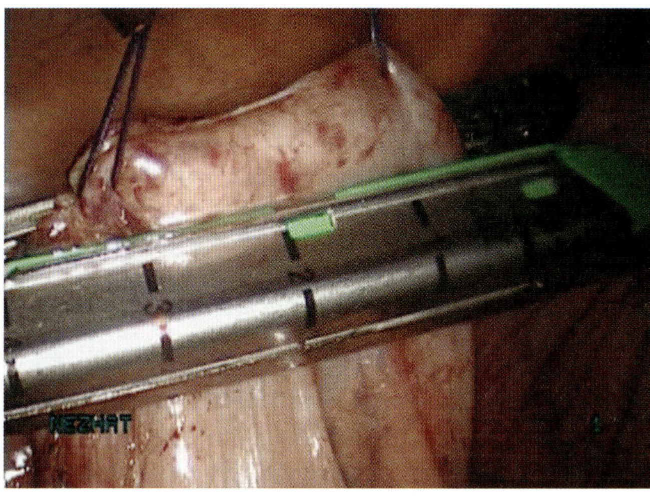

Figure 9.17 Linear stapler applied to excide the diseased bowel (*video*).

9.6.5 Segmental Resection

Laparoscopic segmental resection is performed for lesions larger than 3 cm, multifocal lesions, or in the presence of narrowing of the bowel lumen [19,20]. Segmental resection is performed with a circular stapling device, such as the EEA stapler as follows:

1. Adhesiolysis of the affected adnexal regions, uterine fundus, posterior cul-de-sac, uterosacral ligaments, and bowel is performed.
2. The sigmoid colon is released from the left lateral abdominal wall, opening the retroperitoneum with identification of the left ureter and opening of the mesosigmoid.
3. Dissection of the anterior wall of the rectum from the posterior surface of the cervix is performed. The healthy distal part of the rectosigmoid is skeletonized. A linear stapler is applied distally to the area affected by the disease. Care is taken to spare the superior rectal vessels.
4. The proximal portion of divided bowel including the disease portion is exteriorized through a mini-laparotomy incision and transected proximally to the lesion.
5. The anvil of the circular stapler is placed inside the stump and a purse-string suture is placed.
6. The bowel containing the anvil is reintroduced into the abdominal cavity and an EEA circular stapler (range 21–34 mm in diameter) appropriately sized to the proximal lumen of the bowel so that it conforms with the diameter of the two ends of the bowel for anastomoses (usually 31 or 34 mm) is introduced through the anus and connected to the anvil.
7. The stapler is activated to form the EEA. The donuts obtained after stapling are checked to confirm that complete rings have been obtained.
8. The anastomosis is tested for leaks by placing the patient in the reverse Trendelenburg position and filling the pelvis with saline. A rigid sigmoidoscope may be passed through the anal canal to enable direct visualization of the anastomosis. The colon is compressed proximal to the anastomosis, and air is then insufflated into the rectum via the sigmoidoscope.
9. The colon is checked for adequate distention with air and for any bubbles of air in the pool of saline in the pelvis. The presence of a stream of bubbles indicates a positive leak test, in which case an attempt must be made to identify and over sew the leak. In rare cases, a complete revision of the anastomosis is required.
10. A dilute solution of methylene blue may be introduced into the rectum to assess the thickness and integrity of the area of dissection.

9.6.5 Appendectomy for Endometriosis

Examination of the appendix should be conducted routinely (Figure 9.8). Incidental appendectomy (IA) might be a surgical option worth considering during laparoscopic treatment of endometriosis [21,22]. Nezhat et al. reported on the safety and utility of incidental appendectomy during laparoscopic surgery in the early 1990s [20]. Mean operating times were at 12 minutes with endometriosis diagnosed in 2.2% of incidental appendectomy and appendicitis present in 4.3% of specimens [21]. An additional study in women with ovarian endometriomas demonstrated appendiceal pathology in 35% of the removed appendices with endometriosis present in 13% of IA specimens [22]. The carcinoid tumor of the appendix is reported in 0.3–0.9% of incidental appendectomies [23]. Based on the available evidence, safety of the technique and short procedure times, it appears that IA should be considered in all patients with endometriosis and pelvic pain, particularly patients with ovarian endometriomas. Technically, laparoscopic appendectomy is a relatively simple technique:

1. Once the ileocecal junction has been identified, the appendix is elevated and placed on gentle traction.
2. The meso-appendix is transected utilizing a variety of the available laparoscopic instruments, keeping in mind the presence of appendiceal vessels and the need to control potential bleeding from the site (Figure 9.18).
3. Once hemostasis is achieved, the base of the appendix can be separated from the cecum by either the placement of endoloops and cutting, placement of a stapler, or clips based on surgeon's preference and experience (Figures 9.19 and 9.20).
4. The appendix is then easily removed by holding the transection line with laparoscopic grasper to prevent inadvertent "milking" of the appendiceal contents into the abdominal/pelvic cavity or placed in a bag and removed.
5. The abdomen and pelvis are then copiously irrigated and suctioned, assuring the removal of all the intraluminal material and debris.

9.6.6 Genitourinary Endometriosis

9.6.6.1 Ureter Endometriosis

Ureteral endometriosis has two histologic types: extrinsic (Figure 9.21) and intrinsic (Figure 9.22) [24–26]. Intrinsic

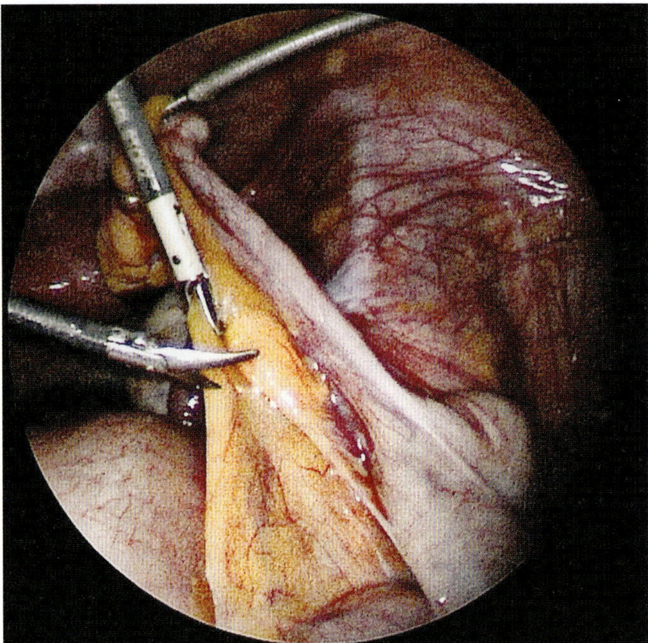

Figure 9.18 Meso-appendix being transected (*video*).

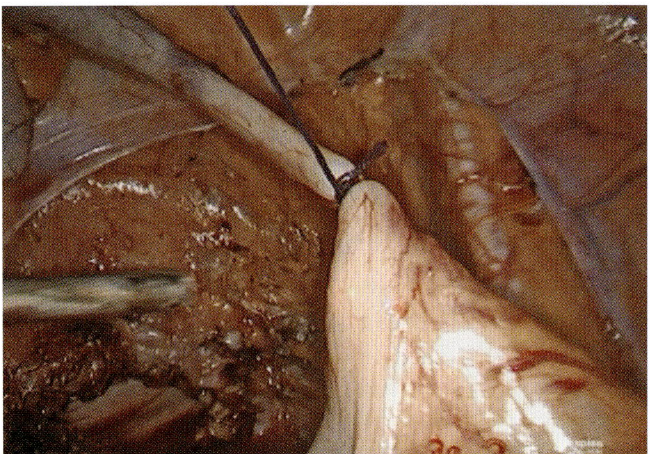

Figure 9.19 Securing the base of the appendix with an endoloop (*video*).

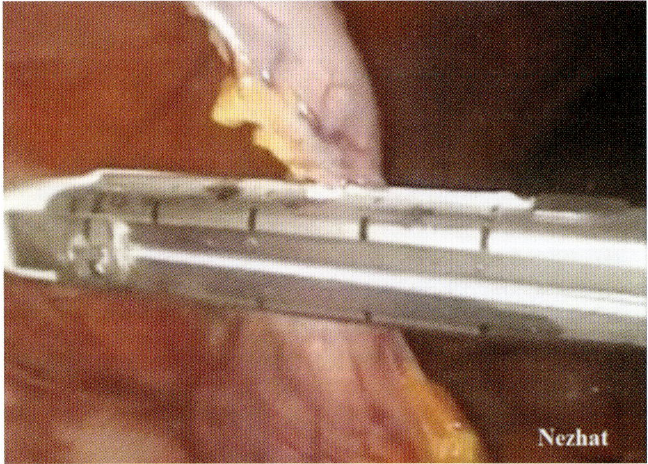

Figure 9.20 Securing the base of the appendix with a linear stapler (*video*).

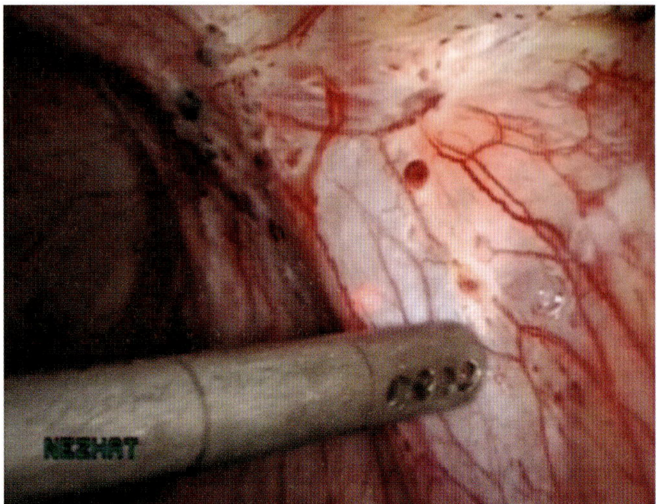

Figure 9.21 Extrinsic endometriosis of the ureter (*video*).

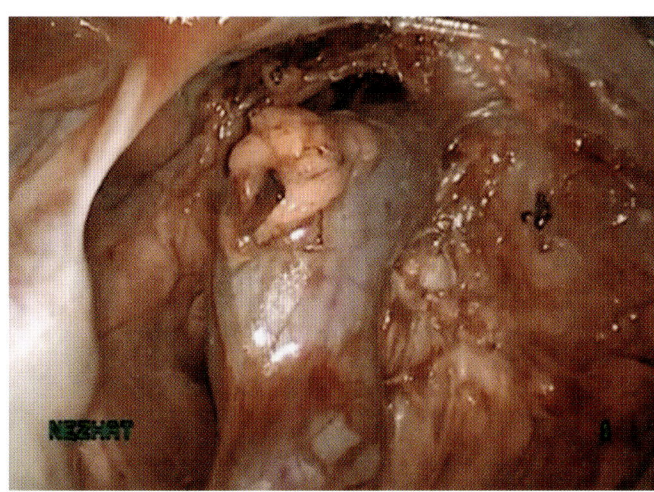

Figure 9.22 Intrinsic endometriosis of the ureter (*video*).
Video link: www.fertstert.org/article/S0015-0282(14)00202-7/ abstract [27].

ureteral endometriosis is histologically defined as infiltrating lesions involving the ureter wall and muscular layer [27]. Extrinsic endometriosis is characterized by infiltrating endometriosis and ureteral obstruction without involvement of the muscular layer [28,29].

In cases where the endometriosis lesion is located in close proximity to the pelvic ureter, ureterolysis is performed. Depending on the extent of the disease in the pelvis and associated adhesions such cul-de-sac obliteration, identification of the ureter is performed at the level of the pelvic brim using common iliac vessels as the landmark. Ureterolysis and assessment of the extent of invasion to the wall is of utmost importance.

Just visualization of ureteral vermiculation might not provide the safety zone required for peri-ureteral endometriosis resection as often the lesion will involve the adventitia of the ureter, or be in such close proximity that damage to the ureter will occur with resection. To safely and successfully perform ureterolysis, the ureter is traced all the way up to the bifurcation of the iliac vessels;

1. The peritoneum of the pelvic sidewall is tented up with a laparoscopic grasper in order to avoid the iliac vessels and peritoneal incision is made laterally to the course of the ureter (Figure 9.23).
2. The incision is extended medially and caudally, parallel to the course of the ureter and by opening the retroperitoneal space, the ureter remains in the medial leaflet of the open peritoneum. It is then traced down and into the insertion into the Wertheim canal, if pathology requires such distal dissection.
3. Any endometriosis adjacent to the ureter can now be resected utilizing traction countertraction technique and laparoscopic instruments, with the ureter being observed at all times (Figure 9.24).

In case of the endometriosis invading the ureter and not allowing the separation of the lesion from the ureter, laparoscopic ureter resection and anastomosis is performed (Figure 9.25):

1. Paraureteral disease is treated and ureter is mobilized to isolate the infiltrative lesion and prepare for approximation without tension. Care is taken to avoid devascularization (Figure 9.26) *(video)*.

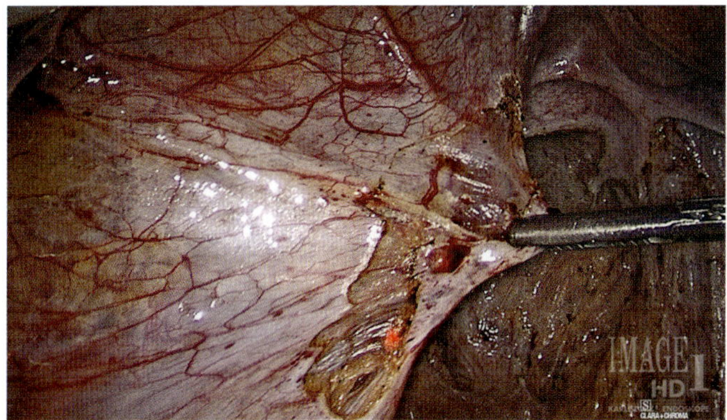

Figure 9.23 Peritoneum surrounding the ureter being tented up with a laparoscopic grasper.

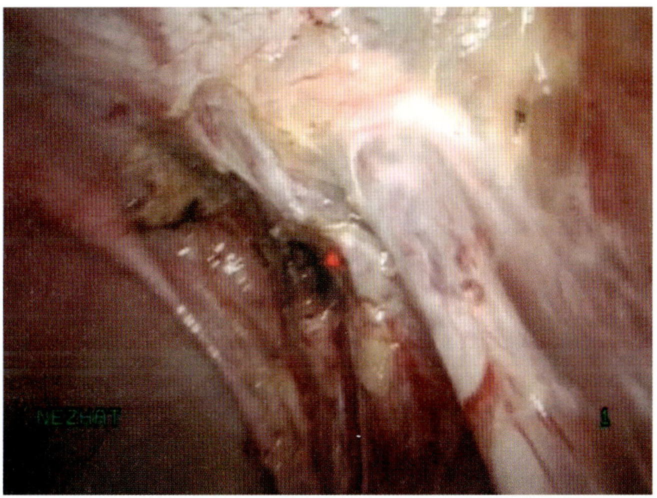

Figure 9.24 View after complete excision of diseased peritoneum surrounding the ureter *(video)*.

2. Placement of a ureteric catheter, later exchanged for a stent, is done prior to the resection or during the procedure – it facilitates the visualization of the ureter's lumen and aids in the placement of the sutures and anastomosis.
3. Once the nodule is resected (Figure 9.27), distal and proximal ends of the ureter are spatulated (Figure 9.28) and anastomosed with multiple interrupted sutures in one layer using 4-0 or 5-0 absorbable suture placed at 6, 9, 3, and 12 o'clock position respectively with either intracorporeal or extracorporeal knot tying. The stent is further advanced prior completing the anastomosis (Figure 9.29). The goal is approximation without tension or strangulation (Figure 9.30).
4. A pelvic drain, such as a Jackson–Pratt, may be placed through one of the port sites for a few days; however, it is rarely required.
5. Ureteric stent is removed 6–10 weeks later. An intravenous pyelograhic (IVP) or computed tomographic (CT) urogram 2 or 3 weeks later is performed to assess the anastomosis site for potential stricture, or rarely, extravasation. A mag-3-renal scan may be performed to assess renal function based on individual indication. Our experience has shown that EEA can be performed without tension in cases of mid- and upper-ureter lesions, while the ureteroneocystectomy with either psoas hitch or Boari flap is reserved for resection in the distal and lower part of the ureter [25–30].

9.6.6.2 Bladder Endometriosis

Endometriosis of the bladder is treated with ether resection or ablation. Primary bladder endometriosis is considered a retroperitoneal adenomyotic nodule, which is the consequence of metaplasia of the Mullerian system and can be resected by a laparoscopic approach [30]. Moderate retrograde distention of the bladder might be helpful, particularly with a stained solution (e.g., methylene blue in normal saline). Superficial lesions, not involving bladder muscularis, can be removed with the help of hydrodissection technique and superficial ablation, such as monopolar electrosurgery, CO_2 laser, or argon plasma.

Deep endometriosis of the bladder will require resection with ureteric catheter placement in areas away from the bladder dome and close to the posterior wall and the trigon prior to the closure of the bladder wall defect (Figures 9.31 and 9.32).

Multiple techniques can be utilized and have been described over the years, all appearing to provide good postoperative results as far as multilayer vs. single-layer closure and the choice of suture material avoiding nonabsorbable sutures [31–33]. If the bladder wall is repaired, the Foley catheter is left in situ for 7–14 days with retrograde cystogram performed to confirm bladder integrity prior to removal. The steps of bladder endometriosis are as follows:

1. Lesion involving full thickness of the bladder is resected by creating intentional cystotomy (Figures 9.33 and 9.34) and excising circumferentially with healthy tissue margins (Figure 9.35).

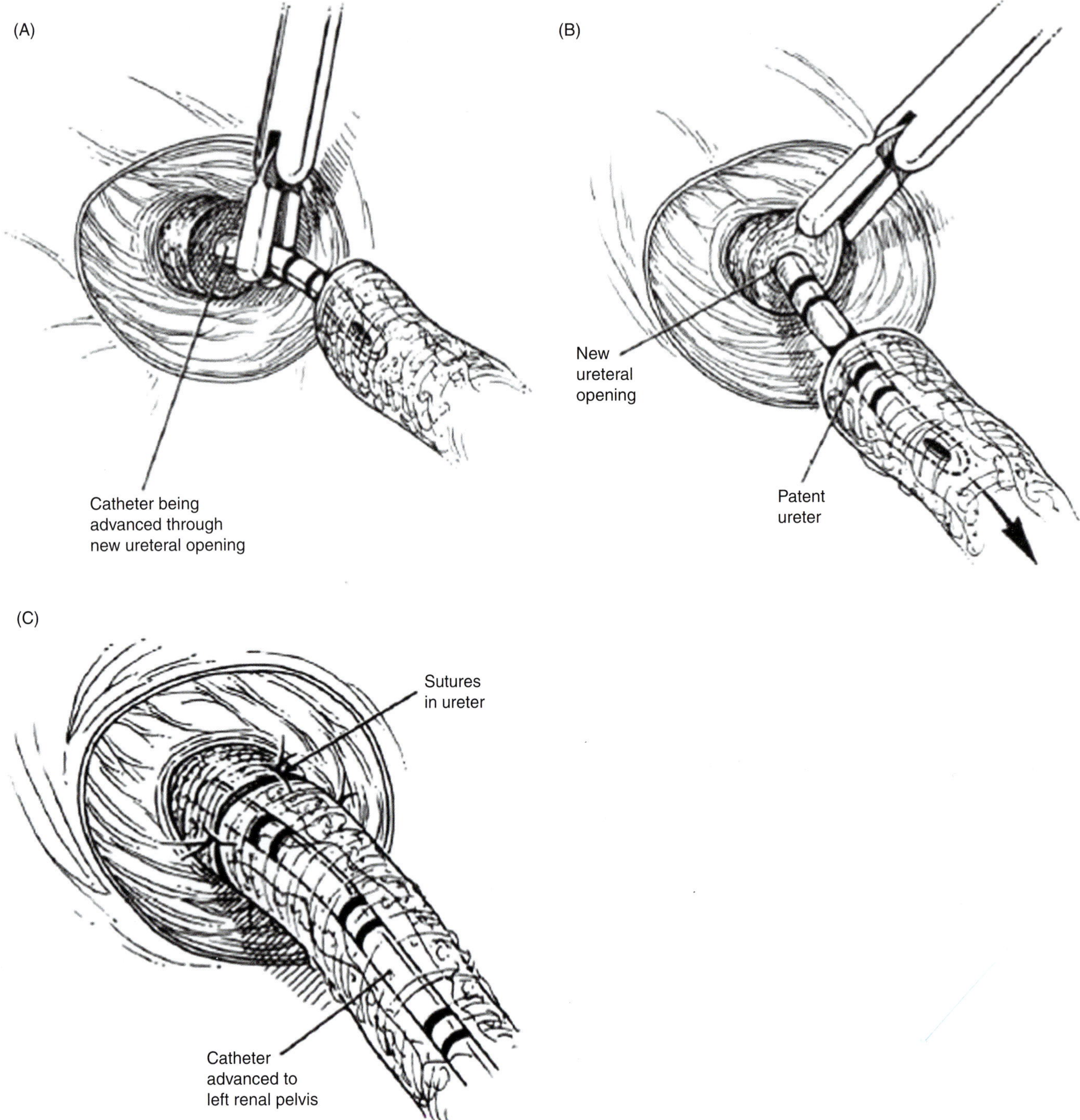

Figure 9.25 Technique of laparoscopic ureter resection with end-to-end anastomosis.

2. Multiple laparoscopic instruments can be utilized based on surgeon's preferences: from sharp scissors to monopolar electrosurgery, CO_2 laser, or ultrasonic technology.

3. The cystotomy is closed utilizing single- or double-layer closure, irrupted or continuous suturing, depending on the location and size of the defect. Delayed absorbable suture material is used (Figure 9.36).

4. Once the cystotomy is repaired, the integrity of the bladder wall and repaired site is assessed by cystoscopy and supra-pubic or trans-urethral catheter is placed. As an alternative, retrograde instillation of 300–400 cc of diluted methylene blue can be utilized (Figure 9.37).

5. If leaks are detected, the area is repaired with single interrupted suture.

Intraoperative cystoscopy is strongly recommended for both the ureterolysis and bladder endometriosis treatment – the procedure is inexpensive, carries minimal morbidity risks, and can potentially detect urinary system damage that, if not

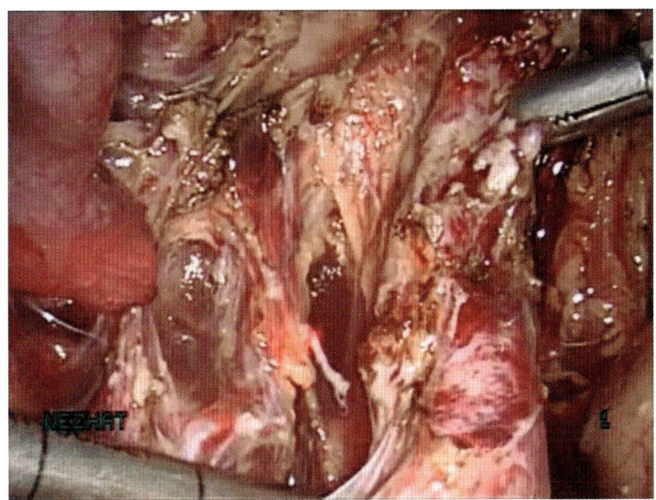

Figure 9.26 Ureter is initially mobilized with laparoscopic scissors (*video*).

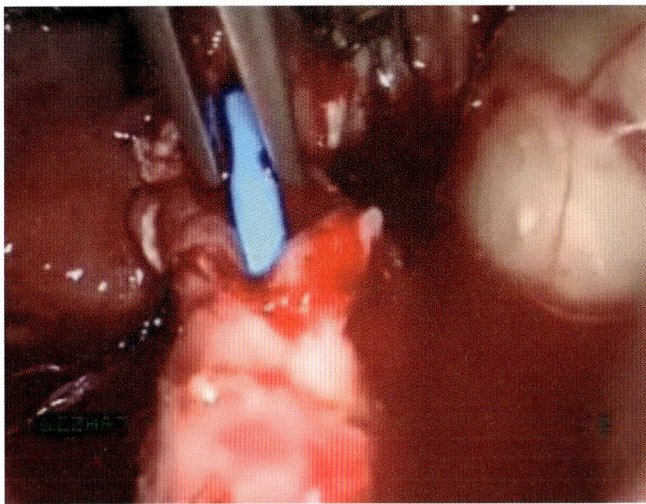

Figure 9.29 Placement of the ureter stent prior to completing the anastomosis (*video*).

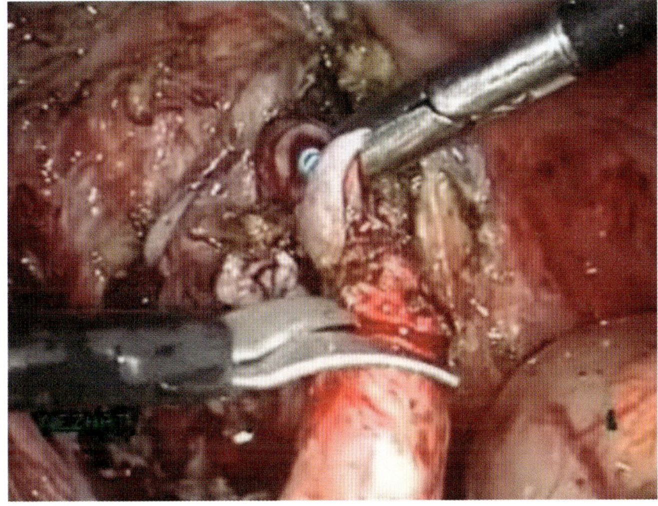

Figure 9.27 Diseased portion of the ureter being resected with laparoscopic scissors (*video*).

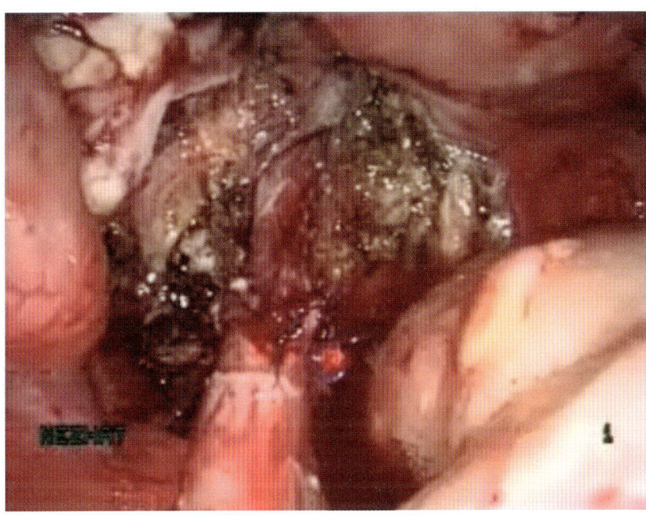

Figure 9.30 Tension-free repair of ureter (*video*).

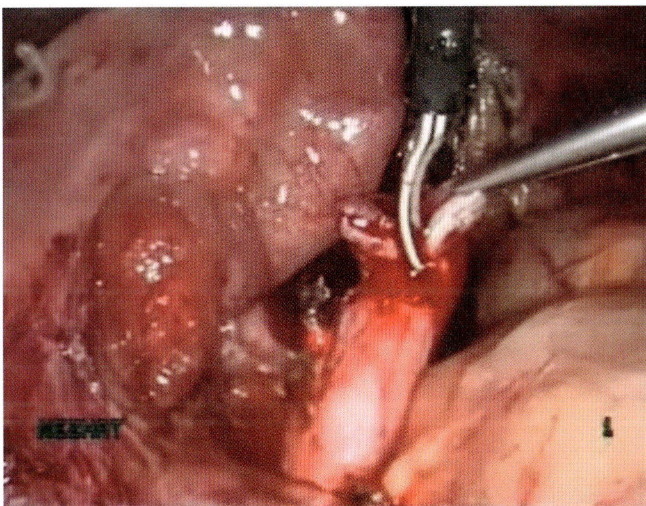

Figure 9.28 Proximal and distal ends of the ureter are spatulated (*video*).

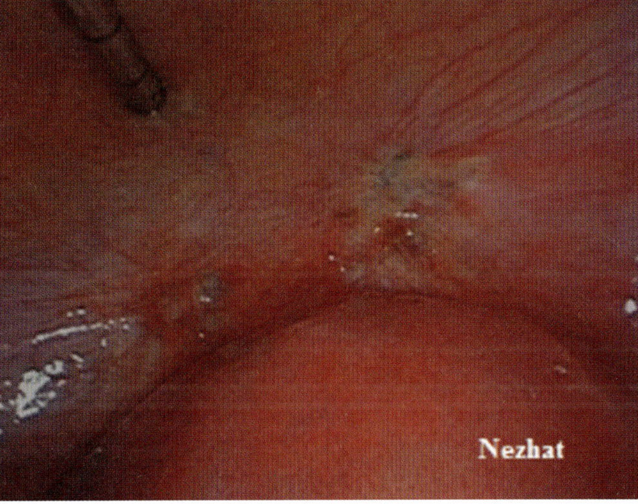

Figure 9.31 Laparoscopic view of DIE of the bladder wall.

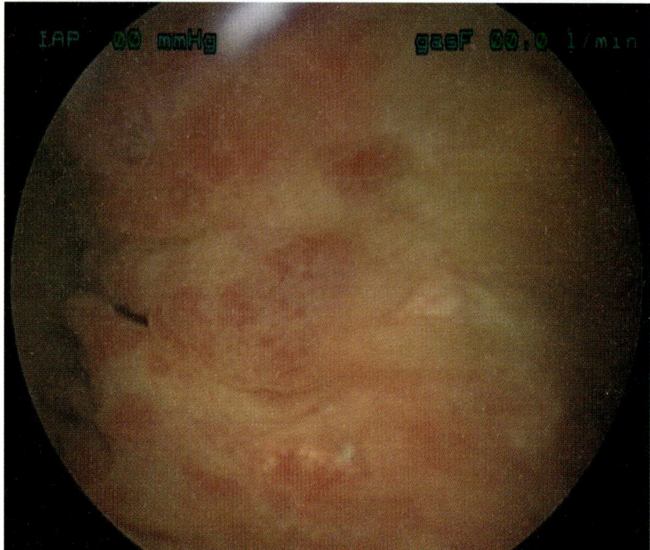

Figure 9.32 Cystoscopic view of DIE of the bladder wall.

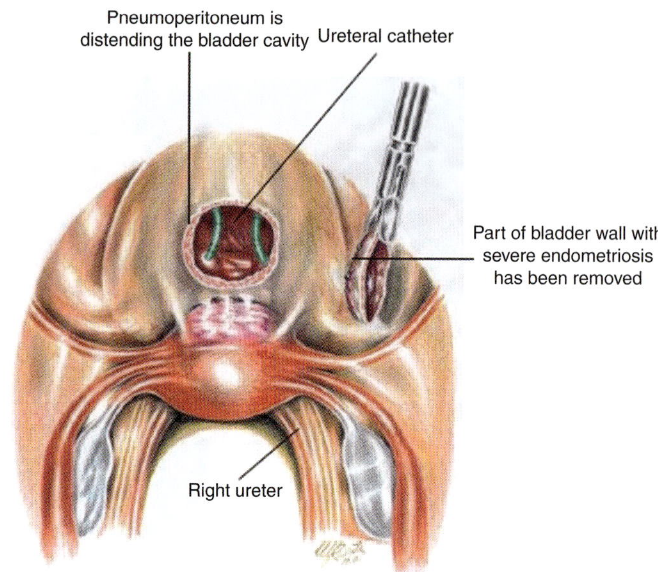

Figure 9.34 Portion of the bladder wall excised.

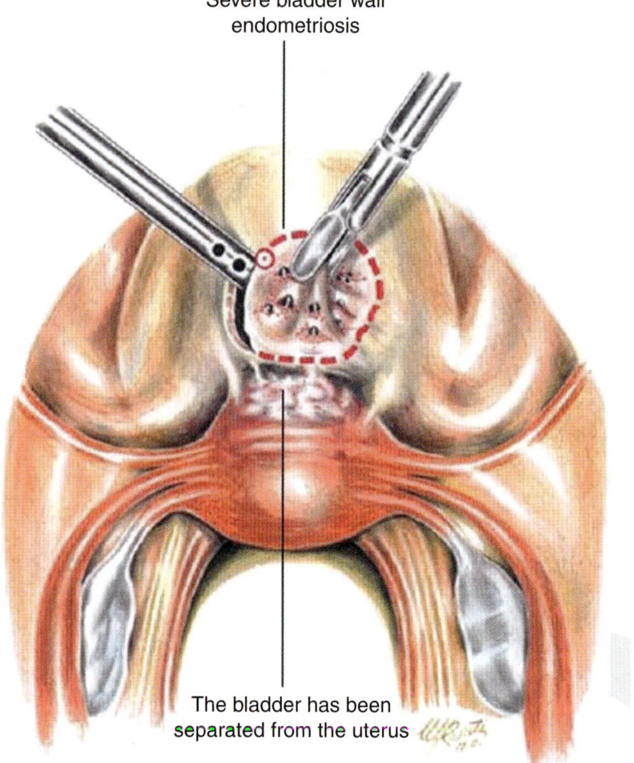

Figure 9.33 Intentional cystostomy for excision of the endometriosis lesion.

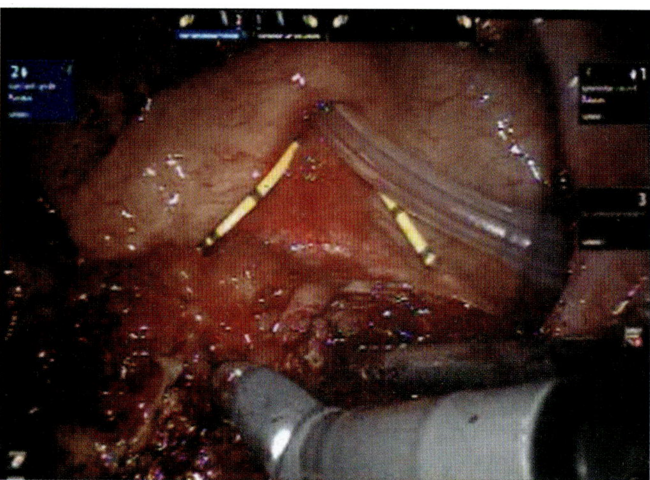

Figure 9.35 Excised portion of bladder wall will Foley catheter balloon visible.

properly recognized, can lead to the long-term complications and sequelae [34].

9.6.7 Computer-Assisted Technology

In the hands of an experienced endoscopic surgeon, both robot-assisted laparoscopic and standard laparoscopic treatment of endometriosis have excellent outcomes. The robotic technique requires significantly longer surgical and anesthesia time, as well as larger cannulas. However, as the technology evolves and instrumentation improves, introduction of a robotic platform into the gynecologic surgical field may increase in reproductive surgery for treatment of endometriosis. Studies have shown that robotic surgery for endometriosis is feasible, even in severe endometriosis cases, without conversion to laparotomy [35]. A multicenter LAROSE study (Laparoscopy vs. Robotic Surgery for Endometriosis: a Prospective Randomized Controlled Trial) is currently being conducted for better understanding of the long-term outcomes in robotic approaches in treatment of endometriosis [35]. Otherwise, complex and suture-intense laparoscopic surgeries can be facilitated by the use of robot-assisted technique.

References

1. Abbas S, Ihle P, Köster I, Schubert I. Prevalence and incidence of diagnosed endometriosis and risk of endometriosis in patients with endometriosis-related symptoms: findings from a statutory

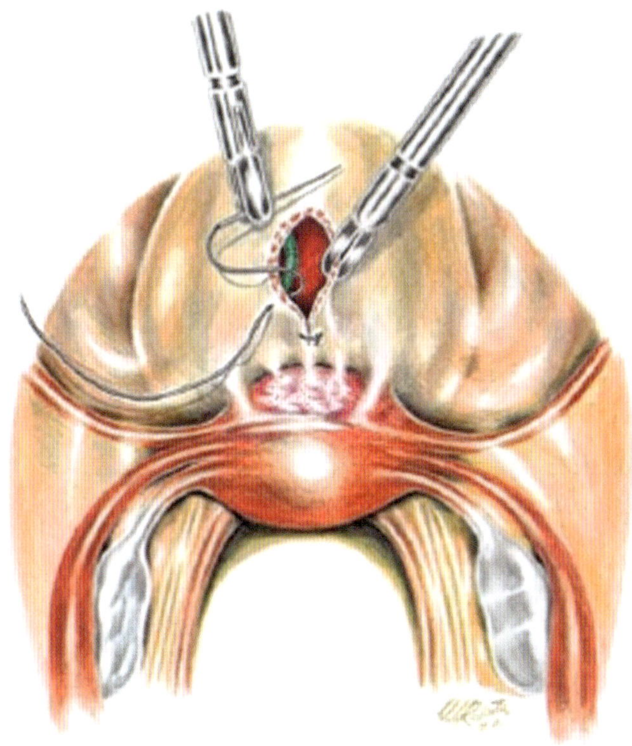

Figure 9.36 Cystotomy repair.

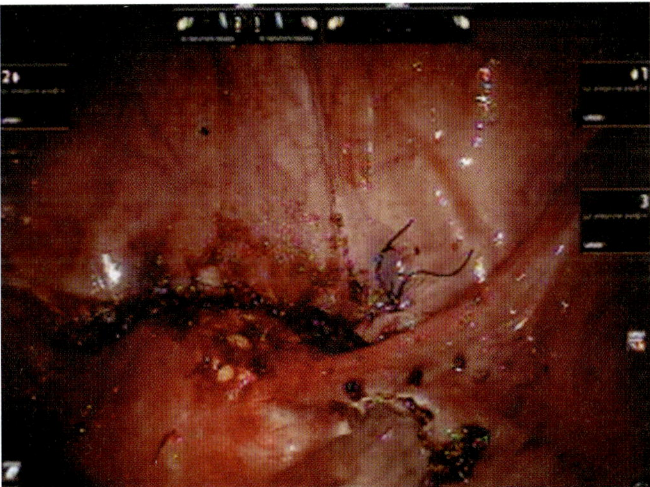

Figure 9.37 Final outcome of repaired bladder wall.

health insurance-based cohort in Germany. *Eur J Obstet Gynecol Reprod Biol.* 2012;160(1):79–83.

2. Langan KL, Farrell ME, Keyser EA, Salyer BA, Burney RO. Endometriosis: translation of molecular insights to management. *Minerva Endocrinol.* 2014; 39(3):141–54.

3. Ahangari, A. Prevalence of chronic pelvic pain among women: an updated review. *Pain Physician.* 2014;17(2):141–7.

4. Sutton CJ, Ewen SP, Whitelaw N, Haines P. Prospective, randomized, double-blind, controlled trial of laser laparoscopy in the treatment of pelvic pain associated with minimal, mild, and moderate endometriosis. *Fertil Steril.* 1994;62(4):696–700.

5. Howard H. Endometriosis and mechanisms of pelvic pain. *J Min Invas Gynecol.* 2009;16(5):540–50.

6. Nezhat C, Santolaya J, Nezhat FR. Comparison of transvaginal sonography and bimanual pelvic examination in patients with laparoscopically confirmed endometriosis. *J Am Assoc Gynecol Laparosc.* 1994;1(2):127–30.

7. Dun EC, Wong S, Lakhi NA, Nehzat CH. Recurrent massive ascites due to mossy endometriosis. *Fertil Steril.* 2016;106(6):e14.

8. Abbott J, Hawe J, Hunter D, Holmes M, Finn P, Garry R. Laparoscopic excision of endometriosis: a randomized, placebo-controlled trial. *Fertil Steril.* 2004;82:878–84.

9. Nezhat C, Nezhat FR. Safe laser endoscopic excision or vaporization of peritoneal endometriosis. *Fertil Steril.* 1989;52(1):149–51.

10. Brown J, Farquhar C. Endometriosis: an overview of Cochrane Reviews. *Cochrane Database Syst Rev.* 2014, March 10.

11. Nezhat C, Pennington E, Nezhat F, Silfen SL. Laparoscopically assisted anterior rectal wall resection and reanastomosis for deeply infiltrating endometriosis. *Surg Laparosc Endosc.* 1991;1(2):106–8.

12. Nezhat F, Nezhat C, Pennington E. Laparoscopic proctectomy for infiltrating endometriosis of the rectum. *Fertil Steril.* 1992;57(5):1129–32.

13. Nezhat F, Nezhat C, Pennington E, Ambroze W Jr. Laparoscopic segmental resection for infiltrating endometriosis of the recto sigmoid colon: a preliminary report. *Surg Laparosc Endosc.* 1992;2:212–16.

14. Nezhat C, Nezhat F, Pennington E. Laparoscopic treatment of lower colorectal and infiltrating rectovaginal septum endometriosis by the technique of videolaseroscopy. *Br J Obstet Gynaecol.* 1992;99:664–7.

15. Messori P, Faller E, Albornoz J, Leroy J, Wattiez A. Laparoscopic sigmoidectomy for endometriosis with transanal specimen extraction. *J Minim Invasive Gynecol.* 2013;20(4):412.

16. Nezhat C, de Fazio A, Nicholson T, Nezhat C. Intraoperative sigmoidoscopy in gynecologic surgery. *J Minim Invasive Gynecol.* 2005;12(5):391–5.

17. Faller E, Albornoz J, Messori P, Leroy J, Wattiez A. A new technique of laparoscopic intracorporeal anastomosis for transrectal bowel resection with transvaginal specimen extraction. *J Minim Invasive Gynecol.* 2013;20(3):333.

18. de Almeida A, Fernandes LF, Averbach M, Abrão MS. Disc resection is the first option in the management of rectal endometriosis for unifocal lesions with less than 3 centimeters of longitudinal diameter. *Surg Technol Int.* 2014;24:243–8.

19. Haggag H, Solomayer E, Juhasz-Böss I. The treatment of rectal endometriosis and the role of laparoscopic surgery. *Curr Opin Obstet Gynecol.* 2011;23(4):278–82.

20. Jatan AK, Solomon MJ, Young J, Cooper M, Pathma-Nathan N. Laparoscopic management of rectal endometriosis. *Dis Colon Rectum.* 2006;49(2):169–74.

21. Nezhat C, Nezhat F. Incidental appendectomy during video-laseroscopy. *Am J Obstet Gynecol.* 1991;165(3):559–64.

22. Song JY, Yordan E, Rotman C. Incidental appendectomy during endoscopic surgery. *JSLS.* 2009;13(3):376–83.

23. Wie HJ, Lee JH, Kyung MS, Jung US, Choi JS. Is incidental appendectomy necessary in women with ovarian endometrioma? *Aust N Z J Obstet Gynaecol.* 2008;48(1):107–11.

24. Modi P, Goel R, Dodiya S. Laparoscopic ureteroneocystostomy for distal ureteral injuries. *Urology.* 2005;66(4):751–3.

25. Nezhat CH, Malik S, Nezhat F, Nezhat CR. Laparoscopic ureteroneocystostomy and vesicopsoas hitch for infiltrative endometriosis. *JSLS*. 2004;8(1):3–7.

26. Nezhat CR, Siegler A, Nezhat F, Nezhat CH, Seidman D, Luciano A. Laparoscopic treatment of endometriosis. *Operative Gynecologic Laparoscopy: Principles and Techniques*. 2nd ed. New York, NY: McGraw-Hill; 2000:169–209.

27. Lakhi N, Dun EC, Nezhat CH. Hematoureter due to endometriosis. *Fertil Steril*. 2014;101(6):e37.

28. Nezhat C, Nezhat F, Green B. Laparoscopic treatment of obstructed ureter due to endometriosis by resection and ureteroureterostomy. A case report. *J Urol*. 1992;148:865–8.

29. Nezhat CH, Nezhat F, Freiha F, Nezhat C. Laparoscopic vesicopsoas hitch for infiltrative ureteral endometriosis. *Fertil Steril*. 1999;71:376–9.

30. Donnez J, Spada F, Squifflet J, Nisolle M. Bladder endometriosis must be considered as bladder adenomyosis. *Fert and Steril*. 2000;74(6):1175–81.

31. Nezhat CH, Siedman DS, Rottenberg H. Laparoscopic management of intentional and unintentional cystotomies. *J Am Assoc Gynecol Laparosc*. 1996; 3(4, Supplement):S34.

32. Taskin O, Wheeler JM. Laparoscopic repair of bladder injury and laceration. *J Am Assoc Gynecol Laparosc*. 1995;2(2):227–9.

33. Esparaz AM, Pearl JA, Herts BR, LeBlanc J, Kapoor B. Iatrogenic urinary tract injuries: etiology, diagnosis, and management. *Semin Intervent Radiol*. 2015;32(2):195–208.

34. Sadik S, Onoglu AS, Mendilcioglu I, Sehirali S, Sipahi C, Taskin O. Urinary tract injuries during advanced gynecologic laparoscopy. *J Am Assoc Gynecol Laparosc*. 2000;7(4):569–72.

35. Carvalho L, Abrão Mauricio S, Deshpande A, Falcone T. Robotics as a new surgical minimally invasive approach to treatment of endometriosis: a systematic review. *J Med Robotics Comput Assist Surg*. 2012;8(2):160–5.

36. Falcone T. The Cleveland Clinic. Laparoscopy vs. Robotic Surgery for Endometriosis (LAROSE): a Prospective Randomized Controlled Trial. In: ClinicalTrials.gov [Internet]. Bethesda, MD: National Library of Medicine (US). 2000 [cited January 29, 2015]. Available from: http://clinicaltrials.gov/show/NCT01556204 NLM Identifier: NCT01556204.

Female Fertility Preservation Surgery

Sara Arian, Rebecca Flyckt, and Tommaso Falcone

10.1 Introduction

Cancer continues to remain a leading cause of death in the United States and can have life-changing impacts. According to the National Cancer Institute statistics, about 10% of new cases of invasive cancer are diagnosed in women of reproductive age [1]. Although patient survival has shown a significant improvement over the last decade, many cancer treatment options including chemotherapy and radiation therapy can negatively affect a women's reproductive health and her ability to bear children. Therefore, there is considerable interest in fertility preservation options for women of reproductive age who are planning cancer treatments. However, having fully informative conversations on fertility preservation can often be challenging for clinicians, especially in the highly emotional context of a new cancer diagnosis. For this reason and others, physician–patient discussions of fertility preservation are still far from universal. Furthermore, for young women who do receive fertility preservation counseling, only a few actually undergo fertility preservation procedures due to social, financial, cultural, or technical limitations [2]. Providing answers and increasing the availability of fertility preservation options to women who seek these services in the setting of a cancer diagnosis would remain a challenge for health-care providers in the coming years.

The majority of cancer treatments including chemotherapy (specifically the use of alkylating agents such as cyclophosphamide), pelvic radiation, surgery, bone marrow transplantation, or a combination of these treatments can have a harmful impact on a woman's reproductive capacity, ovarian reserve, and uterine function. Given these documented negative effects on a woman's reproductive system, ovarian function, and subsequently her quality of life, fertility preservation options appropriate to each of these settings should be discussed. Hematologic cancers and breast cancer are the most frequent indications for fertility preservation [3].

There are currently three major fertility preservation strategies that can be used either singly or in combination. These include medical options, surgical options, and assisted reproductive technologies (including oocyte and embryo cryopreservation as the standard options) available to preserve the fertility of young women with cancer. In this chapter, we will focus on three fertility-preserving surgical techniques. Procedures to be discussed include ovarian transposition, ovarian tissue harvesting for cryopreservation, and ovarian autotransplantation.

10.2 Ovarian Transposition

Pelvic irradiation is indicated for the treatment of some malignancies including Hodgkin's lymphoma and genitourinary cancers; it is known that this type of radiation can result in ovarian follicular damage and subsequent loss of ovarian function. Radiation doses as low as 2 Gy can result in the loss of half of human oocytes [4]. Ovarian transposition is a surgical approach that has been developed to minimize radiation damage to the ovaries without having to remove them. This procedure can be done laparoscopically or via laparotomy. The goal of ovarian transposition is to reposition the ovaries outside of the radiation field. The ovaries can be transposed to a variety of different locations, and transpositions have been described anywhere from the base of the round ligament to the level of the kidneys. The exact location for ovarian transposition depends on patient's anatomy and the planned radiation field. Patients are usually marked on the skin for the radiation field. When deciding the level of transposition, the amount of radiation outside the field should be calculated. The ovaries are commonly transposed to the high lateral abdominal wall above the pelvic brim and outside of the radiation field cases of mid-pelvic irradiation such as what is recommended for vaginal, rectal, and cervical cancers. Another site for ovarian transposition is medially behind the uterus. This is the preferred location in the cases of planned abdominal radiation. The ovaries can also be transposed to distant locations [5–13]. Ovarian transposition can be performed laparoscopically or via laparotomy, as discussed in the following section.

10.3 Ovarian Transposition via Laparotomy

Ovarian transposition via laparotomy often requires a large abdominal incision and can be performed at the same time as a primary staging surgery or as a separate procedure [14]. Transposition via laparotomy has been reported to be associated with a successful preservation of ovarian function in approximately 83% of patients undergoing pelvic radiation [14]. Transposing the ovaries by laparotomy is associated with a longer hospital stay and postoperative recovery, as well as increased risks of adhesion formation and post-op intestinal obstruction. Furthermore, initiation of therapies is often delayed. For this reason, unless performed as part of a concomitant staging surgery, most centers now perform ovarian transposition via a minimally invasive approach.

10.4 Laparoscopic Ovarian Transposition

Laparoscopic ovarian transposition is accompanied by decreased postoperative discomfort due to smaller incisions, shorter hospital stay, more rapid recovery, and return to planned radiotherapy [15]. Laparoscopic transposition is therefore the preferred and more effective method for ovarian transposition and has been described using conventional laparoscopy, single-port methods, or robotic surgery. Laparoscopic ovarian suspension has been reported to have as high as 88.6% chance of successful ovarian function preservation [16]. As stated earlier, the anatomic positioning of the ovary with transposition depends on the type of radiation planned. Posterior-medial ovarian transposition is accomplished by mobilization of the ovary and fixation of the ovary to the uterosacral ligament. The uterus will then shield the transposed ovaries. Lateral ovarian transposition may be more effective in ovarian protection and is our preferred method for ovarian transposition.

One main consideration is whether to transpose the fallopian tube to the ovary. Various reports have described different strategies to approach the fallopian tubes at the time of oophoropexy. One advantage to leaving the fallopian tube intact is the option of having to avoid the cost of having to undergo in vitro fertilization (IVF) to achieve pregnancy, which may not be available to some patients due to limited financial resources. To enable this, we prefer to keep the tube attached and dissect the tube off the vascular pedicle that binds it to the ovary-mesosalpinx. In the following section we will describe our technique for laparoscopic lateral ovarian transposition.

10.5 Laparoscopic Lateral Ovarian Transposition: Surgical Technique

After induction of anesthesia, the patient is placed in standard dorsal lithotomy position. A Foley catheter is placed into the urinary bladder. A uterine manipulator is also inserted.

Four laparoscopic trocars are placed to facilitate laparoscopic intracorporeal suturing and knot tying. Initially, a small 5 mm infraumbilical skin incision is made using a scalpel. After insertion of the 5 mm optical trocar to introduce the laparoscope and obtaining adequate pneumoperitoneum, three additional 5 mm laparoscopic trocars will be introduced under direct visualization: two on the side of the primary surgeon and one on the other side. In this example, we will place two trocars on the left side. The right trocar will be placed at the level of the iliac crest to serve as a landmark for transposition. After performing a thorough survey of the abdominal and pelvic cavities with attention to metastatic implants on the liver, diaphragm, and omentum, the peritoneum is elevated laterally above the exterior landmark of the iliac crest on the abdominal sidewall and incised with scissors (Figure 10.1). Next, the ovary is grasped and the utero-ovarian ligament is electrocoagulated and transected (Figure 10.2). In order to be able to extend and fix the ovary as high and as lateral as possible, it has to be detached from the uterus by taking the utero-ovarian ligament. The blood supply to the ovary is then isolated by incising the peritoneum medially and laterally to

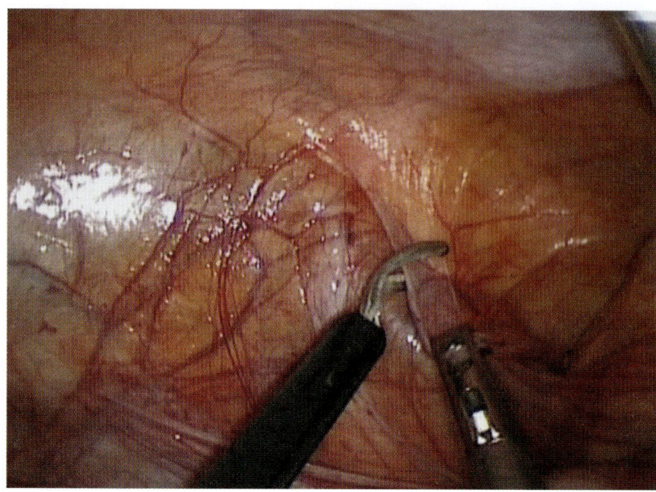

Figure 10.1 Using laparoscopic scissors, a small peritoneal incision is made in the lateral wall above the pelvic brim.

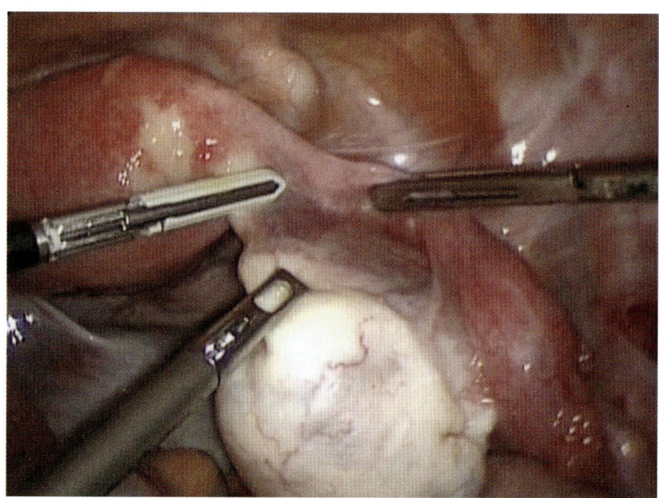

Figure 10.2 Transection of the utero-ovarian ligament.

the infundibulopelvic ligament. The infundibulopelvic ligament is isolated and mobilized away from the ureter. The peritoneal incisions are extended along the length of the ovarian vessels until the ovary is reached (Figure 10.3). Next, the ovary is separated from the fallopian tube (Figure 10.4). When the ovary is completely mobilized, a blunt grasper is used to create a tunnel in the retroperitoneum from the initial defect above the pelvic brim to the secondary defect in the area of the infundibulopelvic ligament (Figure 10.5). The ovary is gently grasped and guided through the retroperitoneal channel out through the superior defect in the peritoneum (Figure 10.6). In so doing, the ovary will now be positioned above the iliac crest with ovarian vessels coursing superiorly in the retroperitoneal space. It will therefore be mobilized laterally and cephalad to the level of the anterior-superior iliac spines and lateral to the psoas muscles. Retroperitoneal tunneling of the ovary is a unique surgical feature. Ovarian vessels are retroperitoneal structures that travel into the pelvic cavity without any turns. When the vessels are dissected off, they become intraperitoneal and make a sharp turn into the area where the

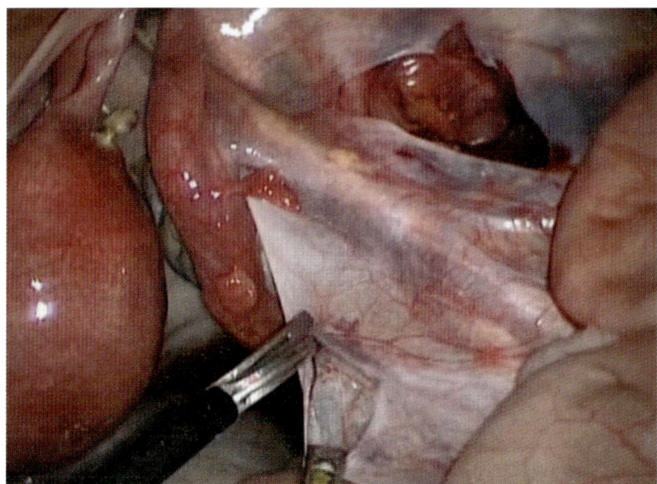

Figure 10.3 Using the scissors, the peritoneum is incised medially and laterally along the length of the ovarian vessels to isolate the infundibulopelvic ligament and mobilize it away from the ureter.

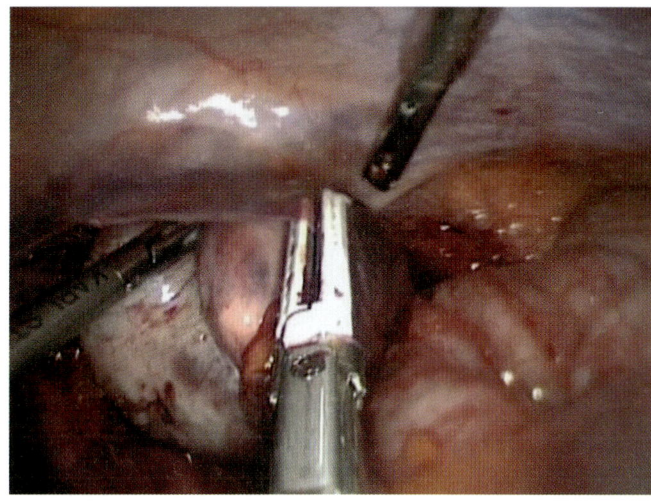

Figure 10.6 The ovary is gently grasped and guided through the retroperitoneal channel.

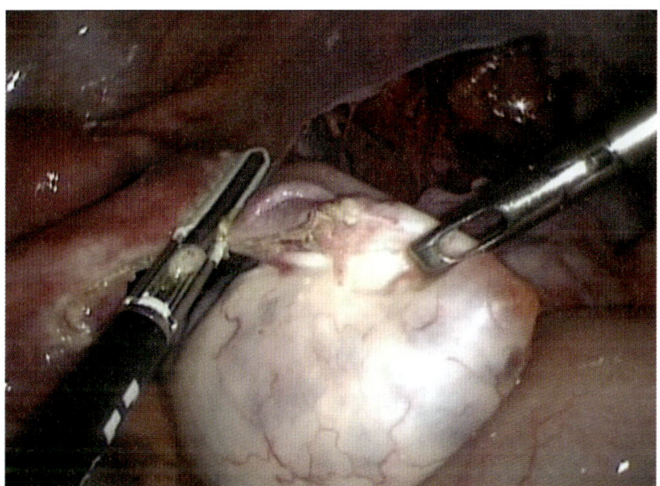

Figure 10.4 Separation of the ovary from the fallopian tube.

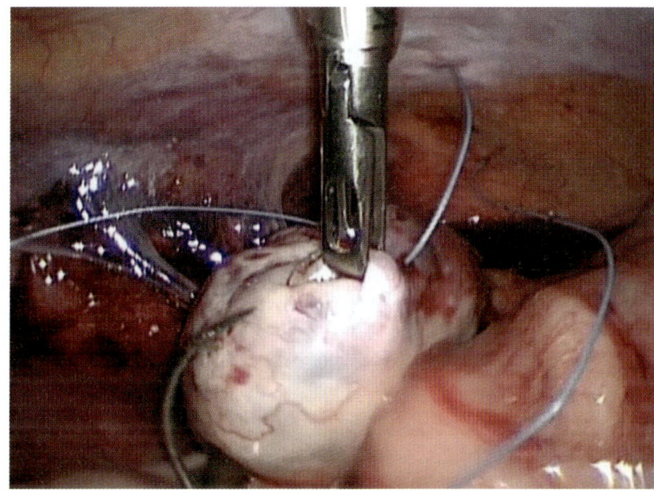

Figure 10.7 Anchoring of the transposed ovaries to the peritoneum and the underlying fascia.

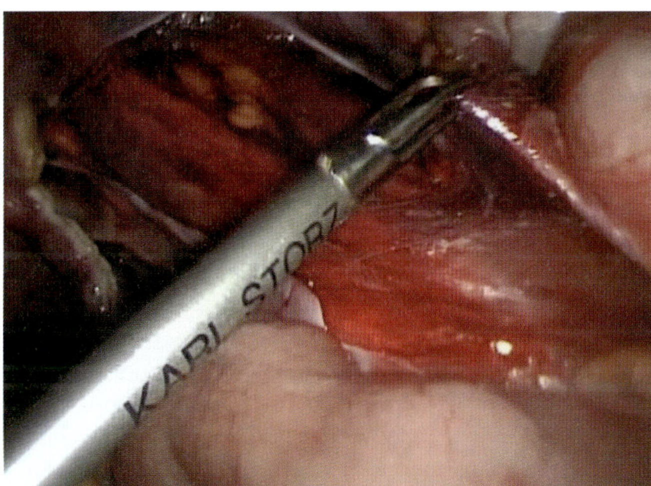

Figure 10.5 Using a blunt grasper a tunnel is created in the retroperitoneum from the initial defect above the pelvic brim to the secondary defect in the area of the IP ligament.

ovary is attached. It is thought that ovarian blood flow can potentially be altered because of this anatomical change. By creating this tunnel, the ovarian vessels will be maintained in their retroperitoneal position, preventing from their sharp turn into the pelvis [17]. The left lower port can be enlarged to 10 mm to introduce the needle. However, a 5 mm port can also be used. This requires removing the trocar and introducing the needle through the incision. The ovary is then sutured to the abdominal sidewall anteriorly using a nonabsorbable suture. In order to prevent the "drift" of the transposed ovaries back into the pelvic cavity, the transposed ovaries should be anchored securely to the peritoneum using transfixing nonabsorbable sutures [18] (Figure 10.7). In a case report of ovarian transposition wherein the ovaries were attached to the peritoneum using hemo-clips only, the ovaries were noted to slip back inside the pelvic cavity and the patient became menopausal following completion of pelvic radiation [8]. Surgical clips should however be placed on the ovarian boundaries after suture fixation for radiographic identification to map

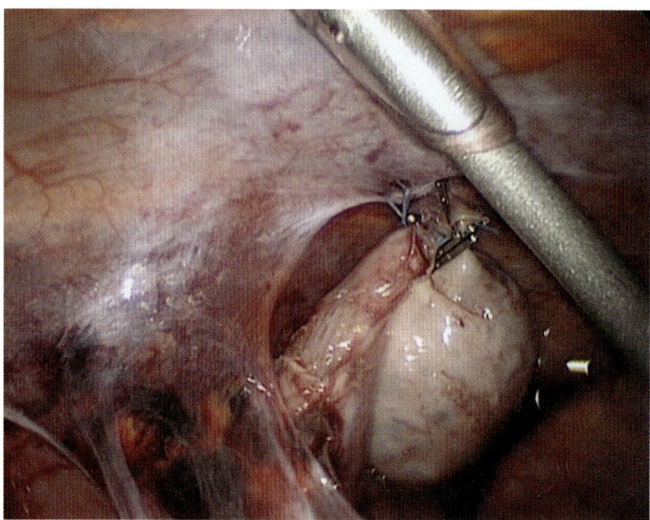

Figure 10.8 Ovarian transposition with placement of surgical clips after suturing that will help in radiographic identification in the future. Note that the vessels are under the peritoneal reflection.

out the ovaries during radiotherapy (Figure 10.8). The procedure is then completed after inspection of the pelvic cavity for hemostasis, irrigation, and removal of all debris and blood.

Both ovaries can be transposed above the level of the anterior-superior iliac spines without having to transect the fallopian tubes from their uterine origin. This allows for the possibility of spontaneous conception.

Some of the potential complications of laparoscopic ovarian transposition include possible damage to the ovarian blood vessels, ovarian or fallopian tube infarction, abdominal pain, and ovarian torsion. There is also a small risk of possible radiation-induced cancer or metastasis of gynecological malignancies in the transpositioned ovaries [14,19]. Due to high rate of ovarian failure, ovarian transposition is not usually recommended in women older than 40 years. We also recommend ovarian suppression after transposition to avoid cyst formation, as this procedure may promote some ovarian dysfunction and cyst development.

After ovarian transposition, there is typically no need to reposition the ovaries for pregnancy to occur. However, additional surgery may be indicated to return the ovaries to their normal anatomic position to facilitate access for transvaginal oocyte retrieval for in vitro fertilization, as the procedure may complicate future oocyte retrieval.

10.6 Ovarian Tissue Harvesting and Cryopreservation

Ovarian tissue cryopreservation (OTC) is an emerging fertility preservation option for prepubertal girls and pediatric female patients with cancer, as controlled ovarian hyperstimulation is challenging in this population. The ovaries may not yet be as responsive to the exogenous gonadotropins used for controlled ovarian stimulation as part of assisted reproductive technologies (ART). OTC is also an evolving alternative for reproductive-aged women with cancer or benign conditions such as autoimmune diseases (e.g., multiple sclerosis and severe rheumatic diseases) or aplastic anemia, who may also need to undergo high doses of gonadotoxic chemotherapy or bone marrow transplant [20]. This promising investigational option may also be used for adult female cancer patients with hormone-sensitive malignancies who are advised against controlled ovarian stimulation associated with in vitro fertilization, or in patients who cannot delay cancer treatment in order to undergo standard fertility preservation options including oocyte or embryo cryopreservation.

10.6.1 Ovarian Tissue Harvesting

Harvesting and cryopreservation of ovarian tissue prior to initiation of sterilizing chemotherapy has been developing over the past 20 years, initially in animal models and now with successful application to humans as well. Pregnancy and live birth rates following this procedure have continued to increase steadily, with an exponential rise. The number of reported live births as of June 2017 have exceeded 130 worldwide following transplantation of ovarian tissue [21–23].

OTC in the United States can currently only be offered under Institutional Review Board (IRB)-approved experimental protocols, and the technique is still considered experimental, but it may move toward broader clinical implementation with the use of appropriate selection criteria. At our institution, under an IRB-approved tissue registry, women desiring OTC undergo extensive counseling prior to the procedure. Recently a pediatric IRB has allowed children with cancer and other conditions whose treatments threaten future fertility to bank ovarian tissue as well. The experimental nature of this procedure is discussed with patients or families prior to signing a consent form. Harvesting of the ovarian tissue can be performed laparoscopically or via minilaparotomy and can involve a complete oophorectomy versus removing a portion of the ovary (a process known as ovarian decortication). In the prepubertal child, due to the small size of the ovaries, we recommend oophorectomy rather than decortication. The increased number of eggs in pre-pubertal children underscores the fact that smaller ovarian size in this population does not preclude ovarian tissue banking. In the following section, we outline our technique for laparoscopic ovarian tissue harvesting prior to OTC.

10.6.2 OTC: Surgical Technique

After induction of anesthesia, the patient is placed in standard dorsal lithotomy position. A Foley catheter is placed into the urinary bladder and a uterine manipulator is also placed. After creating an adequate infraumbilical skin incision, a 10 mm optical trocar is placed to introduce the laparoscope. Three additional 5 mm laparoscopic trocars are then introduced under direct visualization. After performing an intra-abdominal survey, attention is turned to the ovaries. One entire ovary is decorticated and the other is left intact to preserve the potential for ongoing ovarian function after chemotherapy and

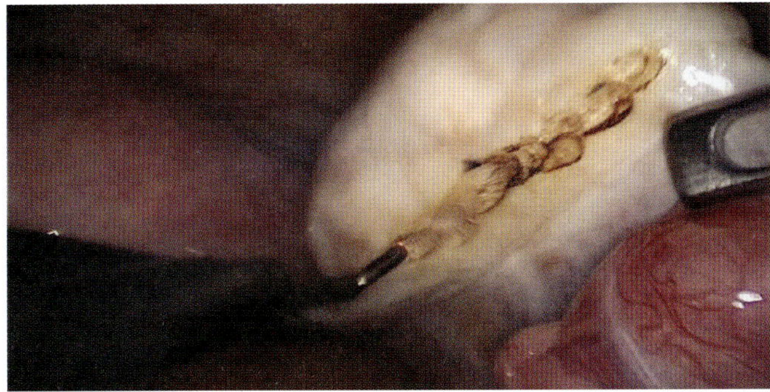

Figure 10.9 A longitudinal incision is made along the ovarian cortex.

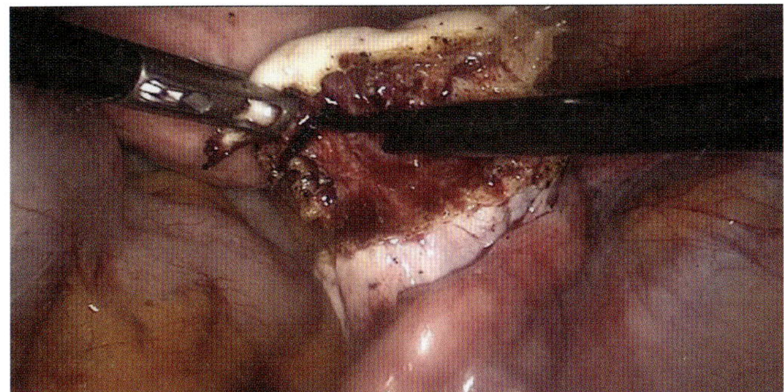

Figure 10.10 Dissection of the ovarian cortex away from the medulla.

spontaneous pregnancy. This ovary can also be transposed in cases of concomitant radiation to the pelvis.

Vasopressin is injected into the ovary for hemostasis. A longitudinal incision is made along the ovarian cortex using monopolar electrocautery on low voltage or using harmonic scalpel (Figure 10.9). The ovarian cortex is then carefully dissected away from the medulla on either side of the incision line (Figure 10.10). Preservation of the medulla allows a site for future reimplantation of cryopreserved tissue. Using a laparoscopic grasper, the ovarian cortex can then be removed through the umbilical port and prepared for cryopreservation. The ovarian bed is evaluated for hemostasis and irrigation is performed prior to concluding the case. The ovarian cortex is divided on a side table into strips measuring approximately 1 cm in length, 5 mm in width, and 1–2 mm in thickness, according to previously described methods [24] (Figure 10.11). These strips are then transported to our embryology laboratory in culture media on ice, and will be cryopreserved within an hour of procurement. Some surgeons simply perform an oophorectomy and decorticate the ovary on the back table. The ovarian tissue can then be frozen using either traditional slow-freezing method or using vitrification technique. To date, the majority of reported live births have resulted from tissue frozen using slow freezing [24], but many groups are electing to vitrify ovarian tissue based on promising data from egg and embryo freezing programs. In regards with the freezing protocols, there is no evidence showing that vitrification of ovarian tissue is superior to slow freezing, since vitrification has resulted in only two live births so far [25].

10.7 Ovarian Tissue Autotransplantation

Following ovarian tissue cryobanking, the restored ovarian tissue can be reimplanted, with hormonal activity habitually resuming within 3–4 months. The ovarian tissue appears to be functional for approximately 5 years [26]. Ovarian tissue reimplantation can therefore be considered once the patient is disease-free and cleared by her medical team to conceive. In 2004, Donnez et al. reported the first successful autotransplantation of cryopreserved ovarian tissue resulting in a live birth. There are now over 130 children worldwide born following this procedure; however, most of the live births are from a small number of prominent international centers [21,27]. The number of attempts at reimplantation that were unsuccessful is unknown, which is one of the limitations of OTC at present.

Once the decision for reimplantation has been made, the cortical tissue can be placed using any number of surgical techniques into either the pelvic cavity (this is known as orthotopic autotransplantation) or into a heterotopic site such the abdominal wall, forearm, or the breast (heterotopic autotransplantation) [28]. Some of the advantages of heterotopic reimplantation of ovarian tissue include easier transplantation procedure and that there is no restriction in the number of ovarian tissue fragments that can be transplanted. However, reestablishment of fertility using this procedure has not yet been unequivocally shown. Furthermore, the effects of the nonovarian environment on follicular development and quality are not well known [28]. Orthotopic ovarian transplantation is therefore the most commonly used autotransplantation technique. Using this technique, the medullary bed or contralateral ovary can provide an ideal environment through satisfactory oxygenation and presence of peritoneal fluid for ovarian follicular development.

It should be noted that some groups have proposed vascular reanastomosis of a whole frozen-thawed ovary; this could avoid theoretical follicular loss caused by graft ischemia. Unfortunately, freezing of whole ovaries is limited by several technical challenges and this method has not yet been widely adopted.

10.8 Orthotopic Ovarian Autotransplantation

Orthotopic ovarian autotransplantation of cryopreserved ovarian tissue has so far resulted in the birth of over 40 healthy infants worldwide [24]. Two techniques have been used for orthotopic ovarian autotransplantation, depending on the presence or absence of a medullary bed.

10.8.1 Presence of a Medullary Bed

This technique starts with laparoscopic decortication of the ovary at the time of the initial harvest and cryobanking of tissue. A large portion of ovarian cortex if not the entire cortex is removed to preserve access to the medulla and its vascular network. When reimplantation is attempted, the ovarian bed can be prepared by incising the fibrotic tissue. The frozen-thawed ovarian strips of large enough size are then placed on the decorticated ovarian medulla and fixed using 7-0 or 8-0 propylene sutures [29]. These cortical strips can also be simply

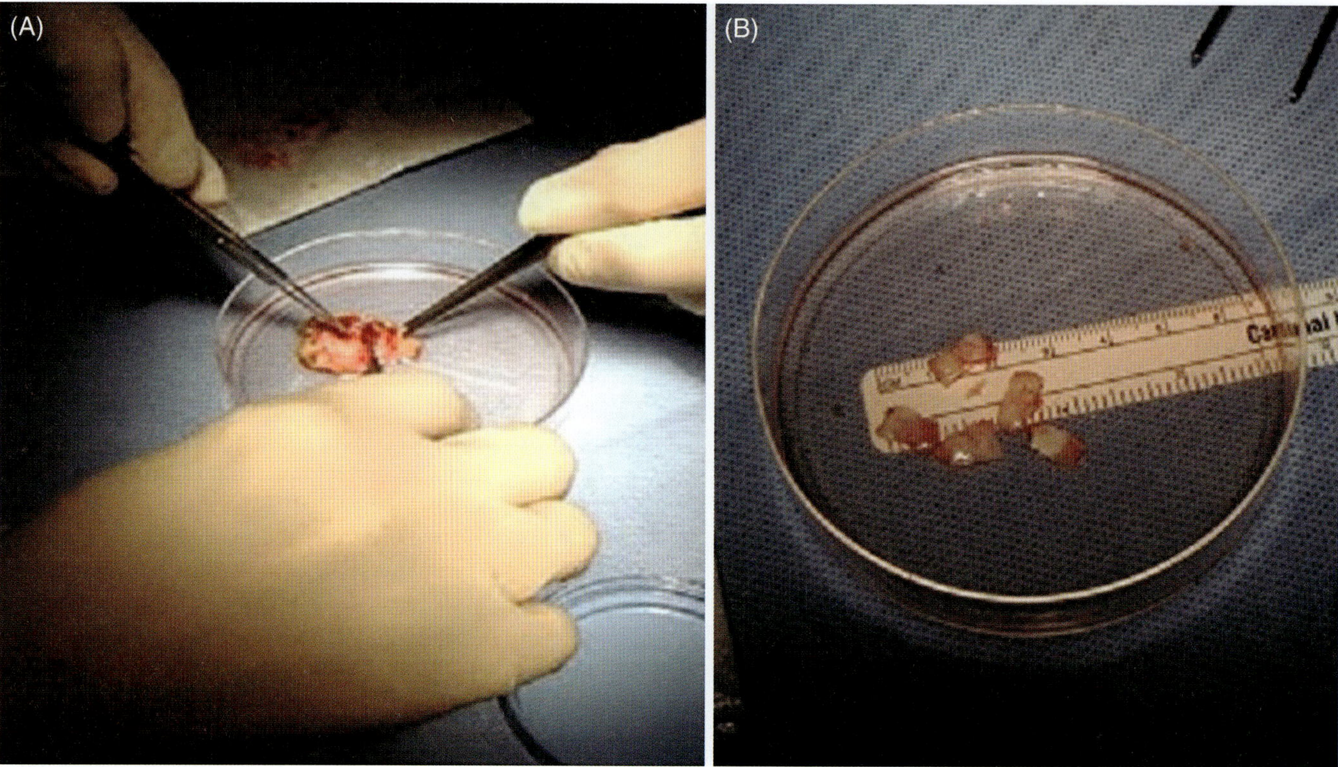

Figure 10.11 Division of the ovarian cortex on a side table into strips measuring approximately 1 cm in length, 5 mm in width, and 1–2 mm in thickness prior to cryopreservation.

placed on the ovarian medulla and fixed by covering the area with Interceed (Johnson & Johnson, Raritan, USA). This is especially effective if the cortical pieces are quite small.

Recently, in a report by Oktay et al., robot-assisted ovarian transplantation approach has been described. This procedure consists of three steps: (1) reconstruction of the ovarian tissue graft, (2) preparation of the contralateral menopausal ovary as the recipient site, and (3) transplantation of the reconstructed graft to the bivalved contralateral ovary [30]. Another technique is to make a small cortical incision on the ovary and push the pieces of thawed ovarian tissue under the cortical capsule. The same surgery can be performed by laparoscopy, robotic surgery, or laparotomy. In 2005, Meirow et al. described a case of live birth after in vitro fertilization following transplantation of thawed cryopreserved cortical ovarian tissue. Autotransplantation was performed via laparotomy in this case. Three sets of 5 mm transverse incisions were made on the ovary through the tunica albuginea. Tunnels were created underneath the ovarian cortex using blunt dissection. Each piece of thawed ovarian tissue was placed inside the tunnel. Using 4-0 Vicryl sutures, the incisions were then closed. After undergoing in vitro fertilization, patient became pregnant, which resulted in a live birth of a healthy appearing female infant [31]. The general observation is that all the techniques work.

10.8.2 Absence of the Ovaries

If bilateral oophorectomy has been performed, then a peritoneal window can be made to accommodate pieces of ovarian tissue. The peritoneal window can be created as either a two-step or a one-step procedure. As described previously by Donnez in 2004, during the two-step procedure a laparoscopy was done a week prior to reimplantation to create a peritoneal window. This window is created by making an incision on the anterior leaf of the broad ligament in the area where the retroperitoneal vessels are visible. The edges of this window are then coagulated. The aim of this procedure is to stimulate neoangiogenesis and neovascularization in the graft area prior to reimplantation. The second laparoscopic surgery was then done a week after creation of this window. The fragments of thawed ovarian tissue were then placed inside the peritoneal window where the neovascularization was clearly notable, without any stitching [32]. Another technique is to cover this window with Interceed in order to fix the ovarian cortical tissue. This procedure can also be used in the presence of a nonfunctional ovary. This technique for ovarian autotransplantation resulted in a pregnancy followed by the live birth of a healthy female infant.

In the one-step procedure, a peritoneal window is created using the same technique as described before via laparoscopy. The ovarian cortical tissue fragments will then be placed in this window during the same laparoscopic procedure [33].

In reviewing the available data on ovarian tissue transplantation techniques, it appears that both ovarian medulla and the peritoneal window technique have been proven to be equally effective sites for ovarian tissue reimplantation.

In a recent meta-analysis, of the 267 reported cases where the surgical technique for ovarian tissue transplantation was described in the literature, 195 were performed laparoscopically (three with robotic assistance) and 72 via laparotomy. Of the 228 transplantations where the grafting site was described, 195 were performed exclusively to an orthotopic site and three to a heterotopic site. Orthotopic and heterotopic sites were combined in 30 cases [22]. After reimplantation of ovarian tissue in the pelvic cavity ovarian activity is restored in more than 95% of cases [24,34]. The mean duration of ovarian function after ovarian reimplantation is 4–5 years, but depending on the density of the ovarian follicles at the time of OTC, this function can last for up to 7 years [27].

References

1. Siegel RL, Miller KD, Jemal A. Cancer statistics, 2015. *CA Cancer J Clin*. 2015;65:5–29.

2. Rodriguez-Wallberg KA, Oktay K. Fertility preservation medicine: options for young adults and children with cancer. *J Pediatr Hematol Oncol*. 2010;32:390–6.

3. Donnez J, Dolmans MM. Fertility preservation in women. *N Engl J Med*. 2017;377(17):1657–65.

4. Wallace WH, Thomson AB, Kelsey TW. The radiosensitivity of the human oocyte. *Hum Reprod*. 2003; 18:117–21.

5. Classe J, Mahe M, Moreau P, et al. Ovarian transposition by laparoscopy before radiotherapy in the treatment of Hodgkin's disease. *Cancer*. 1998;83:1420–4.

6. Clough KB, Goffinet F, Labib A, et al. Laparoscopic unilateral ovarian transposition prior to irradiation: prospective study of 20 cases. *Cancer*. 1996;77:2638–45.

7. Ray GR, Trueblood HW, En Right L, Kaplan HS, Nelson TS. Oophoropexy: a means of preserving ovarian function following pelvic mega voltage radiotherapy for Hodgkin's disease. *Radiology*. 1970;96:175–80.

8. Covens A, Putten H, Fyles A, et al. Laparoscopic ovarian transposition. *Eur J Gynaecol Oncol*. 1996;3:177–82.

9. Gabriel DA, Bernard SA, Lambert J, Croom RD III. Oophoropexy and the management of Hodgkin's diseases. *Arch Surg*. 1986;121:1083–5.

10. Hart R, Sawyer E, Magos A. Case report of ovarian transposition and review of literature. *Gynecol Endosc*. 1999;8:51–4.

11. Howard FM. Laparoscopic lateral ovarian transposition before radiation: treatment of Hodgkin's disease. *J Am Assoc Gynecol Laparosc*. 1997;5:601–4.

12. Williams R, Mendenhall N. Laparoscopic oophoropexy for preservation of ovarian function before pelvic node irradiation. *Obstet Gynecol*. 1992;80:541–3.

13. Kovacev M. Exterioration of ovaries under the skin of young women operated upon for cancer of the cervix. *Am J Obstet Gynecol*. 1968;101:756–9.

14. Husseinzadeh N, Nahhas WA, Velkley DE, Whitney CW, Mortel R. The preservation of ovarian function in young women undergoing pelvic radiation therapy. *Gynecol Oncol*. 1984;18:373–9.

15. Lee CL, Lai YM, Soong YK, Lin TK, Tang SG. Laparoscopic ovariopexy before irradiation for medulloblastoma. *Hum Reprod*. 1995;10:372–4.

16. Bisharah M, Tulandi T. Laparoscopic preservation of ovarian function: an underused procedure. *Am J Obstet Gynecol*. 2003;188:367–70.

17. Arian SE, Goodman L, Flyckt RL, Falcone T. Ovarian transposition: a surgical option for fertility preservation. *Fertil Steril*. 2017;107(4):e15.

18. Tulandi T, Al-Took S. Laparoscopic ovarian suspension before irradiation. *Fertil Steril*. 1998;70:381–3.

19. Anderson B, LaPolla J, Turner D, Chapman G, Buller R. Ovarian transposition in cervical cancer. *Gynecol Oncol*. 1993;49:206–14.

20. Jadoul P, Dolmans MM, Donnez J. Fertility preservation in girls during childhood: is it feasible, efficient and safe and to whom should it be proposed? *Hum Reprod Update*. 2010;16:617–30.

21. Donnez J, Dolmans MM. Ovarian cortex transplantation: 60 reported live births brings the success and worldwide expansion of the technique towards routine clinical practice. *J Assist Reprod Genet*. 2015;32:1167–70.

22. Pacheco F, Oktay K. Current success and efficiency of autologous ovarian transplantation: a meta-analysis. *Reprod Sci*. 2017;24(8):1111–20.

23. Van der Ven H, Liebenthron J, Beckmann M, et al. Ninety-five orthotopic transplantations in 74 women of ovarian tissue after cytotoxic treatment in a fertility preservation network: tissue activity, pregnancy and delivery rates. *Hum Reprod*. 2016;31:2031–41.

24. Harp R, Leibach J, Black J, Keldahl C, Karow A. Cryopreservation of murine ovarian tissue. *Cryobiology*. 1994;31:336–43.

25. Suzuki N. Ovarian tissue cryopreservation using vitrification and/or in vitro activated technology. *Hum Reprod*. 2015;30:2461–2.

26. Donnez J, Dolmans MM. Fertility preservation in women. *Nat Rev Endocrinol*. 2013;9:735–49.

27. Donnez J, Dolmans MM. Fertility preservation in women. *N Engl J Med*. 2017;377(17):1657–65.

28. Donnez J, Dolmans MM. Transplantation of ovarian tissue. *Best Pract Res Clin Obstet Gynaecol*. 2014;28:1188–97.

29. Donnez J, Silber S, Andersen CY, et al. Children born after autotransplantation of cryopreserved ovarian tissue. A review of 13 live births. *Ann Med*. 2011;43:437–50.

30. Oktay K, Taylan E, Sugishita Y, Goldberg GM. Robot-assisted laparoscopic transplantation of frozen-thawed ovarian tissue. *J Minim Invasive Gynecol*. 2017;24(6):897–8.

31. Meirow D, Levron J, Eldar-Geva T, et al. Pregnancy after transplantation of cryopreserved ovarian tissue in a patient with ovarian failure after chemotherapy. *N Engl J Med*. 2005;353:318–21.

32. Donnez J, Dolmans MM, Demylle D, et al. Livebirth after orthotopic transplantation of cryopreserved ovarian tissue. *Lancet*. 2004;364:1405–10.

33. Donnez J, Jadoul P, Pirard C, et al. Live birth after transplantation of frozen-thawed ovarian tissue after bilateral oophorectomy for benign disease. *Fertil Steril*. 2012;98:720–5.

34. Donnez J, Dolmans MM, Diaz C, Pellicer A. Ovarian cortex transplantation: time to move on from experimental studies to open clinical application. *Fertil Steril*. 2015;104:1097–8.

Chapter 11

The Role of Robotics in Reproductive Surgery

Antonio R. Gargiulo

11.1 Background

The goal of reproductive surgery is to cure pathology in a way that maximizes the patient's chance of achieving a healthy pregnancy. Tissue sparing is essential, and strict adherence to microsurgical technique is implicit. However, microsurgery has developed in the age of open abdominal surgery, whereas the modern patient-centered approach to health care compels us to translate most open surgeries to their minimally invasive counterparts. Few surgeons can combine uncommon surgical aptitude with high case volume and can meet this challenge through conventional laparoscopy. The great majority of surgeons in our subspecialty, however, are not able to master laparoscopic microsurgery. Indeed, we are all well aware that practical time-management factors come into play in the field of reproductive surgery. Reproductive surgeons are infertility experts who practice assisted reproductive technologies (ART). The practice of ART is complex, constantly evolving, and requires at least as much time and dedication as our surgical practice. For modern infertility specialists who cannot master laparoscopic microsurgery three alternative practice models exist: (1) to give up reproductive surgery; (2) to continue to offer mostly open surgical options; and (3) to enhance their laparoscopic armamentarium by adopting robot-assisted surgery.

The choice of making the robot one's main surgical tool has implicit value in our field because it engages infertility subspecialists in the comprehensive care of their patients. Outsourcing reproductive surgery to professionals who are not fully in charge of the patient's reproductive endeavor, and do not treat infertility, carries the risks of undertreatment or overtreatment.

Because infertility subspecialists are universally trained in laparoscopy, the additional skills needed for the safe use of surgical robots can be fully acquired (and maintained) on a simulator. This reduces to a minimum the portion of the learning curve that occurs on actual patients. Such a unique safety feature is particularly important for reproductive surgeons who, as a consequence of their minimalistic approach to surgery, tend to experience a relatively low surgical case volume.

In conclusion, as reproductive endocrinologists practising patient-centered medicine, reproductive surgery must remain central to the scope of our practice. If robotic assistance is needed to achieve this goal, then our subspecialty should embrace it. Indeed, recent amendments to the training requirements of the American Board of Obstetrics and Gynecology for reproductive endocrinology and infertility fellowships now include the teaching of robotic surgery [1].

11.2 Port Placement in Robotic Surgery

At the time of this publication, port placement can "make or break" a surgical case in laparoscopy, and even more so in robot-assisted laparoscopy. Two limitations of current robotic platforms can affect optimal instrument triangulation. First, surgical robots operate in only two of the four abdominal quadrants, at any given docking configuration. New generations of robots are easier to reposition, but remain 2/4 quadrant operators. This can represent a challenge when dealing with large pelvic masses extending outside of the lower abdominal quadrants. Second, current robotic arms are relatively bulky, feature a relatively small number of joints, and do not communicate with each other. These features make external collisions an issue. Indeed, such collisions are arguably the main technical limitation of the current generation of robotic platforms, particularly when all four robotic arms are utilized. As a result of this, there is a learning curve in port placement, which is difficult to simulate in a dry lab: the information contained in this propaedeutic paragraph should assist in shortening this specific component of the learning curve.

In current multiport robot-assisted laparoscopy we describe three types of ports: (a) robotic camera port, (b) robotic instrument ports, and (c) nonrobotic (assistant) port.

The robotic camera port can be any 12 mm disposable or nondisposable cannula (for the 12 mm or 8 mm robotic laparoscope), or an 8 mm dedicated steel cannula (for the 8 mm laparoscope). More recent robotic platforms lack a dedicated camera arm, allowing "port-hopping" of an 8 mm laparoscope. With the exception of those scenarios that mandate the choice of Palmer's point as the safest primary, the camera port is placed in the midline, and the umbilical location is preferred. Following the electromechanical morcellation controversy of 2015 [2], the umbilicus has also become a common access route for contained uterine tissue extraction via an open laparoscopy-like access (see the later discussion). When pelvic pathology extends to the upper abdomen, as it is often the case for large uterine fibroids, placing the laparoscope more cephalad on the midline is a wise idea. Because the laparoscope is a wide-angle lens, any length of cephalad shift of the lens will significantly "shrink" pelvic pathology. A recent magnetic resonance imaging (MRI)-based study concluded that placing a laparoscopic port in the midline at 6.5 cm or less above the umbilicus has no chance of interfering with the falciform ligament [3]. However, it may be reasonable to place the camera port as high as 10 cm above the umbilicus in longitype patients. Our review of the literature has yielded no reports of complications related to puncture of the falciform ligament.

Robotic instrument ports are generally limited to two, as this will suffice for most applications. However, three robotic instrument ports should be employed when all of the following circumstances apply: (a) the surgical team is experienced; (b) the pathology at hand is complex; and (c) the patient's abdomen is wide (or long) enough to accommodate two robotic instruments on one side without predisposing to external collisions. These criteria can be relaxed with recently introduced platforms that offer computer assistance to reduce the risk of external collisions.

The two basic robotic instrument ports are placed symmetrically to the right and to the left of the midline, either in the mid-abdomen or in the lower quadrants. We will describe specific scenarios and choice of port placement for each operation in the following paragraphs. In a mid-abdomen port configuration the points of entry are made roughly at the same height of the umbilicus, between 8 and 10 cm lateral from the camera port. In the lower-quadrant port configuration the points of entry are at the height of the anterior-superior iliac spines (ASIS), and about 2–3 cm medial to them. All generations of robots beyond the original 2005 model are perfectly capable of operating in a lower-quadrant configuration, either with center docking or with lateral docking of the patient-side cart. Instrument triangulation in the lower-quadrant port configuration is different from that achieved with a mid-abdomen configuration: the instrument shafts form an obtuse, rather than an acute, angle. Consequently, this lower-quadrant port setup must be practised on a pelvic trainer before it is employed on patients.

We recommend that the assistant port (the nonrobotic port) in reproductive surgery should be placed as close to the pelvis as possible. In a classic mid-abdomen port configuration we place the assistant port in one of the lower quadrants, just medial to the ASIS, on the side where the assistant will stand (i.e., opposite to the location of the patient-side robotic cart, if side-docking is chosen). In the lower-quadrant configuration, we place the assistant port in a suprapubic location.

The rationale for a caudal placement of the assistant port in reproductive surgery is based on several considerations. First, reproductive surgery is suture-intensive, and needles must travel in and out of the abdomen in full view: losing a needle between loops of bowel in the upper abdomen with the patient in Trendelenburg (which can happen if the assistant port is situated out of the most cephalad reach of the laparoscope) is not an excusable mistake. Second, the lower quadrant as well as the suprapubic port locations for the assistant port are part of the classic laparoscopic training of gynecologists, and avoid vascular and muscular structures that can be encountered instead if the assistant port is placed in a paramedian location of the upper abdomen. Third, when the mid-abdomen port

configuration is chosen, the lower-quadrant assistant cannula forms a classic "vertical zone" setup with the ipsilateral robotic port; this allows an ideal instrument triangulation that has been safely utilized in advanced gynecologic laparoscopy for decades [4]. As a result, if any portions of the surgery are to be performed via conventional laparoscopy, the team will have an ideal port configuration. Indeed, this is the basis of our "hybrid" approach to very large myomas, which includes both conventional laparoscopic and robot-assisted laparoscopic techniques. Finally, an incision performed suprapubically (or medial to the ASIS) when the abdomen is distended by pneumoperitoneum will fall below this landmark when the abdomen is desufflated; this avoids one extra visible scar in the upper abdomen. A genuine concern with cosmetic port placement is appropriate in reproductive surgery. If it is true that the overarching intent of reproductive surgeons is to facilitate our patient's reproductive endeavor, then we cannot deny the impact of body image on human reproduction. Recent studies have polled prospective surgical patients, asking them to rank drawings of scars in order of their cosmetic preference. Upper abdomen scars (except for scars within the umbilicus) were ranked consistently low by prospective gynecologic patients, even when compared to full laparotomy by Pfannestiel incision [5–7]. Because of the common utilization of upper abdominal entries, robot-assisted surgery has been criticized by some as a setback in the realm of cosmetically conscious laparoscopy. However, surgeons' experience and new applications have brought about the ability to perform most of our complex robot-assisted reproductive surgery operations in the absence of any visible scar above the line connecting the ASIS. Most myomectomies, adenomyomectomies, excisions of endometriosis, and tubal reanastomoses can be safely performed in this fashion. In other words, robot-assisted laparoscopy can outperform conventional laparoscopy in most reproductive surgery applications where cosmetic considerations are an issue.

Figure 11.1 describes, in a schematic fashion, all of the port placement options available to the reproductive surgeons. Note that not all placements include an assistant port. However, we recommend the use of an assistant port by default; only cases with pathology of limited complexity (such as small myomectomies) can be confidently approached without an independent assistant port. In those cases, the bedside assistant should be an expert laparoscopist, able to promptly withdraw a robotic instrument, use the empty 8 mm robotic port to grasp specimens, suction-irrigate or introduce adhesion barriers, and safely replace the appropriate instrument.

11.3 Robotic Myomectomy and Adenomyomectomy

Myomectomy represents one of the first clinical applications of robot-assisted laparoscopy, with the first case series reported as early as 2005 [8]. This is not surprising, given that conventional laparoscopic myomectomy (LM) has been adopted only by a minority of gynecologic surgeons, even after decades of its introduction [9]. The safety and efficacy of robotic myomectomy (RM) is well established: perioperative outcomes

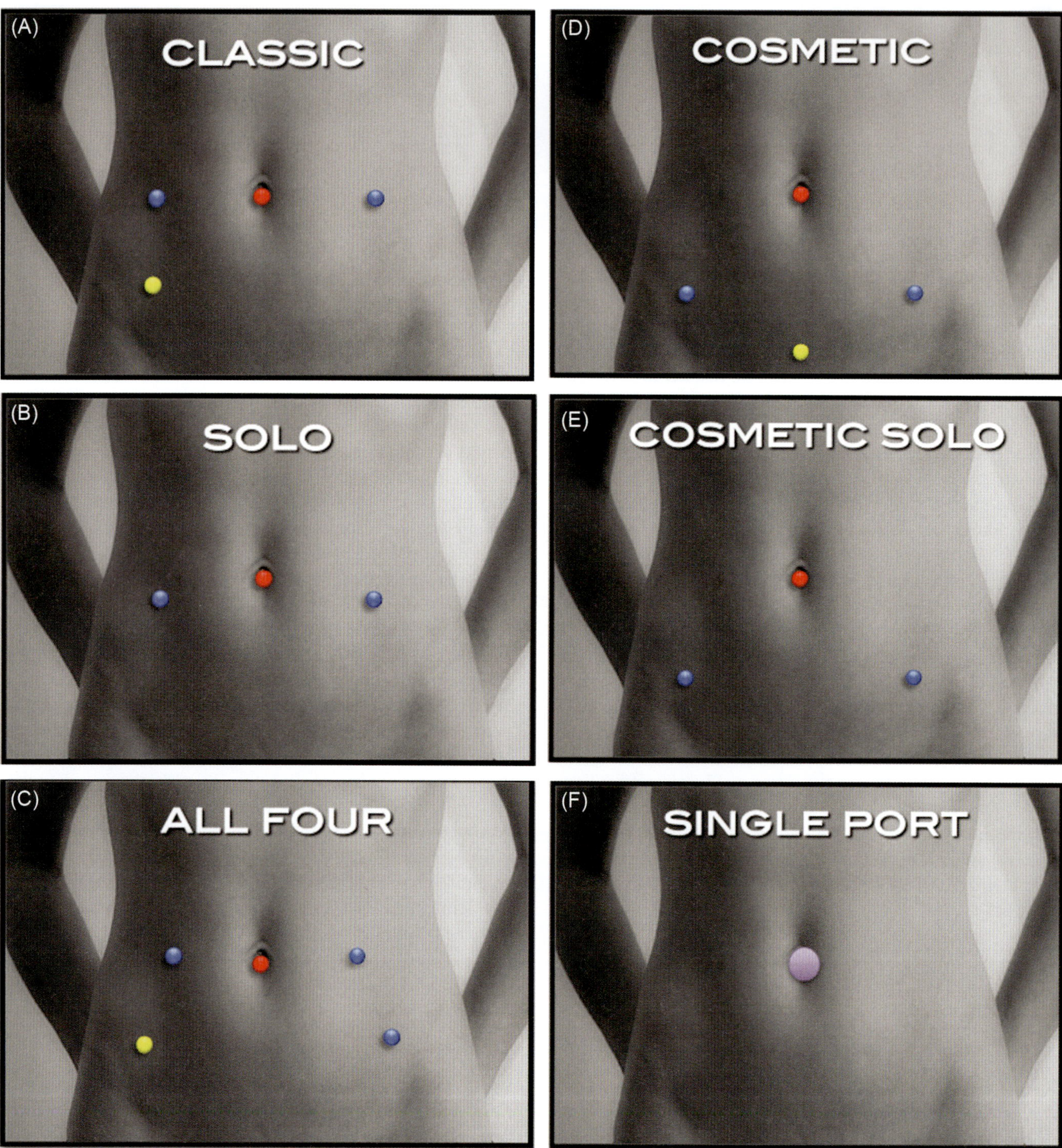

Figure 11.1 Port placement in robotic reproductive surgery: (A) standard multiport; (B) standard multiport solo; (C) multiport for large pathology; (D) cosmetic multiport; (E) cosmetic multiport solo, and (F) single site.

are superior to those of open myomectomy and mirror those of LM, and long-term reproductive and symptomatic outcomes are excellent [10–15].

Our team has recently reported preliminary data on our first 600 consecutive robot-assisted myomectomies, which include a rate of conversion to laparotomy of 0.1% [16]. This series includes our entire robotic learning curve. As it is the case for any new surgical technique, careful patient selection has been an essential component of our clinical success.

Successful robotic adenomyomectomy has been described by our team [17]. Recently, a small case series with good long-term clinical outcome has also been published [18]. The surgical indications for adenomyosis remain controversial at best; currently acceptable indications include patients who have not completed childbearing and have failed medical treatment for symptomatic disease [19]. However, a recent cohort study suggests that focal laparoscopic adenomyomectomy can be advantageous for women aged 39 or younger with a history of recurrent implantation failure in IVF [20]. If confirmed, such new evidence will bring adenomyomectomy front and center into the realm of reproductive surgery.

11.3.1 Preoperative Considerations

Myomectomy is a technically demanding and potentially dangerous operation. It has been traditionally associated with high rates of perioperative transfusions, postoperative adhesions, and even the rare risk of unplanned hysterectomy. Every effort must be taken to secure ideal conditions before embarking on this elective surgery. We will focus on preoperative considerations that are particularly germane to the robot-assisted approach. We will not cover general preoperative considerations such as preoperative iron treatment, management of blood products, and cell savers.

11.3.1.1 Simulation

Speed is the essence of this procedure; blood flows in the hourglass of myomectomy. Fortunately, top technical proficiency at the robotic console can be achieved outside of the operating room, through one of the many available digital simulation options. This is an ethical imperative for every aspiring robotic surgeon and surgical trainee [21]. Until a specific simulation protocol for myomectomy comes about, we recommend passing the validated protocol published by Culligan et al. [22] as a prerequisite for attempting robotic myomectomy. Moreover, the makers of the only currently available robotic console have developed specific simulator exercises combinations to hone one's console skills in preparation for specific gynecologic operations, including myomectomy.

11.3.1.2 Case Selection

Reproductive surgeons transitioning to robotics should adhere to the recently published AAGL credentialing criteria to identify basic robotic myomectomy (a maximum myoma number of 4 and a maximum myoma size of 6 cm) [23]. This case selection should be in place for the first 15 cases, at a minimum. Expert surgeons will rapidly increase their comfort zone in terms of myoma size and number once they move beyond the robotic learning curve. Current top single myoma size at our institution lies between 15 and 20 cm. Current top myoma number is at 15. Final assessment is made on a case-by-case basis, and depends on the location and cumulative uterine size, among other general preoperative considerations.

11.3.1.3 Magnetic Resonance Imaging

When the goal is extraction of deeply situated tumors of uncertain nature that lie adjacent to irreplaceable anatomical structures, high-quality preoperative imaging is essential. One could say that this is particularly relevant when we operate in the absence of haptic feedback. However, the superiority of imaging over direct tactile feedback in myomectomy has been proven even for the open technique [24]. Hence, myoma mapping through imaging has more clinical impact than any degree of tactile feedback in myomectomy. The ability of MRI to detect and locate smaller (but potentially clinically significant) fibroids is superior to ultrasound, and so is its accuracy in ruling out adenomyosis, a condition that changes indications, counseling, and execution of surgery (see Section 11.3.1.9) [25,26]. Additionally, MRI has a developing role in the screening for leiomyosarcoma. In addition to morphological features (namely peripheral margins and necrosis), diffusion-weighted imaging (DWI) is a useful tool in defining the benign or malignant nature of large uterine lesions, particularly when high signal intensity is seen on T2-weighted images [27].

In our robotic operating rooms, a large video display is dedicated to the display of key MRI images at all time during our operations. The TilePro™ function of current robotic platforms allows the direct visualization of the MRI images through the robotic operator console. We have not found this technology to provide a real advantage though, because both the laparoscope feed and the MRI images become too small to be of real assistance.

11.3.1.4 Timing

The timing of surgery in relation to phases of the menstrual cycle has only been addressed at the level of expert opinion. In the absence of strong evidence, avoidance of surgery in the perimenstrual phase can be considered, but it is not strictly recommended.

11.3.1.5 GnRH Agonists

Known benefits of pretreatment with GnRH agonists (GnRHa) in myomectomy include a decrease in intraoperative blood loss and a lower risk for perioperative blood transfusion (largely based on better preoperative hematocrit). Indeed, the only Food and Drug Administration (FDA)-approved use of depot leuprolide in the treatment of uterine fibroids is preoperative. Patients with fibroid-induced anemia and large fibroids are ideal candidates for the use of these drugs. In these cases we administer a quarterly Depot dose and plan the surgery for 3 months later. The expected shrinking of most fibroids is between 30% and 40% of the original volume. Fibroids that are poorly vascularized or frankly necrotic at MRI may not shrink, and should probably be addressed with minimal delay. The preoperative use of GnRHa is ill-advised in cases where small myomata are present. A potential risk in such scenarios is that of missing fibroids in surgery because they have become too small; this can result in a rapid postoperative recurrence once the patient is off GnRHa.

11.3.1.6 Misoprostol

Misoprostol induces uterine contractions and vascular constriction. Preoperative administration of misoprostol (vaginal or rectal) has been shown to decrease intraoperative bleeding in abdominal myomectomy. We currently administer a single 400 mcg rectal dose of misoprostol at the time of patient positioning in the operating room, following induction of anesthesia. A double dose (400 mcg 3 hours before and 1 hour before surgery) has been shown to be more effective, but it is less practical in the setting of a day surgery protocol, because it can cause diarrhea and cramping by the time of patient admission [28,29].

11.3.1.7 Tranexamic Acid

This antifibrinolytic agent is an excellent therapeutic option in patients with abnormal uterine bleeding. It is generally well tolerated and very safe (available over the counter in the European Union for the treatment of menorrhagia). Its role in the treatment of symptomatic fibroids is emerging. However, its role to decrease intraoperative blood loss in myomectomy is not established. The only randomized study employing intravenous tranexamic acid has not found a significant advantage in terms of blood loss during open myomectomy [30].

11.3.1.8 Informed Consent

There is no question that the recent controversy surrounding the use of electromechanical morcellation in laparoscopic myomectomy [2] has impacted the practice style of many surgeons in terms of the informed consent process. We recommend that a surgical consent for robot-assisted laparoscopic myomectomy should be delivered at a sixth-grade language level, and in the format of a detailed contract between the patient and the operator. It should always be stored in the electronic record and should contain (at a very minimum) the following sections:

(a) self-explanatory name for the planned surgery (no acronyms)
(b) indication(s) for surgery
(c) alternatives discussed and declined (always including hysterectomy)
(d) concise review of the preoperative testing performed, as well as the limitations of such preoperative testing in detecting all uterine cancer
(e) conservative risk assessment of the prevalence of uterine cancer among patients undergoing myomectomy [31]
(f) specific mention of the current limitations imposed by the FDA (or other regulatory agency or hospital administrative body) on the use of electromechanical morcellation
(g) specific mention of the planned use of robotic devices in the upcoming surgery, and the specific level of FDA approval for their use.

11.3.1.9 Special Considerations for Adenomyomectomy

The modern reproductive surgeon must never face unexpected adenomyosis. Rather, he or she should take active steps to diagnose it radiologically and plan accordingly. High-quality imaging is the starting point of therapeutic success in adenomyosis. In the early days of robotic surgery, I agreed to proctor a very experienced reproductive surgeon on his first robotic myomectomy. An oblong 8 cm anterior intramural myoma had been identified by an expert sonographer. An MRI was ordered, per our protocol, which identified diffuse adenomyosis infiltrating the entire anterior myometrium, but no fibroid. The robotic case was canceled, and an alternative management was planned for this patient. The MRI saved the day on that occasion, as it has done for my patients many times before and since. Recent technological developments in three-dimensional high-definition ultrasonography have made it an acceptable alternative to MRI, provided that one understands the limitations of an operator-dependent modality such as ultrasound, as opposed to the operator-independent nature of MRI. There is an added value to the surgeon reading the preoperative MRI, or performing the three-dimensional ultrasonography: surgeons enjoy a unique visual feedback of the actual pathology during surgery, and therefore are in a unique position to build exceptional diagnostic imaging skills over time. Without exception, an expert reproductive surgeon should never operate without having studied the images; radiology reports should not be overlooked, but they should never guide our decisions.

Once adenomyosis is correctly diagnosed, a complex patient counseling follows, the scope of which is vastly beyond that of this chapter. A concise take-home message from the robotic surgeon's standpoint is the following. There is no doubt that robotic platforms empower gynecologists to address adenomyosis laparoscopically as effectively as they would at laparotomy: this fact however does not broaden the surgical indications for adenomyomectomy, and restraint must be observed. With a few exceptions, surgery should be limited to focal adenomyosis, because adenomyomectomy implies loss of myometrium, whereas myomectomy, when performed with intracapsular technique (discussed later in section 11.3.2.1), does not result in any tissue loss [32]. High-complexity conservative surgical procedures for diffuse uterine adenomyosis have been described, and the long-term follow-up of these operations is reportedly good [33,34]. However, it should be stressed that these are open microsurgical procedures that have not been replicated laparoscopically or robotically and should not be performed outside of an experimental protocol for the foreseeable future.

11.3.2 Intraoperative Procedure

Reproductive endocrinologists agree that there is only one correct technique to perform a myomectomy in respect of microsurgical principles; this technique must not adapt itself to the current limitations of the operator. Robot-assisted myomectomy offers the realistic option to consistently fulfill all microsurgical criteria while operating in a laparoscopic environment.

11.3.2.1 General Technical Considerations

Hemostasis is, obviously, paramount. A Trendelenburg angle of 20–25° and an intraabdominal pressure of 15 mmHg will help decrease uterine arterial pressure, but judicious use of dilute vasopressin causes a very effective vasoconstriction. We infiltrate 5 IU of vasopressin in the myometrium (note that no untoward events have ever been reported with doses under 5 IU) and repeat the injection every 30–60 minutes, if needed. A recent randomized study has demonstrated with finality that the degree of dilution has no effect on the efficacy of vasopressin [35]. We dilute a standard 20 IU ampoule of vasopressin in 40 cc or 100 cc of normal saline; a 5 IU infiltration would therefore employ 10 cc or 25 cc of the above solutions, respectively.

The choice of energy is important for hemostasis, also to limit the risk for adhesion formation and uterine rupture. Our energy tools of choice are the ultrasonic scalpel and the CO_2 laser. We do not employ monopolar electrocautery in women of reproductive age but have done so occasionally in postreproductive myomectomy cases. The dramatic reduction in collateral thermal damage obtained by avoiding monopolar energy is well documented. When monopolar cautery is used, it should exclusively be used in the cutting mode, as the coagulation mode results in even more significant uterine tissue damage [36]. To date, all reported uterine ruptures following laparoscopic and robotic myomectomy have occurred following monopolar or bipolar electrocautery use [14]. We are unaware of any reports implicating the use of ultrasonic scalpel or CO_2 laser in a subsequent uterine rupture.

Regardless of the type of energy chosen for the hysterotomy, one should always remember that the surface of the hysterotomy must be completely free of char and should ideally be oozing from transected myometrial vessels. Hemostasis in myomectomy is achieved with suturing.

The type of uterine incision for myomectomy remains a matter of personal preference, as arguments have been proposed in support of both transverse and sagittal incisions (relative to the axis of the uterus). In robot-assisted myomectomy, the type of incision can influence the speed and accuracy of myometrial repair. In general, the triangulation achieved by the most common robotic port placements (see earlier discussion in Section 11.2) facilitates the repair of transverse uterine incisions in particular. Elliptical incisions should be reserved for FIGO 7 myomata, and some FIGO 6 myomata covered by a very thin layer of uterine serosa, because these incisions cause loss of native uterine tissue. Elliptical incisions are also more technically difficult to repair compared to any linear incision. When addressing FIGO 7 myomas, it is important that the elliptical incision be performed at the equator of the mass, lest the tissue should retract and result in a more challenging closure of the defect. Also with FIGO 7 myomas, vasopressin should be injected away from the tumor pedicle, to avoid intravascular injection (which is both ineffective and dangerous).

Effective myoma enucleation is based on three cardinal principles:

(a) planning the location of the incision(s) and the vector(s) of the enucleation based on preoperative imaging

(b) entering the pericapsular space

(c) applying steady traction to the myoma(s) with a tenaculum, while proceeding with gentle detachment of the pseudocapsule (and its all-important neurovascular bundle) using mechanical counter-traction and minimal thermal energy application [32].

Chromopertubation with methylene blue or indigo carmine (depending on availability) is performed in most of our myomectomies to identify any breach into the uterine cavity in a timely fashion. Early identification of a breached endometrial cavity is very helpful in limiting further damage and guiding repair (see discussion later in this section). Even though it can be reassuring to observe tubal fill and spill at the time of such chromopertubation, one should remain cognizant of the fact that the fallopian tubes may scar after myomectomy and that failures of the tubes to fill and spill during myomectomies can be for reasons independent of the actual anatomical compartment (tissue edema, low injection pressure from points of leak, etc.). Hence, chromotubation at the time of myomectomy is done to recognize endometrial entry.

Repair in layers is an essential feature of myomectomy. This is where the increased dexterity offered by robotic assistance has been shown to generally improve the operators' ability to proceed with an uncompromised technique. A recent study reports that a single-layer suturing represents the prevailing type of repair in conventional laparoscopic myomectomy, in contrast to a two- and three-layer suturing in robotic myomectomy [37]. The number of layers depends on the size and depth of the incision; we use between one and five layers. When the endometrial cavity is breached, we carefully approximate the edges of the endometrial tear, and proceed with a running closure of the layer of myometrium immediately above it, so that no suture comes close to the endometrium itself. Reapproximation of an endometrial tear is the only situation in which we occasionally use a nonbarbed suture in myomectomy. Other than that, a delayed absorbable 2.0 barbed suture is considered the optimal choice in the modern approach to minimally invasive myomectomy [38]. A barbed suture can be used all the way to the serosal layer (be it a subserosal closure or a classic imbricating "baseball stitch"). Because of case reports of postoperative bowel obstruction associated with the use of barbed sutures, it is important to avoid leaving exposed barbs on the serosal surface; a simple running suture on the outermost layer of the uterine repair is never acceptable.

The choice of adhesion-prevention barriers is a personal one, and a review of the vast literature on this aspect of reproductive surgery is not immediately relevant to this chapter. We universally apply oxidized regenerated cellulose to cover all of the uterine incisions and all deperitonealized areas. Some surgeons suture the mesh in place. Although this can easily be accomplished robotically with a 4.0 or 6.0 Vicryl suture, we have noticed that suturing the mesh in pace can result in its staining with blood from the suture points. Because this is known to increase the chance of postoperative adhesions in studies employing this type of barrier, we do not suture this barrier in place. We take particular care in suctioning all blood and irrigation fluid from the abdominal cavity before the end of the case, in order to avoid a postoperative flooding of the pelvis which is likely to wash away the barrier.

11.3.2.2 Techniques for Small Myomas (<7 cm Diameter)

Please refer to Section 11.2 on port placement for a general explanation of the positioning described here. Myomas of this size are universally addressed with fully cosmetic approach, which means that they can either be completed through single-site surgery or through a cosmetic multiport approach.

Our single-site approach has been recently published in full detail [39,40]. The main steps can be summarized as follows. Please refer to Figure 11.2 for illustrations of the following operative steps:

1. The patient is anesthetized in supine position on a disposable memory foam pad and then positioned in dorsal lithotomy on Allen stirrups with both arms tucked along her sides in clear plastic toboggans. Foam padding is placed to protect the arms, thighs, and face. Standard surgical preparation is performed following the exam under anesthesia and the placement of rectal misoprostol (see Section 11.4.1.6).

2. A uterine manipulator with chromopertubation capacity and without cervical delineator is placed. A standard Foley catheter is placed. An 8.5 mm primary cannula of the da Vinci Surgical System is placed in the umbilicus. The 8 mm robotic laparoscope is inserted to confirm an atraumatic entry before Trendelenburg position (20–25° angle) is obtained. A full inspection of the pelvis, facilitated by the use of the uterine manipulator, is made to confirm that the patient is a candidate for single-site surgery. If not a candidate, then a cosmetic multiport technique is chosen (see later in this section).

3. While keeping the primary steel cannula in the umbilicus, the primary skin incision is extended cephalad and caudad to a final length of 2.5 cm. The cannula is a backstop to the knife so that the widening of the umbilical incision is safe and fast. The skin incision is then carried down to the fascia with a knife and with curved Mayo scissors (similar to the classic technique for open laparoscopy). The index finger is used to perform a 360° palpation around the inner margin of the incision to rule out the presence of bowel or omental adhesions. Sutures are introduced in the abdominal cavity within a closed endoscopic specimen bag connected to a lifeline. Between three and five sutures (20 cm long, 2.0 barbed) are placed in the bag. Alternatively, a Gelpoint Mini (single-incision-laparoscopy port) is placed at this point; this is particularly useful when the abdominal wall is unusually thick (obese patients), or if there are upper abdominal adhesions that need to be removed with single-incision conventional laparoscopy technique.

4. The da Vinci Surgical System's multilumen silicone port is set within the umbilical incision (or within the mini Alexis retractor of the GelPoint Mini, if used as described in the previous paragraph, for obese patients) and the abdominal cavity is insufflated again. A camera cannula is placed through the dedicated lumen of the silicon port, the robotic patient-side cart is docked in a central position, and the camera arm secured to cannula. The robotic laparoscope is inserted. Two 250 mm instrument curved cannulas inserted under continuous laparoscopic guidance and connected to robotic arms #1 and #2. We have found the 5 mm and 10 mm assistant ports provided in this instrument kit to be of limited use in this particular operation. The 5 mm port is too small and the 10 mm port does not allow for a smooth use of arm #2. Hence, an 8 mm bariatric (long) robotic instrument cannula is placed through the dedicated assistant cannula lumen of the silicon port.

5. Two semirigid 5 mm wristed robotic needle drivers are loaded through the curved cannulas. A flexible laser fiber is inserted through the 8 mm assistant port. The tip of the fiber (in its armored guide) is grasped and operated with either of the wristed needle drivers.

6. Dilute vasopressin is injected with a spinal needle inserted suprapubically. CO_2 laser is set at 20 W. A nonwristed monopolar cautery hook can be used for this technique, with all the limitations implicit in monopolar energy and nonwristed instrumentation. Incision of the myometrium is made to reach the intracapsular space. The free avascular surface of the myoma is then grasped by the surgical assistant with 5 mm laparoscopic tenaculum to provide traction. The main operator pushes the muscle fibers away from the exposed area of the tumor using the wristed needle drivers and the tip of the laser guide. A known limitation of current single-site technology is that the operator is restricted to a range of distance above which the cannulae restrict movement, and below which the semirigid instruments are too flimsy to operate. Several tricks can be adopted to circumvent this limitation: (1) cannulae can be pushed in or retracted for up to a couple of centimeters, without affecting instrument function; (2) the patient's Trendelenburg angle can be changed with the robot docked (steeper Trendelenburg brings the target closer to port and less Trendelenburg brings the target farther from port). This is the only case in robotics where it is safe to change the Trendelenburg angle without undocking and redocking (unless one uses the synchronized robotic bed available for the da Vinci Xi system).

7. The enucleated myomas are placed in posterior cul de sac for later retrieval. In case of multiple myomas, a formal "myoma count" is kept by the surgical technologist at bedside. Using one of the 20 mm barbed sutures introduced originally, all enucleated fibroids are placed onto a single "safety line." Suturing of each incision is performed after each myoma enucleation to limit blood loss. Suturing follows standard microsurgical technique (see Section 11.3.2.1).

8. There are two modalities of specimen extraction for this technique, depending on the specimen size. For smaller specimens, all enucleated fibroids and all needles are placed in the original endoscopic specimen bag. Oxidized regenerated cellulose is placed to cover uterine incisions. The multilumen port is removed from the umbilical incision and the specimen bag is pulled to the incision by its lifeline. Needles and fibroids are carefully removed and counted. A number 10 blade is used to cut larger myomata and to allow their passage in strips through the 2.5 cm umbilical incision. Towel clips or Kocher clamps are used for traction on the specimen to be extracted. The endoscopic bag is extracted and confirmed to be intact. For larger specimens, needles used in the case are placed back into the endoscopic pouch and retrieved separately with the pouch upon removing the multilumen port. A Mini Alexis self-retaining wound retractor (part of the

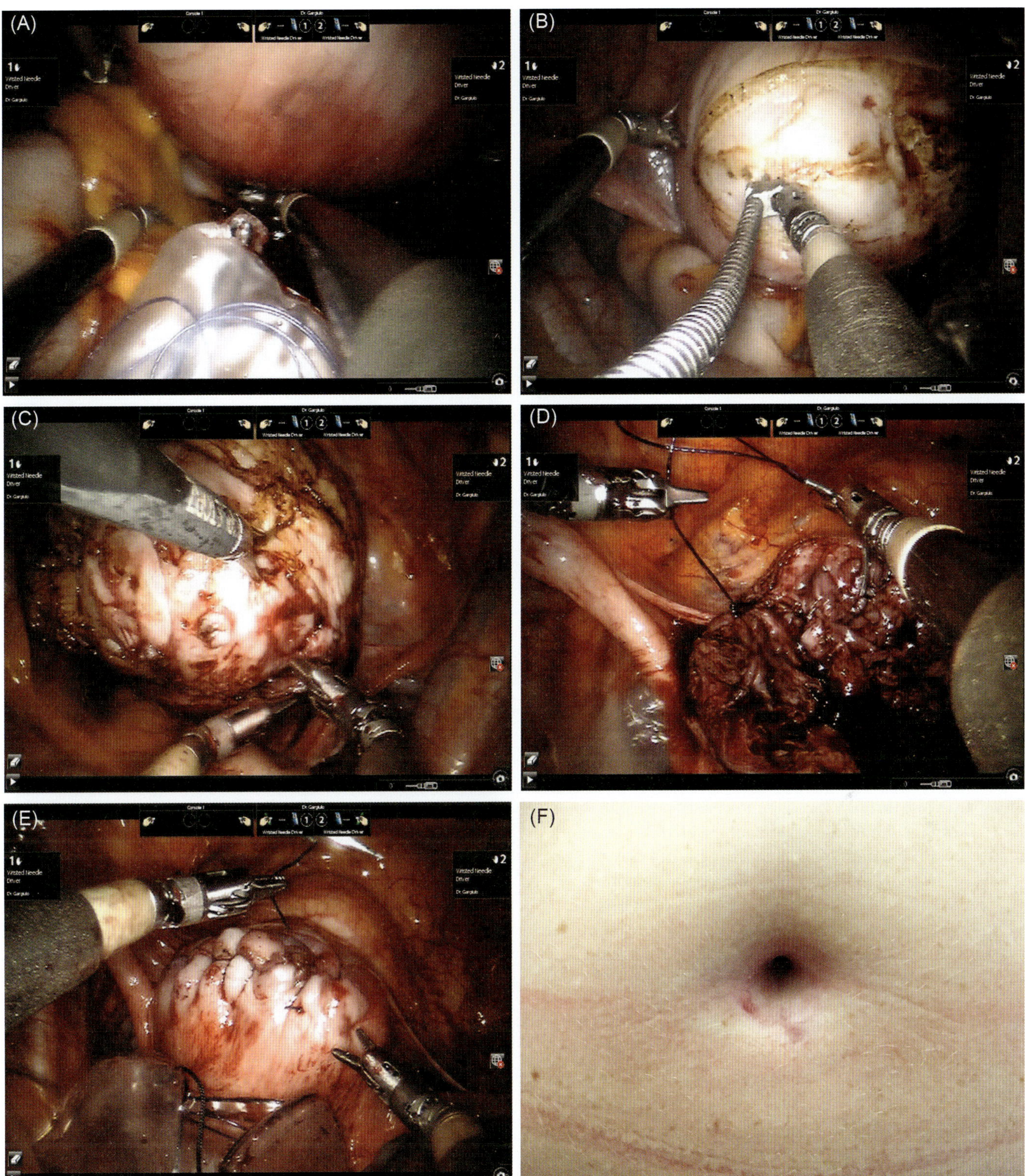

Figure 11.2 Single-site robotic myomectomy. (A) Specimen extraction has to be planned in advance; for small pathology we drop a specimen bag (containing needles) on a lifeline at the beginning of the case. (B) Two wristed needle drivers are the only robotic instruments needed in our technique; a flexible CO_2 laser fiber is used as the only energy device. (C) A skilled bedside assistant will be able to manage the very limited instrument movements allowed by the setup; it is the assistant's tenaculum that actually makes the enucleation possible. (D) We recommend 20 cm long barbed sutures for this technique, given the small range of movement allowed by the single-site port and cannulas. (E) A complete, uncompromised uterine reconstruction is always possible with the single-site setup. (F) Cosmetic outcome at 4 weeks makes every technical effort worthwhile; in well-selected patients, this procedure results in a completely hidden scar.

Gelpoint Mini single-incision-laparoscopy port) is set in the umbilical incision, if not already set at the beginning of the case. A separate, larger endoscopic specimen bag is placed in the abdominal cavity through the umbilical incision. Myomas are loaded into the endoscopic bag with conventional single-incision laparoscopy technique. The bag is retrieved through the Alexis retractor. The same sharp tissue extraction technique as described earlier in Section 11.3.2.2 is employed.

9. The single incision is closed with mass closure (peritoneum and fascia together in a running fashion) using 0 Vicryl on UR-6 needles. The dead space in the dermis is closed with running 3-0 Monocryl and the closure is completed with interrupted subcuticular skin sutures of 4-0 Monocryl.

Our cosmetic multiport procedure has been recently described [41]. The main steps can be summarized as follows (all steps already mentioned for other robotic myomectomy techniques will be omitted). Please refer to Figure 11.3 for illustrations of the following operative steps.:

1. See port placement in Figure 11.1. A primary disposable 12 mm camera port is placed in the umbilicus. Two 8 mm robotic cannulas are placed 3 cm medial and 3 cm cephalad to the left and right ASIS. A 5 mm port is placed in the suprapubic area (this can be omitted in easier cases). Camera arm and robotic arms #1 and #2 are used in this setup; occasionally using arm #3 instead of #2 will allow a more functional angle. The patient-side cart docked at a 45° angle from either right or left side.

2. An 8 mm robotic needle driver is loaded on arm #1 and an 8 mm robotic tenaculum on arm #2. A flexible laser fiber within its metal guide is inserted alongside the 8 mm laparoscope through the 12 mm primary port. The tip of the armored guide is grasped and operated by the robotic needle driver. Alternative energy instrument choices are also allowed by this configuration: robotic monopolar curved shears or robotic ultrasonic scalpel can be used, though each present unique disadvantages (the monopolar shears have more thermal spread, while the current ultrasonic scalpel does not allow wrist movements).

3. Barbed sutures (2-0 Stratafix, 20 cm length) are introduced through the 12 mm primary port by temporarily removing the laparoscope and pushing the suture in with a laparoscopic needle driver. Alternatively, they can be inserted and retrieved with conventional technique through the suprapubic incision.

4. There are two modalities of specimen extraction, depending on the specimen size.

   For smaller specimens: A standard 10 cm laparoscopic specimen bag is introduced through the 12 mm primary port. In some cases the best choice is a 15 cm endoscopic bag, in which case the primary port is removed and the 15 cm bag introducer is placed directly through the umbilical incision. Myomas are introduced into the deployed endoscopic bag. While keeping the 12 mm trocar (or the 15 cm bag introducer) in place through the

umbilicus, umbilical skin incision is extended cephalad and caudad to a final length of 2.5 cm. This skin incision was then carried down to the fascia with a knife and with curved Mayo scissors, in a fashion similar to the classic Hasson technique for open laparoscopy. The specimen bag is pulled to the incision. The same tissue extraction technique described for single-site myomectomy is employed.

For larger specimens: While keeping the primary trocar in place through the umbilicus, the umbilical skin incision is extended cephalad and caudad to a final length of 2.5 cm. A Mini Alexis self-retaining wound retractor (part of the Gelpoint Mini single incision laparoscopy port) is set in the umbilical incision. An endoscopic specimen bag is placed in the abdominal cavity through the umbilical incision. Myomas are loaded into endoscopic bag with conventional laparoscopic technique. The bag is retrieved through the Alexis retractor. The same tissue extraction technique as above is employed.

11.3.2.3 Techniques for Larger Myomas (7–10 cm Diameter)

Myomas in this size range can be easily addressed with a completely robotic approach, though port location is different than for the smaller ones. The main steps can be summarized as follows (all applicable steps already mentioned above will be omitted). Please refer to Figure 11.4 for illustrations of the following operative steps.

1. See port placement in Figure 11.1. A disposable 12 mm primary camera port is placed in the umbilicus. Two 8 mm robotic cannulas are placed 8–10 cm to the right and to the left of the camera port, or slightly caudal to it. A 5 or 12 mm assistant port is placed in the right lower quadrant. The camera arm and robotic arms #1 and #2 are used in this setup. Arm #3 is usually not necessary. Patient-side cart is docked at a 45° angle from either the right or left side.

2. An 8 mm robotic needle driver is set on arm #1 and an 8 mm robotic tenaculum on arm #2. A flexible laser fiber within its steel-armored guide is inserted alongside an 8 mm laparoscope through the 12 mm primary port. Alternatively, the laser fiber can be introduced through the 12 mm lower-quadrant assistant port. The tip of the laser guide is grasped and operated by the robotic needle driver. Alternative energy instrument choices are allowed by this configuration; robotic monopolar curved shears or robotic ultrasonic scalpel can be used, though each present unique disadvantages (monopolar has more thermal spread, while the ultrasonic scalpel allows no wrist movement).

3. Barbed sutures (2-0 Stratafix, 20 cm length) are introduced and removed through the lower-quadrant assistant port with a laparoscopic needle driver. Alternatively, the sutures are inserted through the primary 12 mm port, while temporarily removing the camera.

4. The best current modality of specimen extraction for large uterine masses is the Alexis Contained Extraction System (Applied Medical, Rancho Santa Margarita, CA, USA).

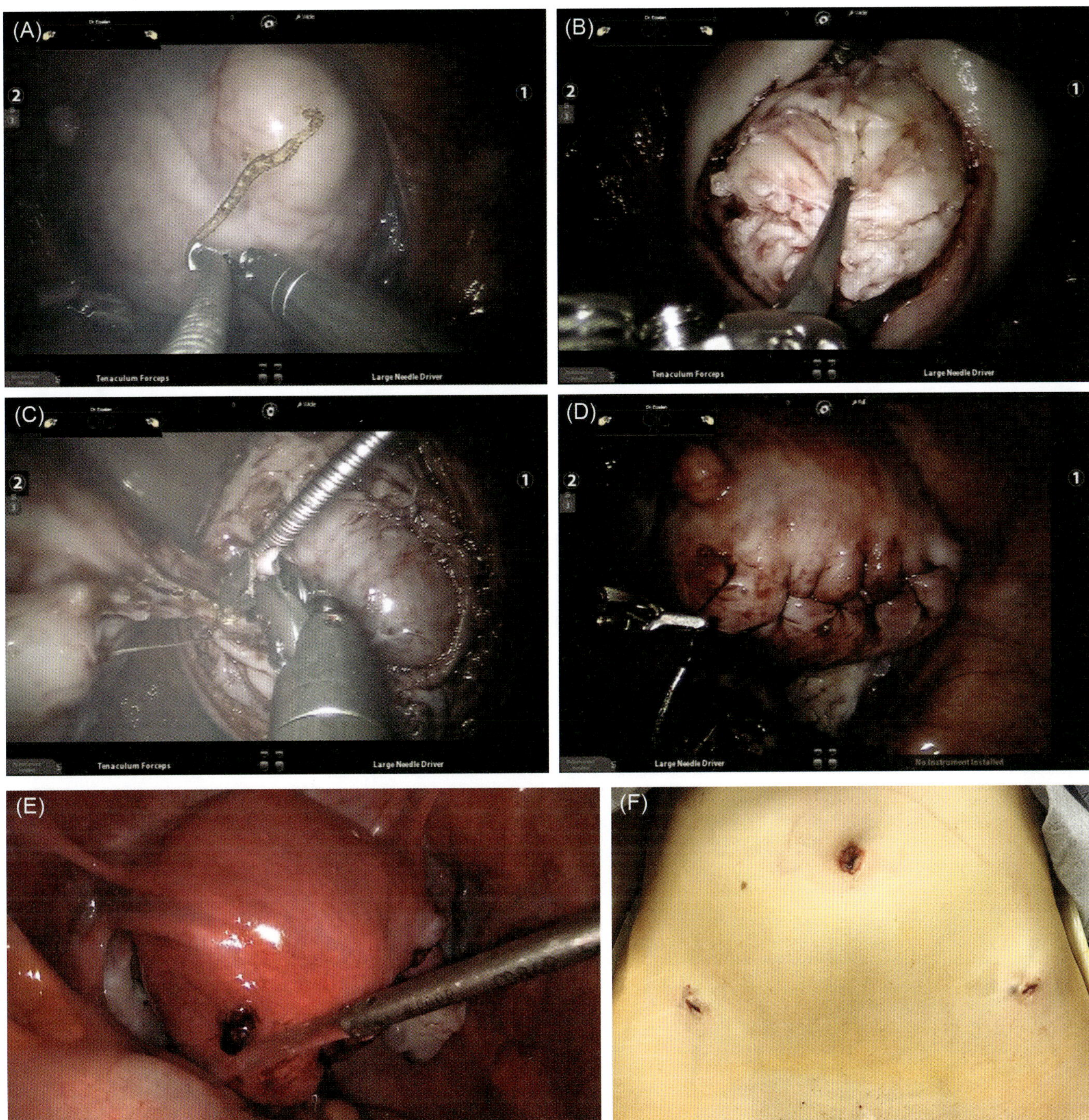

Figure 11.3 Multiport robotic myomectomy, cosmetic approach, solo (no assistant port). (A) Only two ports are placed, medial to the ASIS on each side. Note the obtuse angle of triangulation of the instruments. An oblique incision is made over the two myomata. (B) Intracapsular location is reached and the plane developed. (C) The myoma is enucleated. The endometrium is peeled off the large FIGO 2–5 myoma and not entered. (D) Repair in layers is achieved. Needles are loaded through the 12 mm primary port. The last layer is always imbricating so that no suture is exposed. (E) Irrigation and other assistant functions can be performed through one of the robotic ports. (F) The three incisions as they appear at the end of surgery (note: umbilical tissue extraction performed in containment system).

At the time of this publication, this is the only specimen extraction system specifically approved by the FDA for extracorporeal uterine tissue extraction. While keeping the primary 12 mm trocar in place through the umbilicus to act as a guide and to protect the underlying tissues, the original umbilical skin incision is extended cephalad and caudal to a final length of 2.5 cm. This incision is then carried down to the fascia with curved Mayo scissors, in a fashion similar to the classic Hasson technique for open laparoscopy.

The Alexis Specimen Containment Bag (a dedicated large specimen bag for extracorporeal tissue extraction) is introduced in the abdomen through this umbilical incision. A dedicated Hasson Cannula (Applied Medical,

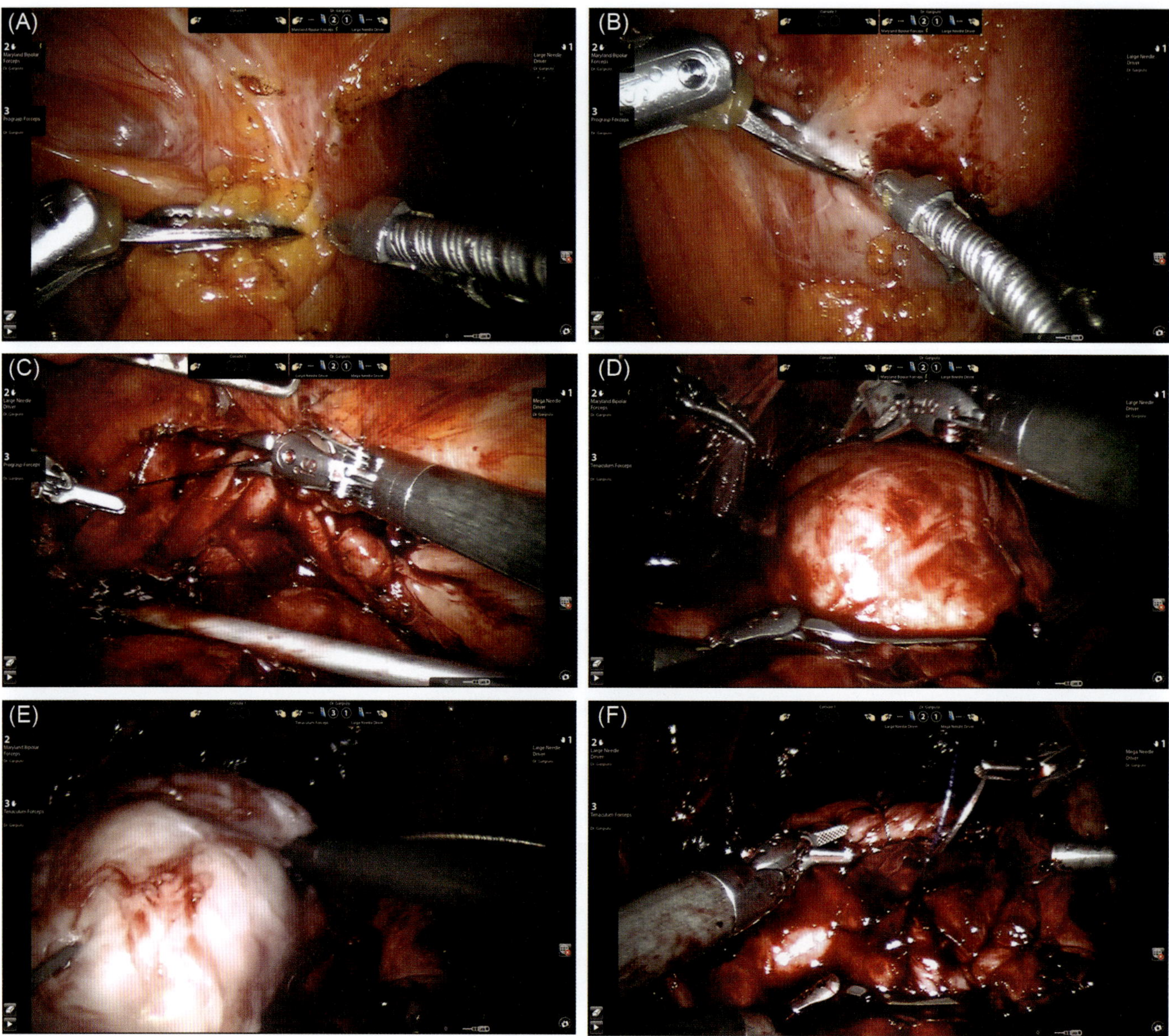

Figure 11.4 Multiport robotic myomectomy, standard approach. (A) Recurrent anterior lower segment myoma following a prior open myomectomy; the entire anterior uterine wall is densely adherent to the abdominal wall and bladder. Continuous low-wattage CO_2 laser energy, delivered through a flexible device driven by a robotic needle driver, is used to perform a complete adhesiolysis. (B) Maryland bipolar graspers act as a safe backstop for the laser beam, and maintain tissue tension, essential for safe and effective adhesiolysis. (C). Repair of the anterior bladder peritoneum at the end of the extensive adhesiolysis. (D) A large FIGO 2–5 myoma is eventually identified, distending the anterior lower segment. (E) Once the intracapsular space is entered, the myoma is immobilized with a robotic tenaculum (lower left) while a blunt instrument pushes away myometrial fibers surrounding the tumor. (F) Repair of the deep incision in layers in this deep pelvic location is made possible by the coordinated work of three instruments, with the robotic tenaculum continuously exposing the correct planes for the needle drivers to suture.

Rancho Santa Margarita, CA, USA) is secured in place to cover the umbilical incision, and the pneumoperitoneum is again created.

The enucleated myomas are placed in the bag and the upper rim of the bag is carefully exteriorized. At this point, a dedicated guard is placed inside the opening to the bag to allow for the safer use of sharp instruments in the removal of the myomas. The specimen is grasped with towel clips and lifted at the level of the umbilical incision. A number 10 blade is used to undermine the specimen to allow for passage through the 2.5 cm umbilical incision, with great care as to not damage the bag. It is essential to always aim for the myoma edge and proceed with either U-shaped or V-shaped cuts while applying traction with the towel clip; the goal is to attempt to roll the myoma while excising a long strip of its outer layer. Allowing some space for the tumors to roll within the bag is essential for the success of this technique. After the entire specimen is removed, the bag itself is extracted and confirmed to be intact. The dedicated Hasson cannula is again secured in place and the pneumoperitoneum is created. Copious irrigation with sterile Ringers lactate is performed and hemostasis is confirmed. Adhesion barrier is placed to cover the uterine incision(s). At this point the dedicated Hasson cannula is removed for the last time and the umbilical fascia is identified and closed with mass closure (see in Section 11.3.2.2). Please note: the extraction technique is the same for very large myomas (see later).

11.3.2.4 Techniques for Very Large Myomas (>10 cm in Diameter)

Current teleoperators are less-than-ideal instruments to tackle very large myomectomies. First, the robotic tenaculum is quite delicate, to the point of not allowing substantial traction on a heavy tumor. Second, the patient-side carts of current robotic platforms (both da Vinci Si and Xi) are designed to work as two-quadrant operators. A laparoscopic myomectomy where the uterine size reaches or surpasses the umbilicus (i.e., the abdominal midpoint) is a four-quadrant operation. Differently from the more common hysterectomy, where most of the surgical targets are fixed (the uterine vessels in the deep pelvis, the round ligaments at the inguinal rings and the ovarian vessels, usually at the pelvic brim), in myomectomy there is a "hourglass effect" of the enucleated myoma that rises over the bulky uterus, which once contained it.

This is not to say that the robot cannot be used to tackle very large myomata. Most expert robotic surgeons can manage to reliably complete these operations, even with the aforementioned limitations. Three fundamental intraoperative steps are essential for success in these scenarios.

1. The primary port must be supraumbilical; the fastest way to "shrink" a large myoma is to move the laparoscope in the upper abdomen. See our considerations in Section 11.2 and refer to Figure 11.1 for our port placement for very large myomata.
2. The only practical energy source in these cases is the robotic monopolar curved shears (always in cutting mode, never in coagulation mode, to limit delayed myometrial thermal injury). The robotic ultrasonic scalpel and the laser are absolutely impractical when dealing with these very large myomas.
3. The bedside surgical assistant must be very well trained with the concomitant use of the uterine manipulator and the laparoscopic tenaculum, in order to provide optimal exposure and to keep the cleavage plane low enough in the abdomen to allow the robotic arms to function properly. This is achieved mainly by lateralizing the uterus so that it lies at a right or left angle in the abdomen, which keeps the operative focus more caudal.
4. The third instrument arm provides a definite advantage during the reconstruction stage of the myomectomy. The robotic tenaculum is an ideal instrument in this part of the operation, allowing positioning of the delicate structures for repair.

As pointed out earlier in Section 11.3.2.3, our team prefers to avoid the use of monopolar energy in myomectomy. Because of this, and because of the limitations discussed at the beginning of this section, we perform our robotic myomectomies for very large myomas with a hybrid technique that entails a first step of conventional laparoscopic myoma enucleation with handheld ultrasonic scalpel, followed by rapid docking of the robotic patient-side cart to proceed with microsurgical reconstruction in multiple layers as described in Section 11.3.2.1. In our hands, this technique allows the best results, because both techniques (conventional laparoscopy and robot-assisted laparoscopy) are used for the steps where they confer an actual advantage. Conventional laparoscopy provides a sturdy tenaculum and an unobstructed four-quadrant technique; robot-assisted laparoscopy provides better visualization and unrestricted intuitive wrist movement for pristine reconstruction in layers [42].

Tissue extraction, also in these cases, occurs through an umbilical incision. Our current preference in terms of equipment goes to the Alexis Contained Extraction System, described earlier in Section 11.3.2.3 in full detail.

11.3.2.5 Special Considerations for Adenomyomectomy

Adenomyosis has no definite planes. Focal adenomyosis is sometimes found in association with myomas, so that what begins as a classic intracapsular myomectomy (see Section 11.3.2.2) soon turns into a struggle, with the surgeon looking for a tissue plane that truly does not exist.

As we have discussed in Section 11.3.1.9, the most important intraoperative advantage when dealing with adenomyosis is that it should not constitute a surgical surprise. When adenomyosis is expected, the surgeon can strategize in advance. Please refer to Figure 11.5 for illustrations of the following operative steps. The basic clinical pearls for focal robotic adenomyomectomy are the following:

1. Focal adenomyosis bleeds just as much as the surrounding myometrium (cystic adenomyosis is often an exception): get a suction-irrigator ready and instruct the assistant to use it aggressively. As a corollary, prefer an insufflation system that keeps the intraabdominal pressure constant in spite of the aspiration. Also, don't skimp on vasopressin use. Also, this is a special situation in which we would not agree to operate during menses.
2. Adenomyosis is friable and no plane exists: the robotic tenaculum and the robotic ultrasonic scalpel are not recommended. The first will mince the tissue while providing grip, and the second has no wristing ability and cannot carve out the abnormal tissue. Robotic Prograsp is ideal to firmly grasp the friable tissue. Flexible laser fibers and the robotic monopolar curved shears are both excellent energy choices.
3. Because no plane exists, it makes no sense to try to enucleate the adenomyoma "intact." Slicing up the adenomyotic tissue and removing it from the field improves visualization and provides better clues as to when to stop the excision (i.e., when normal myometrium reappears).
4. Because adenomyosis is often found in continuity of the endometrial cavity, breaching the cavity is common.

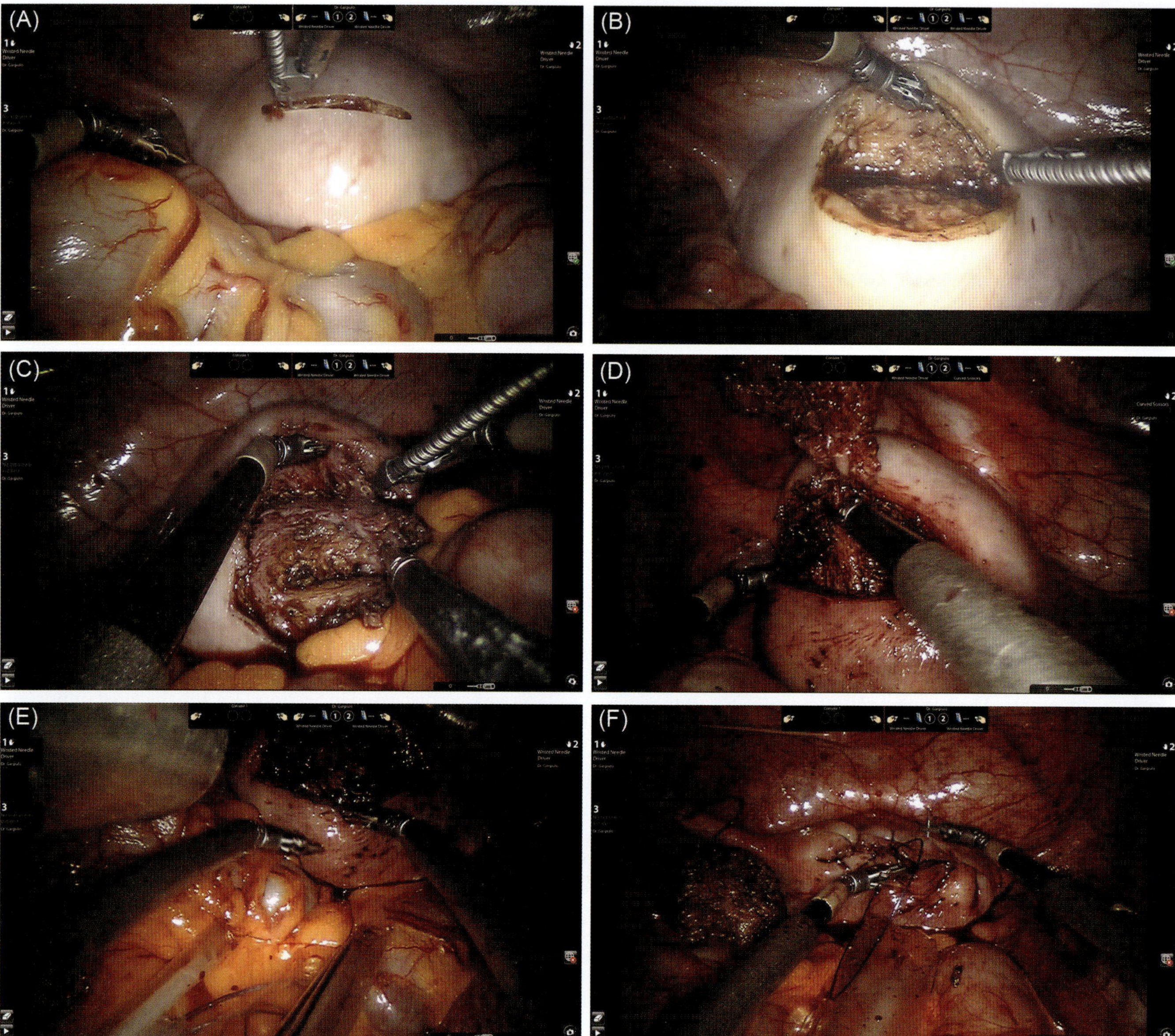

Figure 11.5 Single-site robotic adenomyomectomy. (A) A small focal adenomyoma is located thanks to preoperative MRI and the hysterotomy if performed on the anterior uterine wall. Delineation of the lesion based on visual clues is difficult. (B) Incision with continuous high-wattage CO_2 laser confirms absence of a pericapsular space. No spontaneous plane of cleavage is found. (C) The line of demarcation between healthy myometrium and adenomyoma is traced with the laser beam and the tumor is carved out of its location. (D) A plane is developed sharply between the adenomyoma and the surrounding myometrium; excision is completed by the semirigid instruments while the bedside assistant keeps steady traction on the tumor. (E) The cavity is usually entered in adenomyomectomy, given the intimate relationship between the adenomyosis and the basal endometrium. In this case the defect is estimated to be <5 mm in diameter. (F) Repair completed in layers by placing several sutures in the defect before tying them.

Chromopertubation is essential in adenomyomectomy. One must be careful not to damage the cavity irreparably in this operation (particularly if monopolar shears are used, which produce lateral thermal spread).

5. Excision of a focal or cystic adenomyoma will leave a defect in the myometrium that does not have a tendency to collapse on itself (as the pseudocapsular space of a myoma does instead). Repair of this defect in layers can be challenging. Robotic assistance allows placement of multiple deep sutures that can then be tied in parallel later, in order to avoid dead spaces in the suture planes.

11.3.3 Postoperative Considerations

11.3.3.1 Normal Postoperative Course

Patients can be discharged home on the day of surgery provided that they meet the standard requirements of all laparoscopic operations. As part of a preoperative strategy aiming at promoting day surgery, all patients receive 1,000 mg of acetaminophen and 400 mg of Celebrex on admission to the day surgery preop area, 30 cc of local infiltration on port sites before skin incision, and 30 mg of iv Toradol before emergence from anesthesia.

Patients usually employ mild narcotic analgesics for 1 to 7 days postoperatively; these are alternated with acetaminophen and ibuprofen, to achieve maximum analgesia with minimum use of narcotics.

Pyrexia (noninfectious fever during the first 72 hours postoperatively, typically associated with open myomectomy) is rare in robotic myomectomy likely due to the high quality of uterine closure that does not allow dead spaces and intramyometrial hematoma formation (a cause of pyrogen absorption and pyrexia). Consequently, any report of high fever should be considered a sign of infection until proven otherwise.

While very early ambulation is promoted, pelvic rest and limited lifting (no more than 10 lb/5 kg) is recommended for 2–3 weeks. At 2–3 weeks patients return for their final surgical postoperative visit.

Our standard recommendation for barrier contraception after a robotic myomectomy or adenomyomectomy is 6 months. For small (<7 cm) single tumors we usually recommend 3 months of contraception.

11.3.3.2 Counseling on the Mode of Delivery

We recommend a cesarean delivery for all adenomyomectomy cases and for most intramural myomectomies. We recommend vaginal delivery for small FIGO 5 and for most FIGO 6 and 7 myomata. Although a recent multicenter study reported a 1% chance of uterine rupture following robotic myomectomy [14], one should note that in the only patient in that series who experienced a rupture the surgeons had used monopolar energy. Our personal experience after 700 robotic myomectomies with up to 9 years of patient follow-up has not identified a single uterine rupture. As expected of an IVF unit, our patient pregnancy mix includes many sets of twin and triplet pregnancies. We ascribe the safety of our technique to the choice of energy for hysterotomy, as discussed in Section 11.3.2.1.

Whether the cavity was entered or not is unlikely to affect the structural resilience of the uterine wall in subsequent pregnancies. A breach in the cavity can affect the risk of intrauterine synechiae however, and we recommend a second-look office hysteroscopy of sonohysterogram in those women who plan fertility treatment or spontaneous conception following myomectomy.

11.4 Robotic Resection of Endometriosis

The application of robotic technology to the treatment of pelvic endometriosis is a rapidly evolving field. At the time of this publication there is no demonstrated advantage of robotic assistance in the treatment of superficial peritoneal endometriosis; the evidence of its safe use for this indication amounts to sparse case reports. In the absence of any significant mechanical advantage afforded by the robot in this technically simple procedure, some attention has been given to identifying potential technical advantages at the intraoperative diagnostic level. For example, FireFly fluorescence imaging is an enhanced video feature of some robotic systems, which allows surgeons to better appreciate areas of hypervascularity by means of a laser-excitable tracer dye (indocyanine green). FireFly has been available on robotic platforms since 2012 and has been shown to assist gynecologic oncologists in pelvic lymph-node dissections; however, it has not found any convincing applications in endometriosis surgery to date. Similarly, early reports of improved visual diagnostic abilities afforded by the high-definition stereoscopic view of the robotic platform have not yet amounted to publishable data. Once equipment cost and time considerations are made, it is hard to justify the use of robotic technology in the treatment of peritoneal endometriosis. The combination of a good-quality transvaginal ultrasound and an expert pelvic examination can identify those patients with suspected endometriosis who do not have ovarian or deep infiltrating endometriosis (DIE) and therefore are less likely to benefit from a robotic operation.

The robotic platform does confer technical advantages in the stripping of ovarian endometriomas. We will discuss the special case of ovarian endometriomas in the section on ovarian cystectomy.

Until recently, the involvement of robotic surgeons with DIE has been timid if compared to the high rates of adoption seen for other gynecologic applications of this technology. Nonetheless, safety data (noninferiority studies) for robotic DEI surgery are now available [43,44]. My prediction is that these type of studies are all that we are going to see in the literature until image fusion technology becomes available that can differentiate DIE from surrounding healthy tissue. Safety data is particularly relevant in the case of DIE. This is because the current generation of robotic platforms does not include tactile feedback. The ability to differentiate healthy retroperitoneal tissue from endometriotic tissue, not only visually but also by indirect palpation with laparoscopic instruments, has been an essential feature of DIE surgery in conventional laparoscopy. The value of trading-off tactile feedback (conventional laparoscopy) for improved vision and dexterity (robotics) has never been accepted a priori, even by robotic surgery enthusiasts. At this time however, one can attest that robotic surgery for DIE is a technique of proven safety. In spite of this reassuring data, we would recommend against operating on DIE within the robotic learning curve (i.e., within the first 75–100 surgeries) [45]. This said, as an experienced robotic and laparoscopic operator, I would no longer agree to operate on DIE without robotic assistance.

11.4.1 Preoperative Considerations

11.4.1.1 Simulation

Speed is not essential in this surgery; however, millimetric precision and full command of the console is paramount when resecting lesions that can literally envelop vital organs. As mentioned in Section 11.3.1.1, completion of a formal simulation protocol, such as the one by Culligan et al. [22] is recommended for all beginning robotic reproductive surgeons. Involvement of surgical trainees in DIE surgery should be avoided, or limited to subspecialty training in a dual-console teaching environment.

11.4.1.2 Case Selection

Reproductive surgeons who have recently transitioned to robotics must adhere to the recently published AAGL credentialing criteria, and should not operate on DIE [23]. As mentioned above in this section, robotic excision of DIE is an operation that should be tackled beyond the learning curve (75–100 surgeries, depending on case volume).

11.4.1.3 Imaging

If you cannot identify DIE on a conventional pelvic MRI, you are not alone. Adequate imaging of DIE is difficult to obtain without the application of specific protocols. We recommend that reproductive surgeons seek a close partnership with radiologists who share a specific interest in endometriosis. As already mentioned for the treatment of fibroids, this aspect of preoperative care is particularly relevant when we operate in the absence of haptic feedback. MRI and ultrasound can both be very helpful in identifying areas of interest for surgical exploration, as well as the expected extent of retroperitoneal and ovarian lesions. Bowel involvement and the need for a preoperative colonoscopy and the likelihood of an intraoperative colorectal consultation can also be gauged by adequate preoperative imaging. Both MRI and ultrasound can be completely useless if performed and interpreted by less-than-expert teams. This is a large, emerging, chapter of gynecologic imaging, which can only be mentioned here in passing, given the highly specialized nature of this chapter.

11.4.1.4 Informed Consent

Robotic excision of DIE is a high-risk operation. A surgical consent for this procedure should be written in a sixth-grade language level, in the format of a true contract between the patient and the operator. It should always be documented in the electronic record and should contain (at a very minimum) the following sections:

(a) Self-explanatory name for the planned surgery (no acronyms).

(b) Indication(s) for surgery.

(c) Alternatives discussed and declined (including hysterectomy and salpingo-oophorectomy).

(d) Concise review of the preoperative testing performed, as well as the limitations of such preoperative testing in detecting all ovarian or peritoneal cancer.

(e) Specific mention of the risk of decreased ovarian reserve or even premature ovarian failure as a consequence of severe endometriosis, but also as a consequence of the surgery performed to excise severe endometriosis; serum levels of anti-müllerian hormone (AMH) should be obtained routinely in women of reproductive age undergoing surgery for severe pelvic endometriosis, and ideally discussed and documented during the consent process.

(f) Specific consent for all possible complementary intraoperative procedures should be obtained, particularly for ureteral stenting, cystoscopy, colonoscopy, and all possible resections, such as bladder and rectum.

(g) Specific mention should be made of the planned use of robotic devices in the upcoming surgery, and the specific level of FDA approval for their use. Patients need to understand why their surgeons elect to use robotic teleoperators to excise endometriosis, and have to formally agree with this choice. Those surgeons who insist in considering robotic platforms simply as a laparoscopic tool, and exclude patients from this important technical choice, are setting themselves up for medical-legal trouble in the (not unlikely) case of complications.

11.4.1.5 Bowel Preparation and Perineal Access

Bowel preparation for laparoscopic surgery is not universally recommended even for major operations such as myomectomy and hysterectomy [46]. However, severe endometriosis with possible obliteration of the posterior cul de sac is one of those scenarios where a bowel prep should never be omitted. Rectal injury is not a rare occurrence, and colorectal surgeons willing to offer a primary repair of an injury contaminated with feces are still a rare find. Besides, an empty rectal ampulla facilitates the use of a rectal probe to better define the limits of the rectovaginal and pararectal spaces, which may make an injury less likely. Because of the need to access the perineum for rectal and uterine manipulation, a lateral docking, rather than central docking, of the patient-side robotic cart is recommended in all cases of DIE.

11.4.2 Intraoperative Procedure

The main steps can be summarized as follows (steps already mentioned in the myoma section will be omitted in this section).

1. See port placement in Figure 11.1. The camera port is within the umbilicus: either an 8 mm robotic or a 12 mm disposable. Two 8 mm robotic cannulas are then placed 8 cm to the right and to the left of the camera port. A 5 mm port is placed in the right lower quadrant. Camera arm and robotic arms #1 and #2 are used in this setup, and robotic arm #3 is often necessary. The port for this arm should be placed 8 cm lateral and caudal to the one for robotic arm #2 (moving the port for arm #2 more cephalad will minimize external collisions). As mentioned above, newer robotic platforms (da Vinci Xi) can further limit arm collisions by assisting the surgeon in the position of the robotic arms once the surgical target area is selected.

2. Please refer to Figure 11.6 for illustrations of the following operative steps. The robotic instrument choice is dictated in part by the choice of energy. A cutting and a coagulating (bipolar) instrument is needed. We favor a flexible CO_2 laser for cutting, a Maryland bipolar grasper to coagulate, and Cadiere of Prograsp forceps for retraction. In this setup, a large robotic needle driver is placed on arm #1, the robotic bipolar grasper on arm #2, and the retracting instrument in arm #3. The flexible laser fiber is inserted alongside the 8 mm laparoscope through 12 mm primary port; it is grasped and operated by robotic needle driver. Alternatively, the laser fiber can be introduced through

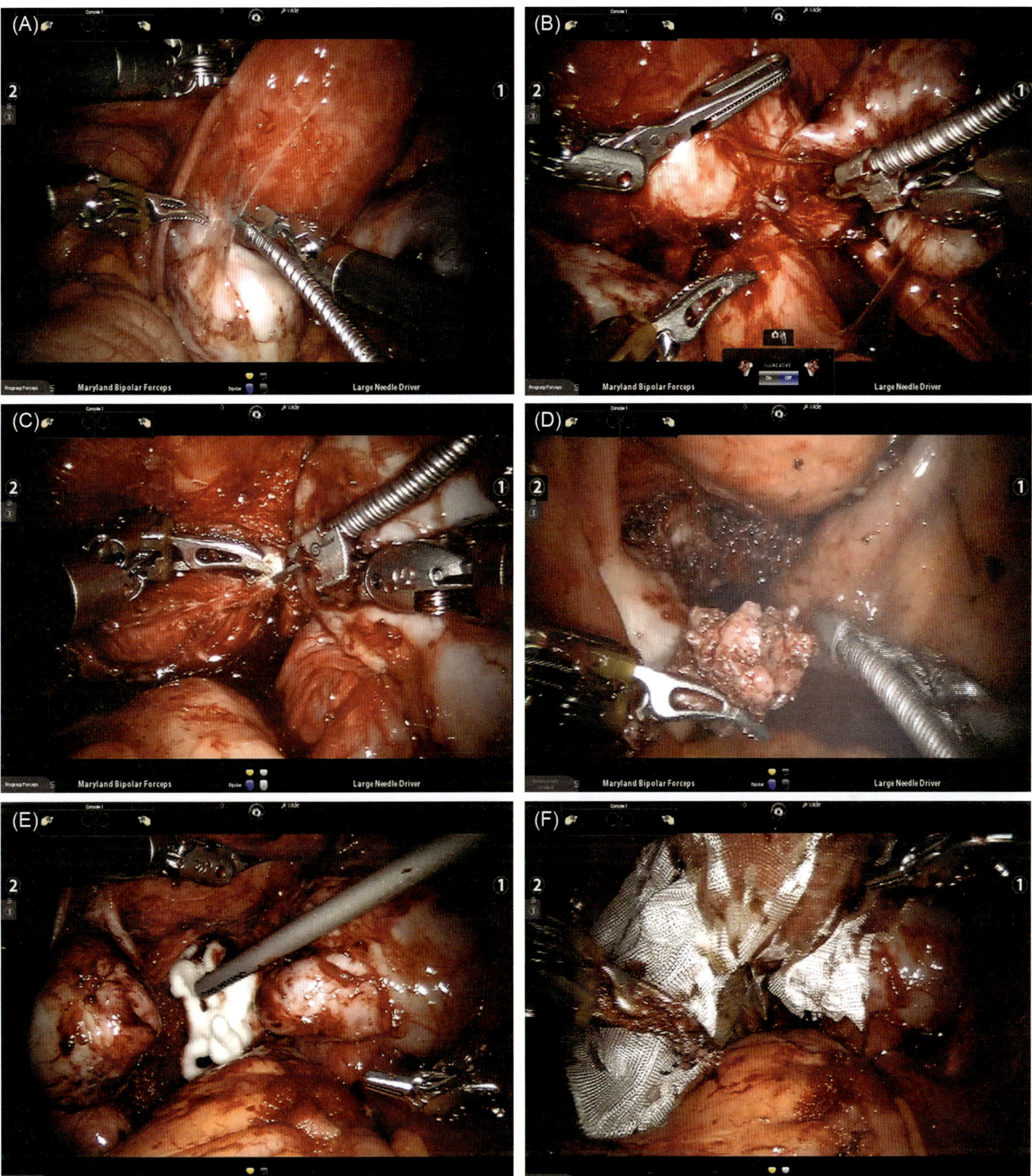

Figure 11.6 Robotic excision of deep infiltrating endometriosis. (A) A standard three robotic arms setup is very helpful in most scenarios of DIE. (B) Lysis of extensive pelvic adhesions is implicit in most DIE operations. (C) Electrocautery is used sparingly in the retroperitoneal spaces, we prefer sharp scissors, or low-wattage CO_2 laser (10 W). (E) An endometriotic nodule is identified and excised. (E) As opposed to uterine and ovarian surgery, hemostasis is rarely achieved by suturing: use of thrombin-containing coagulation gels and powders is a wise option. (F) Extensive use of oxidized regenerated cellulose completes the operation.

a 8–12 mm assistant port. Robotic monopolar curved shears can be used, with particular caution around vital structures, due to their significant thermal spread. Robotic shears can also be used without energy (cold shears), though these semireusable instruments are typically dull past their first use. The robotic ultrasonic scalpel should not be used for this indication, because it does not allow any fine movement at the tip.

3. Cosmetic port-placement options should be offered sparingly in robotic excision of DIE. It is important that the two main robotic instruments can triangulate onto each pelvic sidewall. Robotic ports placed at the level of the ASIS are often inadequate for this operation (they work well for a median target, as in the case of uterine tumors, as discussed in Section 11.3.2.2). Single-site robotics for DIE fulfills the above requirements for triangulation and is an available cosmetic option in some of these cases. However, the lack of wristed movements in most single-site instruments, and the severely limited options for bedside assistance make this technique challenging. An extra assistant port or robotic port (single-site plus 1) can facilitate this technique, albeit partially defeating its purpose.

11.4.3   Postoperative Considerations

At the risk of stating the obvious, patients with severe endometriosis should always be on specific hormonal treatment (with the exceptions being the physiologic states of pregnancy, lactation, and menopause). If infertility is a symptom, high-efficacy treatment modalities should be offered to limit the risk of recurrence. Surgery is an important episode in the chronic medical treatment of endometriosis.

Even if no endometriomas are found, surgery for severe DIE almost invariably includes some degree of adhesiolysis, including periovarian adhesiolysis. Therefore, one should consider remeasuring the serum AMH a few months after the surgery to document whether the patient has sustained a follicular loss compared to her baseline.

11.5   Robotic Excision of Endometriomas and Dermoid Cysts

We begin this section by acknowledging the findings of a recent study aimed at shedding light on the merits and demerits of robotic ovarian surgery [47]. This population-based analysis lumped together all benign oophorectomies and ovarian cystectomies performed by conventional and robot-assisted laparoscopy, and found a higher complication rate and higher cost in the robotic group. However, this study failed to recognize that, particularly in the years before the availability of virtual robotic simulation, gynecologists have consistently performed benign ovarian operations as their introductory cases to robotic surgery. The findings of this study are indeed the result of a highly skewed population sample. In reality, few robotic surgeons would ever perform a simple ovarian cystectomy or a simple oophorectomy with robotic assistance, as it is indeed true that these operations do not justify the added time and cost. Differently, ovarian cystectomies performed for endometriomas or mature cystic teratomas (dermoid cysts) can present unique challenges that are ideally addressed by robotic surgery. The reader is referred to other sections of this manual and to recent peer-reviewed publications on this topic [19] for a review of the indications for ovarian cystectomy in the presence of endometriomas and dermoid cysts.

11.5.1   Preoperative Considerations

Dermoid cysts are the most common benign germ cell tumors of the ovary in women of reproductive age; as a rule, they are remarkably slow-growing (1–2 mm a year) and can be expectantly managed. Most surgeons recommend annual ultrasound follow-up for lesions under 7 cm, and surgical removal only in larger, symptomatic, or radiologically atypical dermoids [48]. Studies have shown that laparoscopic removal of benign mature teratomas is clinically advantageous compared to laparotomy, though laparotomy has been associated with significantly shorter operative times and lower spillage rates of the dermoid contents [49]. Intraoperative rupture carries an extremely low risk of aseptic peritonitis and subsequent adhesion formation, which may impact fertility. The risk of peritonitis, however, has been reported to be extremely low, and at least one study found no long-term implications of intraoperative spillage of benign mature teratomas during laparoscopy on pregnancy rates, in the absence of peritonitis [50–52].

Endometriomas are not real cysts; they are pseudocysts that originate at the level of the ovarian cortex causing it to stretch and invaginate, with net loss of follicles. Endometriomas can be found in a freely moving ovary but are most often associated with significant pelvic adhesions and DIE [53]. There is no question that the type of technique utilized for the excision of endometriomas determines in great part the fate of the ovary [54]. Endometrioma incision and drainage results in unacceptably high recurrence rates, yet conventional endometrioma "stripping" can result in a significant loss of ovarian reserve. There are two concurrent reasons for the loss of ovarian reserve following endometrioma stripping: (1) the physical loss of cortical follicles implicit in the complete removal of the pseudocyst and (2) the thermal damage caused by the use of thermal energy to achieve hemostasis at the base of the endometrioma (adjacent to the ovarian hilum). To limit ovarian tissue loss, techniques of partial stripping followed by base ablation with either CO_2 laser or bipolar cautery have been proposed [55,56]. However, in a recent randomized study, the partial stripping with bipolar ablation of the base has not been shown to protect the ovarian reserve [57]. Finally, a technique of complete stripping with absolute avoidance of thermal energy has also been shown to avoid loss of ovarian reserve [58].

11.5.1.1   Informed Consent

Robotic excision of endometriomas and dermoid cysts is not considered a high-risk operation in terms of blood loss or organ damage; however, a detailed surgical consent for this procedure should address (at a very minimum) the following topics:

(a) The risk of loss of ovarian reserve.
(b) The risk of cyst recurrence. This implies that cystectomy, while providing advantages to reproductive-age women, carries a higher risk of re-operation compared to oophorectomy.
(c) The rare risk of aseptic chemical peritonitis (for dermoid cysts only). Strategies to limit its incidence should be discussed (see technique discussed later in Section 11.5.2).

(d) The rare possibility that the cyst will be malignant in nature (also see baseline testing). Patients should agree on the course of action in those cases where a suspicious ovarian or tubal mass is found during cystectomy. Our current protocol includes sending a specimen for frozen section, and proceeding with unilateral salpingo-oophorectomy if malignancy is suspected by the pathologist. Final oncologic staging and surgical treatment in women of reproductive age should be reserved for patients with a confirmed diagnosis of cancer on permanent section.

11.5.1.2 Baseline Ovarian Reserve Testing

The mere presence of endometriomas and (more rarely) dermoid cysts can determine loss of ovarian reserve. On the other hand, ovarian cystectomy can also the cause loss of ovarian reserve. Given the widespread availability of well-standardized testing for anti-müllerian hormone (AMH), the best current indicator of ovarian reserve, it makes sense to check its levels before proceeding with an ovarian cystectomy. Because AMH levels vary minimally throughout the menstrual cycle, testing will not delay surgical intervention. AMH should be obtained together with HE4 and CA125, as part of all complex ovarian cyst risk assessment [59]. See our section on postoperative considerations for some recent literature on the clinical use of AMH.

11.5.1.3 IVF Considerations

The decision of whether to perform a cystectomy before or after egg retrieval in the case of complex ovarian cysts is a classic conundrum of infertility practice. There are two scenarios that justify removal before IVF: (1) the cyst needs to be removed because a tissue diagnosis is desirable; (2) the cyst needs to be removed as it is expected to significantly impair our ability to retrieve oocytes after stimulation. The second scenario does not give us a choice. In the first scenario, cystectomy can often be deferred to after IVF, because of the risk of decreased ovarian reserve as discussed above. In this case, embryos can be cryopreserved and only transferred after the tissue diagnosis is achieved with surgery.

11.5.2 Intraoperative Technique

The main steps for ovarian cystectomy can be summarized as follows (steps already mentioned in the myoma section will be omitted in this section):

1. See port placement in Figures 11.1–11.6. The camera port is placed within the umbilicus: either an 8 mm robotic or a 12 mm disposable. Two 8 mm robotic cannulas are then placed 8 cm to the right and to the left of the camera port. A 5 mm assistant port is placed in the right lower quadrant. Camera arm and robotic arms #1 and #2 are used in this setup, and robotic arm #3 is often necessary. The port for this third instrument arm should be placed 8 cm lateral and caudal to the one for robotic arm #2 (moving the port for arm #2 more cephalad will minimize external collisions). As mentioned earlier in Section 11.4.2, newer robotic platforms (da Vinci Xi) can further limit arm collisions by self-optimizing the position of the robotic arms once the surgical target area is selected.

2. The robotic instrument choice is dictated by the choice of energy. A cutting and a coagulating (bipolar) instrument are needed. We favor a flexible CO_2 laser for cutting, a Maryland bipolar grasper to coagulate (within limits, see later in this section) and Cadiere (more delicate) of Prograsp (better grasp) forceps for retraction. In this setup, a large robotic needle driver is placed on arm #1, the robotic bipolar grasper on arm #2, and the retracting instrument in arm #3. The flexible laser fiber is inserted alongside the 8 mm laparoscope through 12 mm primary port; it is grasped and operated by robotic needle driver. Alternatively, the laser fiber can be introduced through a 8–12 mm assistant port. Robotic monopolar curved shears are used as an alternative to the laser, with particular caution around vital organs and on ovarian cortical structures, due to their significant thermal spread. Robotic shears should be used without energy (cold shears) when possible. The robotic ultrasonic scalpel finds no use in this indication, because it does not allow any fine movement at the tip.

3. Cosmetic and single-site port-placement options can be offered in robotic excision of those endometriomas that are not associated with DIE (see Section 11.3 on robotic myomectomy for details on these techniques). Our technique for single-site excision of endometriomas is available as an open-access video publication [60].

4. For dermoid cysts, we do not recommend a cosmetic or single-site port placement. It is our preference to excise these tumors in a contained fashion, to avoid spillage of cyst material, to reduce the risks of chemical peritonitis and intraperitoneal dispersion of a possible immature teratoma. Contained cystectomy is accomplished by placing the entire adnexum in an endoscopic specimen pouch, introduced through a lower-quadrant 12 mm port. A flat bottom pouch is preferred over tapered bottom pouch. A 15 cm endoscopic pouch must be used for masses over 10 cm. The bedside assistant keeps the edge of the pouch at an angle that allows the surgeon to operate inside it (thanks to the fully wristed tips of the robotic instruments) but that does not allow the cyst material to overflow. A regular 5 mm suction-irrigator can be inserted through one of the robotic cannulas for the short time need to decompress the cyst at its entry. If needed, a large bore (10 mm) suction cannula can be inserted through a suprapubic port for larger tumors. We have accomplished this technique (for small dermoid cysts) with a single-site plus one configuration, by placing the suction-irrigator through the assistant port of the single port device (Figure 11.7).

5. We do not perform contained cystectomy for endometriomas, because chemical peritonitis following laparoscopic enucleation of these tumors has not been described, and because the oncologic risk of typical endometriomas diagnosed by ultrasound in women

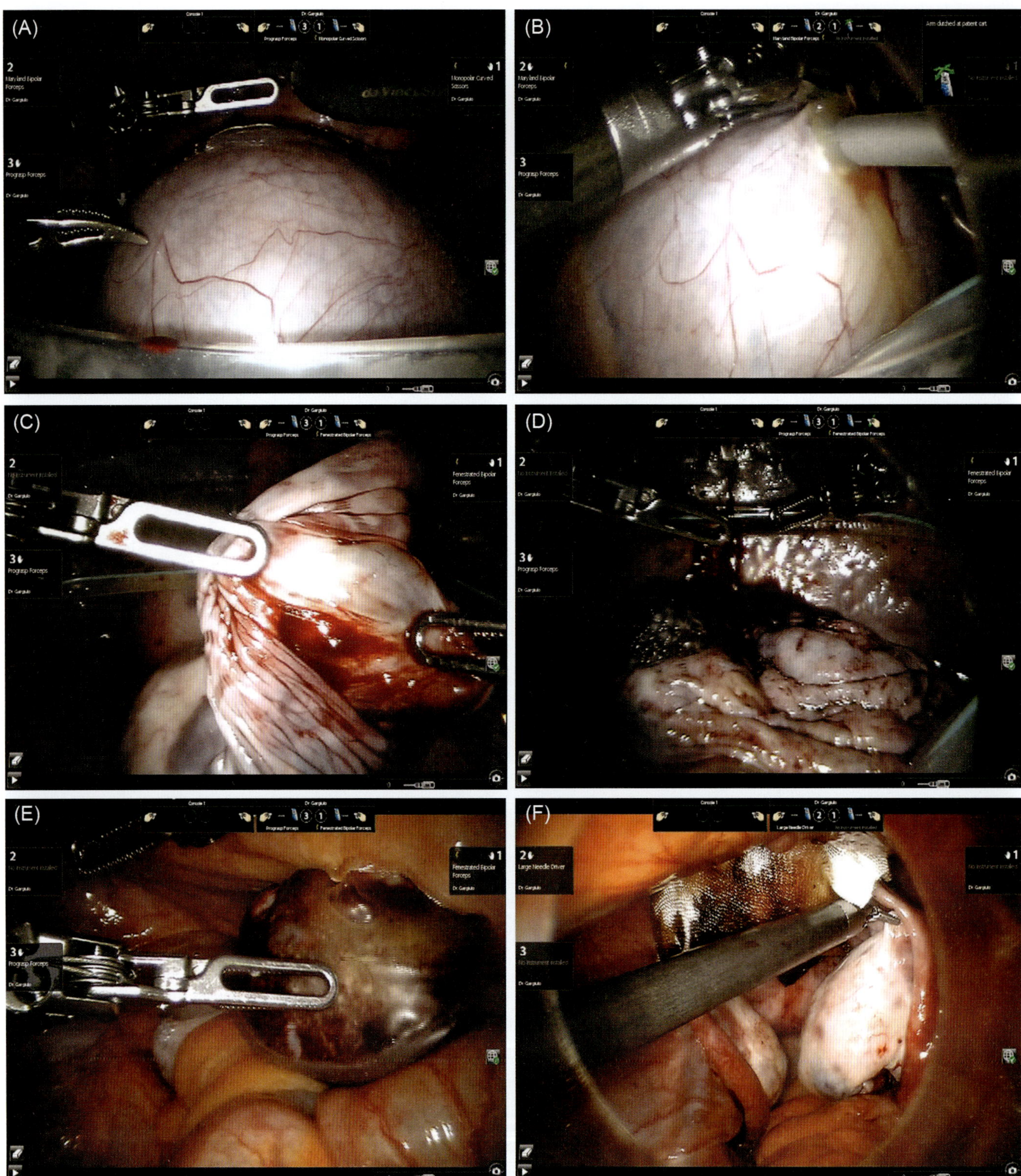

Figure 11.7 Robotic excision of dermoid cyst. (A) A 12 cm right ovarian teratoma is placed in a 15 cm endoscopic specimen bag introduced through the right lower quadrant. (B) The cyst is opened sharply; part of the fluid is aspirated with a suction cannula introduced through one of the robotic ports, and part is collected in the bag. (C) The cyst wall is stripped from the heathy ovarian parenchyma using two graspers. (D) The entire teratoma is in the bag. No fluid is spilled in the abdominal cavity. (E) The cyst is retrieved intact in the bag through a small right lower-quadrant incision. (F) Ovarian hemostasis is confirmed. No electrocautery is employed on the ovarian parenchyma.

of reproductive age is minimal. Indeed, for all but the smallest (and more superficial) endometriomas we routinely apply the technique described by Donnez et al. in which only 90% of the pseudocyst is stripped. The remaining 10% of pseudocyst (that is left adherent to the hilum) is cauterized with superpulse CO_2 laser, to achieve complete destruction of the endometriosis while sparing the ovarian hilum (and preserving the ovarian reserve, as demonstrated by the residual antral follicle count) [55]. We recommend a contained or protected extraction of all endometriomas from the abdominal cavity to reduce the risk to seed endometriosis in the surgical wound (Figure 11.8).

6. Following decompression and enucleation of the cyst, the endoscopic pouch string is synched and the cyst and fluid are removed through a lower-quadrant port. Occasionally, the fascia is gently stretched to allow exit of a larger specimen, by placing and opening a Kelly forceps in a sagittal plane.

7. Hemostasis of the ovarian bed is not always spontaneously achieved following ovarian cystectomy. As already pointed out for the ovarian cortex, electrocautery use (either bipolar or monopolar) should also be avoided on the ovarian stroma, due to the risk is of compromising the ovarian vasculature at the hilum. There are many safe alternatives to the use of cautery. Dropping in a 4 × 4 sterile gauze to apply one or more minutes of steady pressure at the points of bleeding is a quick and easy fix. Several thrombin preparations are also available for local application within the ovary (better if followed by temporary gauze pressure, as mentioned above). Last but not least, robotic surgeons are uniquely equipped to precisely place one or more figure-of-eight sutures; this is a safe and effective technique to completely stop even arterial bleeders without any use of thermal energy.

11.5.3 Postoperative Considerations

All of the principles described for the postoperative management of endometriosis resection also apply for endometriomas (see Section 11.4.3). We reevaluate our patients 2–3 weeks after the operation and usually clear them to resume all activities at that time.

Repeat testing of AMH after ovarian cystectomy should be delayed for 1 year, and patients should be educated about the rationale of this clinical choice. Recent evidence indicates that most of the postoperative drop in AMH is recovered by 12 months after excision of endometrioma [61]. One should expect the most significant drop in women with a high baseline AMH, while women with already decreased ovarian reserve should not expect a large percent change of AMH. Also, excision of endometriomas brings about a significantly more substantial drop of AMH compared to excision of dermoid cysts [62].

Endometriomas and dermoid cysts can both recur after cystectomy. Rogers et al. found that all dermoid recurrences were present within 1 year of surgery, supporting the hypothesis

that incomplete resections might be mislabeled as recurrences. To this end, a single postsurgical ultrasound at 12 months postoperatively may be useful [63]. Endometriomas recur over a more prolonged period of time; a cumulative recurrence rate of 11.7% (with reoperation rate of 8.2%) was documented over a 48-month follow-up study [64]. Yearly ultrasounds should be considered in women of reproductive age who undergo stripping of endometriomas, particularly if any degree of symptomatic recurrence is reported.

11.6 Robotic Tubal Reanastomosis

Regret of voluntary tubal sterilization is still a common scenario in clinical practice. The goal of a tubal reanastomosis is to reestablish the patency of a 1–2 mm tubal lumen; the classic open microsurgical technique employs an operative microscope and ultrafine sutures to produce an anatomically correct, tension-free anastomosis. Very few surgeons have been able to replicate this technique laparoscopically with good clinical result, because the technical challenges posed by a laparoscopic tubal reanastomosis are truly formidable [65]. Even at high-volume centers, the rate of conversion to laparotomy is above 5% [66]. Robotic assistance could help improve the practicality and diffusion of this laparoscopic technique. Several teams have published on the safety, feasibility, and effectiveness of robotic tubal reanastomosis (RTR), while reporting clinical results comparable to those obtained with minilaparotomy [67,68].

11.6.1 Preoperative Considerations

Caillet et al. have provided the most useful data to counsel women regarding their age-dependent chance for success following RTR [69]. This retrospective cohort study analyzed pregnancy outcomes for 97 women aged 24–47 years (median age 37 years) who underwent RTR. All women had normal ovarian reserve and all of the partners had normal spermatogenesis. The overall pregnancy and live birth rates within 2 years of surgery were 71% and 62% respectively. Nearly 88% of women < 35 years old and 44% of women aged 40–42 years delivered at least one child during the follow-up period. These numbers correlate very well with the success rates for assisted reproduction in these types of patients. This is essential information that should be always discussed with prospective patients.

11.6.1.1 Informed Consent

RTR is not considered a high-risk operation in terms of blood loss or organ damage; however, detailed surgical consent for this procedure should address (at a very minimum) the following topics:

(a) The possibility that tubes may scar down and that patency will not be restored in spite of the operation.

(b) The significant risk that pregnancies that result from reversal of tubal sterilization may be tubal ectopics (reported risk between 2% and 10% [70]).

(c) The natural history of tubal ectopics, including the likely need for chemotherapy, the possibility of emergency

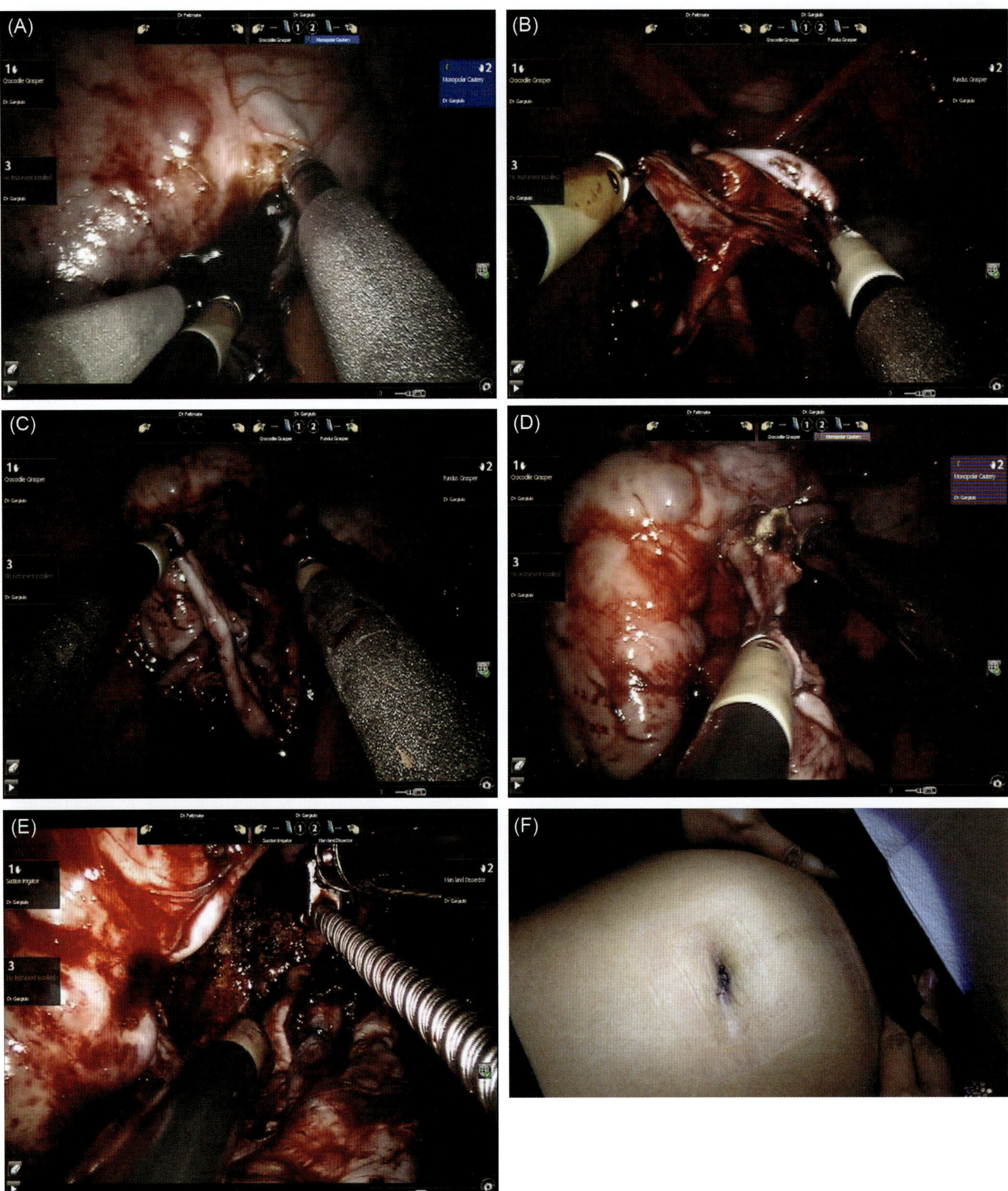

Figure 11.8 Single-site robotic excision of endometrioma. (A) A left ovarian endometrioma is entered sharply and the content is suctioned by the bedside assistant (leftmost instrument). (B) Endometrioma pseudocyst is teased off the healthy parenchyma with classic two-grasper technique (fundus grasper and crocodile grasper employed here). (C) 90% of the pseudocyst has been separated from the ovarian parenchyma. (D) The pseudocyst is cut away from a residual discoid area (estimated at about 10% of the total pseudocyst surface) overlying the ovarian hilum. (E) Superpulse CO_2 laser energy, delivered through a flexible device driven by a robotic grasper, is used to gently vaporize the entire surface of the residual discoid area of pseudocyst overlying the hilum. (F) Patient's wound at the 2-week postoperative visit.

surgery, and even the very rare chance of massive hemoperitoneum and death.

(d) The availability of assisted reproductive technologies as a viable alternative to this surgery (discussed in Section 11.6.1.3).

11.6.1.2 Defining the Type of Sterilization

We require a copy of the operative note for the sterilization procedure to assess the technique employed, the anatomic findings at the time of the operation, and (as much as possible) the expected residual tubal length. Finally, we request a copy of the pathologist report, if applicable, to further corroborate the surgeon's description. A recent study has confirmed the general consensus that the best prognosis is associated with sterilization by clips and rings, the worst prognosis with tubal coagulation, and an intermediate prognosis is associated with ligation and excision [71].

11.6.1.3 IVF Considerations

Patients who are counseled about their reproductive options following tubal sterilization should always be provided with a full and unbiased panorama of the two available alternatives: IVF and RTR. We consider poststerilization regret as a case of classic tubal factor infertility, and proceed with a full evaluation of the couple. At a very minimum, we obtain a semen analysis of the patient's male partner, and an AMH level of the patient, and use both parameters to counsel the couple about their best chance of having a baby. This is another example of how beneficial it is for women to have access to IVF specialists who also perform reproductive surgery. At a very minimum, a reproductive endocrinologist will always keep in mind that the success of sterilization reversal is not the achievement of tubal patency, but rather that of a healthy birth. Indeed, there are many cases in which we recommend IVF over RTR. Such classic scenarios include abnormal spermatogenesis, oligo-ovulation, moderate to severe endometriosis, and sterilization by extensive tubal coagulation or excision (such as a wide Pomeroy).

11.6.1.4 Simulation

Speed is definitely not a factor in this microsurgical operation. However, millimetric precision and dexterity in intracorporeal suturing is paramount when connecting tubal lumina of 1 or 2 mm in diameter. As also discussed earlier in Section 11.3.1.1, completion of a formal simulation protocol, such as the one by Culligan et al. [22], is recommended for all beginning robotic reproductive surgeons. Beyond this basic requirement, however, specific suturing software is now available on most simulator consoles to train the operator's wrist in the many different angles of suturing that are needed for this procedure. Involvement of surgical trainees in robotic tubal microsurgery should be limited to REI fellowships, in a dual-console teaching environment.

11.6.2 Intraoperative Technique

The main steps can be summarized as follows (steps already mentioned in the myoma section will be omitted in this section):

See port placement in Figure 11.1. We use a minimal access, cosmetic approach to RTR. A total of four 8 mm ports are used; none of these require fascial closure, resulting in less postoperative discomfort. A 8-mm robotic camera cannula is placed within the umbilicus, cannulas for robotic arms #1 and #2 are placed 3 cm medial and cephalad to the ASIS, and an 8 mm assistant cannula is placed in a suprapubic midline location. No resulting scars are visible above bikini line once the abdomen is emptied of gas.

Please refer to Figure 11.9 for illustrations of the following operative steps. We dock the patient's side cart in a left side angled position. We load an 8 mm micro bipolar graspers on robotic arm #1 and an 8 mm Potts scissors on robotic arm #2. A concentrated solution of vasopressin (20 units in 20 mL) is injected in the mesosalpinx at the level of proximal and distal tubal stumps (a total of 2.5 units are used for each tube, see our mention earlier in Section 11.3.2.1 of minimal toxic dose of vasopressin being 5 units). We proceed with dissection of the scar at the prior site of tubal interruption using robotic scissors and micro bipolar forceps. We excise the scar and prepare the stumps. We finally decapitate the proximal and distal stumps, exposing healthy tubal luminal epithelium. High-pressure, high-volume chromotubation is performed for the first time, demonstrating full flow of dye from the proximal stumps. All four tubal stumps are prepared at the beginning of the procedure.

We change the robotic instruments to two Black Diamond robotic needle drivers. We place a tapered 3-4-5 French ERCP catheter through the distal portion of the tube and then gently push it into the proximal portion of the left tube. This acts as a stable stent during the procedure. We place a 6-0 Vicryl figure-of-eight suture through the mesosalpinx to take the tension off of the upcoming anastomosis site. We then proceed with placing a minimum of three through-and-through sutures of 8-0 Prolene (entering at the level of tubal serosa wall and skimming the tubal lumen). The sutures are all laid down flat and are only later tied intracorporeally, so as to keep the anastomosis site fully accessible for precise suturing. All 8.0 and 6.0 needles are passed on surgical patties and are directly observed coming in and out of the 8 mm suprapubic assistant port, following a standardized voice confirmation protocol between the operator and the bedside assistant that follows the entire movement of the needle from the instruments' table into the patient and back on the instrument table. A dropped 6.0 needle is usually retrievable in this setup, given the location of the assistant port for exchange. A 8.0 needle is virtually irretrievable, and may well have to be left in the patient's abdomen, with likely minimal, though objectively unknown long-term consequences. Needle management is the main safety concern of this otherwise extremely safe operation.

The ERCP catheter is removed before chromopertubation and immediately removed from the abdominal cavity (a new catheter will be used for the contralateral tube). Gentle, low-pressure chromopertubation is performed at the end of reanastomosis, with filling and spilling of the tube from the distal ampullary portion. Leakage at the anastomosis site is a frequent and technically acceptable finding, as long as distal

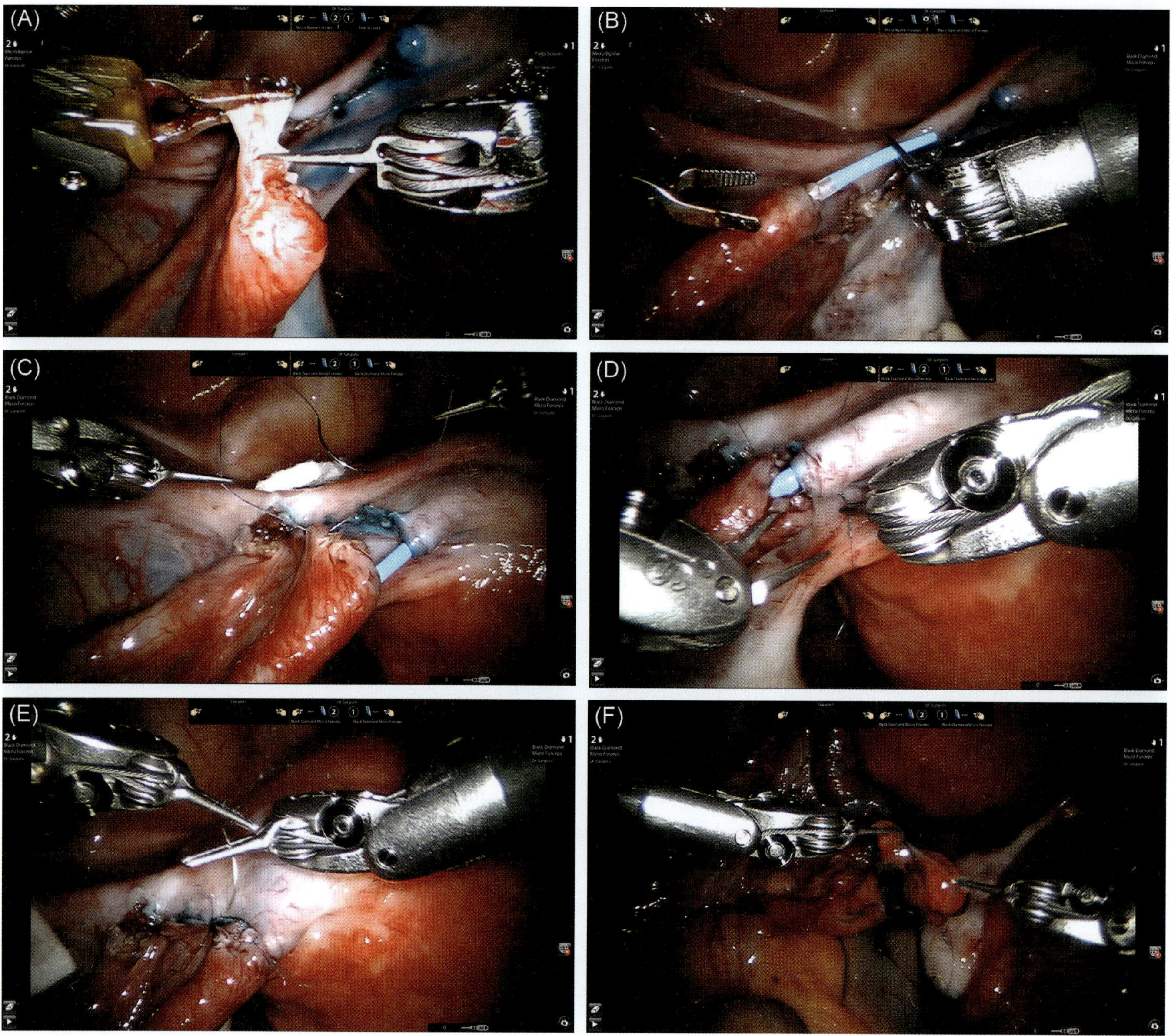

Figure 11.9 Robotic tubal reanastomosis, cosmetic approach. (A) Tubal stumps are identified and prepared bilaterally. Mesosalpinx scar is trimmed; first chromopertubation is performed to confirm proximal stump patency. (B) Tube is cannulated distal to proximal with a tapered 3-4-5 French catheter. (C) Mesosalpinx gap is reapproximation with 6.0 Vicryl. (D) Tubal stumps are reanastomosed with three or four sutures of 8.0 Prolene. (E) Final view, showing both the mesosalpinx gap reapproximation and the isthmic-isthmic tubal reanastomosis. (F) Second chromopertubation is performed, confirming continuity of the reanastomosed tubal lumen.

flow is demonstrated. Indeed, the goal of tubal reanastomosis is not a water-tight junction, but rather a perfectly oriented juxtaposition. A sheet of oxidized regenerated cellulose is carefully wrapped around the re-anastomosed tube and wet with lactated Ringers electrolyte solution in order to protect it from inadvertent damage during the contralateral reanastomosis procedure, as well as to limit the risk for future adnexal adhesions. An identical reanastomosis procedure is performed contralaterally.

At the end of the procedure, the pelvis is gently irrigated with lactate Ringers electrolyte solution, and the patient-side cart of the surgical system is undocked.

A single-stitch robotic tubal reanastomosis procedure has been recently described in a small case series [71]. In this study, surgeons employed a single polyglactin 5.0 suture placed at the 12 o'clock position. In 16 of 17 patients, tubal patency was confirmed in at least one fallopian tube by postoperative HSG and/or subsequent pregnancy. The resulting ongoing pregnancy rate was 41% and the average patient age was 33.7 years. Pregnancy rates in this study are not at par with the results published in the conventional multistitch reanastomosis, reviewed earlier in Section 11.6.1.

11.6.3 Postoperative Considerations

We recommend complete pelvic rest for 1–2 months following tubal reanastomosis, and see our patients 2–3 weeks after surgery to review the important topics mentioned in the following.

Postoperative HSG is an essential component of this surgical procedure, so much so that several surgical practices include this imaging modality in the global payment contract for their patients. A hysterosalpingogram should be deferred to 2 or more months after surgery to allow for adequate healing. All efforts should be taken to avoid involuntary myometrial contractility, including corneal spasm, in these procedures. The procedures should ideally be performed by reproductive surgeons, who – because of their skills in human embryo transfer – are particularly adept in atraumatic cervical cannulation. We employ a 5 French soft silicone balloon catheter, which is placed much in the way of an intrauterine insemination catheter, without the need for a cervical tenaculum. We inflate the balloon very slowly, generally with no more than 5 cc of air. We also recommend a single dose of 10 mg of diazepam and 600 mg of ibuprofen to our patients, 1 hour before the scheduled procedure. Injection of contrast is very slow, and fluoroscopy magnification is high. By employing this technique, we have reversed many "bilateral proximal block" radiology results from outside community radiology centers to "bilateral patency."

Our patients are counseled since before surgery on the fact that a pregnancy following tubal reanastomosis is ectopic until proven otherwise. Patients are encouraged to always use ovulation predictors to time intercourse as well as to use electronic reminders and smartphone applications to remind themselves the expected day of menses, so that they can perform a home pregnancy test on the day of missed menses. When a positive pregnancy test is reported, they contact our office and are instructed to come in for three consecutive serum beta-HCG level checks, 48 hours apart. Ectopic precautions are routinely reviewed with patients at this point. Standard ART ultrasonographic follow-up protocol is followed (with a 5.5 weeks initial ultrasound for location, followed by a 7–8 weeks confirmatory ultrasound for viability).

Particularly with women in advanced reproductive age (40 years and above), the time may come when the question is posed of when to consider IVF as a second-line treatment for clinically failed reanastomosis. The answer to this question is based on multiple considerations, and should be part of the postoperative consultation, so that the biological window of opportunity is not missed.

11.7 Conclusions

Reproductive surgeons own gynecologic microsurgery; this discipline is just as fully integrated within the knowledge basis of the reproductive endocrinology and infertility subspecialty as cancer surgery is with that of gynecologic oncology. Robotic assistance is a timely addition to the surgical armamentarium of reproductive surgeons, allowing more of us to broaden the applicability of our highly specialized operative capabilities. This technology has come of age, following a somewhat tumultuous first decade of alternating enthusiasm and criticism. The unique aspect of integrated, objectively scored, virtual reality simulation adds a substantial layer of safety that commands full attention in a patient-centered age of precision medicine.

Safe robot-assisted laparoscopic techniques are well described for all reproductive surgery applications, many of which have been reviewed in this chapter. The future of robot-assisted reproductive surgery is brighter than ever at a time when concrete prospects of technological alternatives to the single FDA-approved robotic device are at the horizon, with a realistic promise of cost containment and competitive innovation.

Acknowledgments

Robotic surgery has been touted as the technology that allows solo-surgery; in reality, safe and effective robotic surgery is the ultimate team-based surgical endeavor. I would therefore like to acknowledge the invaluable contribution of several colleagues at Brigham and Women's Hospital to the development and/or perfecting of all of the techniques described in this chapter. In particular, I am grateful to surgical technologists Mr. Jackson Sammah and Mr. Diego Martinez for their many contributions, and to our operating room nursing staff for their fastidious commitment to the safe use of robotic technology. I am likewise grateful to generations of our reproductive endocrinology and infertility fellows who have embraced robotic surgery as a valuable complementary tool in the comprehensive care of our infertile couples. Above all, I recognize the essential role of my associate Dr. Serene S. Srouji to a decade of safe robotic trailblazing at Brigham and Women's Hospital.

References

1. *ABOG Program Requirements for Fellowship Graduate Medical Education* for Reproductive Endocrinology and Infertility. 2014. www.abog.org/publications/Program%20Requirements-REI-Sept%202014.pdf#search="special%20requirements" (accessed August 26, 2016).

2. Parker WH, Kaunitz AM, Pritts EA, et al. Leiomyoma morcellation review group. U.S. Food and Drug Administration's guidance regarding morcellation of leiomyomas: well-intentioned, but is it harmful for women? *Obstet Gynecol.* 2016;127:18–22.

3. Bedaiwy MA, Zhang A, Henry D, et al. Surgical anatomy of supraumbilical port placement: implications for robotic and advanced laparoscopic surgery. *Fertil Steril.* 2015;103:e33.

4. Koh C, Janik G. Laparoscopic myomectomy: the current status. *Curr Opin Obstet Gynecol.* 2003;15:295–301.

5. Bush AJ, Morris SN, Millham FH, et al. Women's preferences for minimally invasive incisions. *J Minim Invasive Gynecol.* 2011;18:640–3.

6. Goebel K, Goldberg JM. Women's preference of cosmetic results after gynecologic surgery. *J Minim Invasive Gynecol.* 2014;21:64–7.

7. Yeung PP, Jr, Bolden CR, Westreich D, et al. Patient preferences of cosmesis for abdominal incisions in gynecologic surgery. *J Minim Invasive Gynecol.* 2013;20:79–84.

8. Advincula AP, Song A, Burke W, et al. Preliminary experience with robot-assisted laparoscopic myomectomy. *J Am Assoc Gynecol Laparosc.* 2004;11:511–18.

9. Liu G, Zolis L, Kung R, et al. The laparoscopic myomectomy: a survey of canadian gynaecologists. *J Obstet Gynaecol Can.* 2010;32:139–48.

10. Gargiulo AR, Srouji SS, Missmer SA, et al. Robot-assisted laparoscopic myomectomy compared with standard laparoscopic myomectomy. *Obstet Gynecol.* 2012;120:284–91.

11. Bedient CE, Magrina JF, Noble BN, et al. Comparison of robotic and laparoscopic myomectomy. *Am J Obstet Gynecol.* 2009;201:566 e1–5.

12. Nezhat C, Lavie O, Hsu S, et al. Robotic-assisted laparoscopic myomectomy compared with standard laparoscopic myomectomy-a retrospective matched control study. *Fertil Steril.* 2009;91:556–9.

13. Advincula AP, Xu X, Goudeau St, et al. Robot-assisted laparoscopic myomectomy versus abdominal myomectomy: a comparison of short-term surgical outcomes and immediate costs. *J Minim Invasive Gynecol.* 2007;14:698–705.

14. Pitter MC, Gargiulo AR, Bonaventura LM, et al. Pregnancy outcomes following robot-assisted myomectomy. *Hum Reprod.* 2013;28:99–108.

15. Pitter M, Srouji S, Gargiulo A, et al. Fertility and symptom relief following robot-assisted laparoscopic myomectomy. *Obstet Gynecol Int.* 2015;967568.

16. Choussein S, Srouji SS, Missmer SA, et al. Perioperative outcomes and complications of robot-assisted laparoscopic myomectomy (RALM). *J Minim Invasive Gynecol.* 2015;22:S70.

17. Barton SE, Gargiulo AR. Robot-assisted laparoscopic myomectomy and adenomyomectomy with a flexible CO_2 laser device. *J Robotic Surg.* 2013;7:157–62.

18. Chong GO, Lee YH, Hong DG, et al. Long-term efficacy of laparoscopic or robotic adenomyomectomy with or without medical treatment for severely symptomatic adenomyosis. *Gynecol Obstet Invest.* 2016;81:346–52.

19. Choussein S, Hariton, E, Bortolotto P, et al. Current trends and controversies in reproductive surgery. Epub ahead of print, *Minerva Ginecol.* 2016;68:700–12.

20. Kishi Y, Yabuta M, Taniguchi F. Who will benefit from uterus-sparing surgery in adenomyosis-associated subfertility? *Fertil Steril.* 2014;102:802–7.

21. Gargiulo AR. Will computer-assisted surgery shake the foundations of surgical ethics in the age of patient-centered medicine? In: *OBG Management Supplement: Innovations in Patient Safety for Women's Health: Minimally Invasive Gynecologic Surgery.* 2015;7:S20–4.

22. Culligan P, Gurshumov E, Lewis C, et al. Predictive validity of a training protocol using a robotic surgery simulator. *Female Pelvic Med Reconstr Surg.* 2014;20:48–51.

23. AAGL special article: guidelines for privileging for robotic-assisted gynecologic laparoscopy. *J Minim Invasive Gynecol.* 2014;21:157–67.

24. Angioli R, Battista C, Terranova C, et al. Intraoperative contact ultrasonography during open myomectomy for uterine fibroids. *Fertil Steril.* 2010;94:1487–90.

25. Shwayder J, Sakhel K. Imaging for uterine myomas and adenomyosis. *J Minim Invasive Gynecol.* 2014;21:362–76.

26. Moghadam R, Lathi RB, Shahmohamady B, et al. Predictive value of magnetic resonance imaging in differentiating between leiomyoma and adenomyosis. *JSLS.* 2006;10:216–19.

27. Santos P, Cunha TM. Uterine sarcomas: clinical presentation and MRI features. *Diagn Interv Radiol.* 2015;21:4–9.

28. Celik H, Sapmaz E. Use of a single preoperative dose of misoprostol is efficacious for patients who undergo abdominal myomectomy. *Fertil Steril.* 2003;79:1207–10.

29. Ragab A, Khaiary M, Badawy A. The use of single versus double dose of intra-vaginal prostaglandin E2 "misoprostol" prior to abdominal myomectomy: a randomized controlled clinical trial. *J Reprod Infertil.* 2014;15:152–6.

30. Caglar GS, Tasci Y, Kayikcioglu F, et al. Intravenous tranexamic acid use in myomectomy: a prospective randomized double-blind placebo controlled study. *Eur J Obstet Gynecol Reprod Biol.* 2008;137:227–31.

31. Wright JD, Tergas AI, Cui R, et al. Use of electric power morcellation and prevalence of underlying cancer in women who undergo myomectomy. *JAMA Oncol.* 2015;1:69–77.

32. Tinelli A, Malvasi A, Hurst BS, et al. Surgical management of neurovascular bundle in uterine fibroid pseudocapsule. *J Soc Laparoendosc Surg.* 2012;16:119–29.

33. Osada H, Silber S, Kakinuma T, et al. Surgical procedure to conserve the uterus for future pregnancy in patients suffering from massive adenomyosis. *Reprod Biomed Online.* 2011;22:94–9.

34. Nishida M, Takano K, Arai Y, et al. Conservative surgical management for diffuse uterine adenomyosis. *Fertil Steril.* 2010;94:715–19.

35. Cohen SL, Senapati S, Gargiulo AR, et al. Dilute versus concentrated vasopressin administration during laparoscopic myomectomy: a randomized controlled trial. *Br J Obstet Gynecol.* 2017;124:262–8.

36. Bailey AP, Lancerotto L, Gridley C, et al. Greater surgical precision of a flexible carbon dioxide laser fiber compared to monopolar electrosurgery in porcine myometrium. *J Minim Invasive Gynecol.* 2014;21:1103–9.

37. Pluchino N, Litta P, Freschi L, et al. Comparison of the initial surgical experience with robotic and laparoscopic myomectomy. *Int J Med Robot.* 2014;10:208–12.

38. Tulandi T, Einarsson JI. The use of barbed suture for laparoscopic hysterectomy and myomectomy: a systematic review and meta-analysis. *J Minim Invasive Gynecol.* 2014;21:210–16.

39. Lewis EI, Srouji SS, Gargiulo AR. Robotic single site myomectomy: initial report and technique. *Fertil Steril.* 2015; 103:1370–7.

40. Gargiulo AR, Lewis EI, Kaser DJ, et al. Robotic single site myomectomy: a step by step tutorial. *Fertil Steril.* 2015;104.

41. Choussein S, Srouji SS, Farland LV, et al. Flexible carbon dioxide laser fiber versus ultrasonic scalpel in robot-assisted laparoscopic myomectomy. *J Minim Invasive Gynecol.* 2015;22:1183–90.

42. Quaas AM, Einarsson JI, Srouji SS, et al. Robotic myomectomy: a review of indications and techniques. *Rev Obstet Gynecol.* 2010;3:185–91.

43. Nezhat CR, Stevens A, Balassiano E, et al. Robotic-assisted laparoscopy vs conventional laparoscopy for the treatment of advanced stage endometriosis. *J Minim Invasive Gynecol.* 2015;22:40–4.

44. Magrina JF, Espada M, Kho RM, et al. Surgical excision of advanced endometriosis: perioperative outcomes and impacting factors. *J Minim Invasive Gynecol.* 2015;22:944–50.

45. Lenihan JP Jr. Navigating credentialing, privileging, and learning curves in robotics with an evidence and experienced-based approach. *Clin Obstet Gynecol.* 2011;54:382–90.

46. Zhang J, Xu L, Shi G. Is mechanical bowel preparation necessary for gynecologic surgery? A systematic review and

meta-analysis. Epub ahead of print, *Gynecol Obstet Invest.* 2016;81:155–61.

47. Wright JD, Kostolias A, Ananth CV, et al. Comparative effectiveness of robotically assisted compared with laparoscopic adnexal surgery for benign gynecologic disease. *Obstet Gynecol.* 2014;5:886–96.

48. Multani J, Kives S. Dermoid cysts in adolescents. *Curr Opin Obstet Gynecol.* 2015;27:315–19.

49. Benezra V, Verma U, Whitted R. Comparison of laparoscopy versus laparotomy for the surgical treatment of ovarian dermoid cysts. *Gynecol Surg.* 2005;2:89–92.

50. Templeman CL, Hertweck SP, Scheetz JP, et al. The management of mature cystic teratomas in children and adolescents: a retrospective analysis. *Hum Reprod.* 2000;15:2669–72.

51. Savasi I, Lacy JA, Gerstle JT, et al. Management of ovarian dermoid cysts in the pediatric and adolescent population. *J Pediatr Adolesc Gynecol.* 2009;22:360–4.

52. Pansky M, Shade D, Moskovitch M, et al. Inadvertent rupture of benign cystic teratoma does not impair future fertility. *Am J Obstet Gynecol.* 2010;203:442e1–4.

53. Lafay Pillet MC, Huchon C, Santulli P, et al. A clinical score can predict associated deep infiltrating endometriosis before surgery for an endometrioma. *Hum Reprod.* 2014;29:1666–76.

54. Muzii L, Miller CE. The singer, not the song. *J Minim Invasive Gynecol.* 2011;18:666–7.

55. Donnez J, Lousse JC, Jadoul P, et al. Laparoscopic management of endometriomas using a combined technique of excisional (cystectomy) and ablative surgery. *Fertil Steril.* 2010;94:28–32.

56. Muzii L, Panici PB. Combined technique of excision and ablation for the surgical treatment of ovarian endometriomas: the way forward? *Reprod Biomed Online.* 2010;20:300–2.

57. Muzii L, Achilli C, Bergamini V, et al. Comparison between the stripping technique and the combined excisional/ablative technique for the treatment of bilateral ovarian endometriomas: a multicentre RCT. *Hum Reprod.* 2016;31:339–44.

58. Asgari Z, Rouholamin S, Hosseini R, et al. Comparing ovarian reserve after laparoscopic excision of endometriotic cysts and hemostasis achieved either by bipolar coagulation or suturing: a randomized clinical trial. *Arch Gynecol Obstet.* 2016;293:1015–22.

59. Lokich E, Palisoul M, Romano N, et al. Assessing the risk of ovarian malignancy algorithm for the conservative management of women with a pelvic mass. *Gynecol Oncol.* 2015;139:248–52.

60. Gargiulo AR, Feltmate C, Srouji SS. Robotic single-site excision of ovarian endometrioma. *Fertil Res Pract.* 2015;1:19.

61. Vignali M, Mabrouk M, Ciocca E, et al. Surgical excision of ovarian endometriomas: does it truly impair ovarian reserve? Long term anti-müllerian hormone (AMH) changes after surgery. *J Obstet Gynaecol Res.* 2015;41:1773–8.

62. Lind T, Hammarström M, Lampic C, et al. Anti-Müllerian hormone reduction after ovarian cyst surgery is dependent on the histological cyst type and preoperative anti-müllerian hormone levels. *Acta Obstet Gynecol Scand.* 2015;94:183–90.

63. Rogers E, Allen L, Kives S. The recurrence rate of ovarian dermoid cysts in pediatric and adolescent girls. *J Pediatr Adolesc Gynecol.* 2014;27:222–8.

64. Busacca M, Marana R, Caruana P, et al. Recurrence of ovarian endometrioma after laparoscopic excision. *Am J Obstet Gynecol.* 1999;180:519–23.

65. Deffieux X, Morin Surroca M, Faivre E, et al. Tubal anastomosis after tubal sterilization: a review. *Arch Gynecol Obstet Rev.* 2011;283:1149–58.

66. Yoon TK, Sung HR, Kang HG, et al. Laparoscopic tubal anastomosis: fertility outcome in 202 cases. *Fertil Steril.* 1999;72:1121–6.

67. Rodgers AK, Goldberg JM, Hammel JP, et al. Tubal anastomosis by robotic compared with outpatient minilaparotomy. *Obstet Gynecol.* 2007;109:1375–80.

68. Dharia Patel SP, Steinkampf MP, Whitten SJ, et al. Robotic tubal anastomosis: surgical technique and cost effectiveness. *Fertil Steril.* 2008;90:1175–9.

69. Caillet M Fau, Vandromme J, Vandromme J Fau, Rozenberg S, Rozenberg S Fau, Paesmans M, et al. Robotically assisted laparoscopic microsurgical tubal reanastomosis: a retrospective study. *Fertil Steril.* 2010;94:1844–7.

70. The Practice Committee of the American Society for Reproductive Medicine. Role of tubal surgery in the era of assisted reproductive technology: a committee opinion. *Fertil Steril.* 2015;103:e37–43.

71. Berger GS, Thorp JM Jr, Weaver MA. Effectiveness of bilateral tubotubal anastomosis in a large outpatient population. *Hum Reprod.* 2016;31:1120–5.

72. Kavoussi SK, Kavoussi KM, Lebovic DI. Robotic-assisted tubal anastomosis with one-stitch technique. *J Robot Surg.* 2014;8:133–6.

Vasectomy Reversal

Daniel Greene and Edmund Sabanegh, Jr.

12.1 Background and History

Vasectomy is the safest and least expensive option for permanent sterilization and up to 354,000 men will undergo vasectomy reversal yearly in the United States [1,2]. Although vasectomy is considered permanent, up to 6% of men will ultimately seek a reversal [3]. Change in marital status is cited as the most common reason for seeking a reversal and younger age at time of vasectomy also is predictive of reversal [1]. A case–control study demonstrated that age < 30 years and spousal employment status are significant predictors of those seeking reversal [4]. There was no association with patient's occupation, religion, or number of children [4]. Another indication for vasectomy reversal is postvasectomy pain syndrome, which is a chronic condition of scrotal pain that is estimated to occur after 1 in 1,000 vasectomies [5]. Regardless of the reasons, vasectomy can be reversed with good success rates.

Vasectomy reversal represents a technically challenging and resource-intensive undertaking [1,6]. Vasovasostomy (VV) is the surgical anastomosis of segments of the vas deferens. Vasoepididymostomy (VE), in contrast, is the surgical anastomosis of the vas deferens to a portion of the epididymis. In 1903, Martin et al. reported the first technique for VE by creating a fistulous tract between the cut end of the vas and multiple incised epididymis tubules [6]. In 1919 Quinby reported the first successful VV for vasectomy reversal [7]. A 1948 urological survey revealed that 18% of urologists were performing vasectomy reversals with success rates of about 40% of patients [8]. Minimal advancement in the technique occurred until 1977 when Silber and Owen separately reported the first microsurgical single-tubule vasoepididymal anastomosis with significantly improved success rates [9,10].

12.2 Relevant Anatomy

Vasectomy represents an iatrogenic cause of obstructive azoospermia where a portion of the vas deferens is divided to prevent passage of sperm from the testes to the ejaculatory duct. An understanding of the relevant surgical anatomy is required to understand the surgical bypass procedure needed to restore continuity. Sperm begins its transit from the seminiferous tubules through the rete testis, efferent ductules, epididymis, vas deferens, ejaculatory duct, and then urethra (Figure 12.1). After reconstruction, patency is defined as any sperm in the ejaculate.

12.2.1 Epididymis

The epididymis is composed of a single, continuous, highly convoluted tubule contained within the tunica vaginalis. The lumen of the epididymis has a diameter that varies from 150 to 250 μm. The epididymis is divided into three anatomical segments: (1) the head (caput), (2) the body (corpora), and (3) the tail (cauda). The proximal epididymis is concerned with sperm maturation whereas the distal epididymis is concerned with sperm storage. Vasal anastomosis to the proximal epididymis has a decreased pregnancy rate when compared with those performed to the distal epididymis as it bypasses an area of critical importance for sperm maturation.

12.2.2 Vas Deferens

At the terminal end of the epididymis, a thick muscular wall surrounds the tubule and marks the proximal portion of the vas deferens. The vas deferens travels as a continuous tubule from the tail of the epididymis, through the spermatic cord, into the inguinal canal and into the pelvis where it joins with the seminal vesicles to form an ejaculatory duct. The ejaculatory duct enters the prostate posteriorly where sperms enter the urethra. The lumen of the vas deferens has a diameter of 400 μm, which is nearly twice that of the epididymis.

12.2.3 Blood Supply

The testicular artery emerges directly from the aorta and supplies the majority of the blood flow to the testis. Additional flow derives from the deferential and cremasteric arteries. In patients with history of vasectomy the deferential artery is likely compromised due to the procedure and special care should be exercised to preserve the testicular artery during dissection to avoid testicular ischemia.

The vas deferens receives its blood supply from two sources. The abdominal vas deferens receives its supply from the deferential artery. The testicular side of the vas deferens receives additional blood flow from free anastomosis between the supply to the epididymis, testicle, and vas deferens. After a vasectomy in which the deferential artery is ligated, the distal end of the vas deferens receives its supply from the supply to the testicle and epididymis in a retrograde fashion. If the vas deferens is sectioned in two locations the intervening portion is at risk of fibrosis due to ischemia.

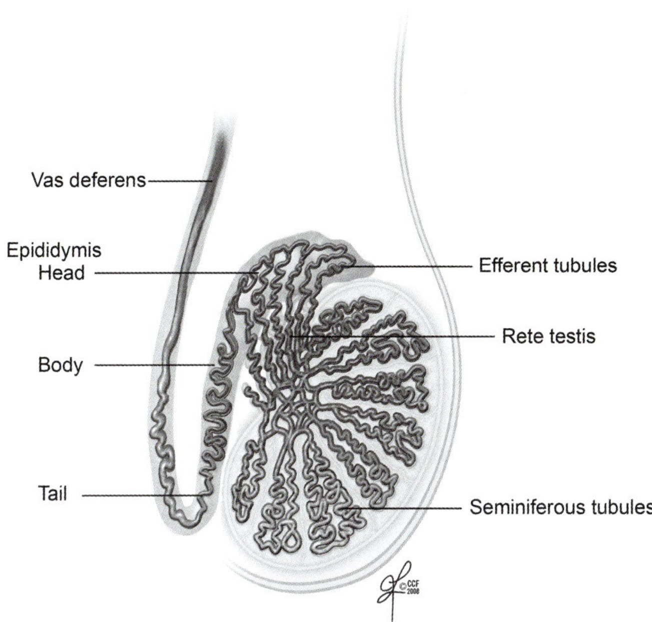

Figure 12.1 Sperm production begins in the seminiferous tubules and progresses through the rete testis, efferent tubules, epididymal head, body, tail, and then into the vas deferens. Reprinted with permission, Cleveland Clinic Center for Medical Art & Photography © 2007–2015. All Rights Reserved.

12.3 Patient Evaluation

Men seeking vasectomy reversal self-refer for surgical evaluation often with the direction of a primary care physician. Men with previous paternity and normal genitourinary exams do not require additional fertility evaluation before proceeding to surgery. Patients should be questioned about previous inguinal, scrotal, or pelvic surgery as these may complicate vasal reconstruction. A number of factors should be explored including the obstructive interval, age, and reproductive status of the female partner and history of previous reconstruction as these have been shown to impact the success rates. More recently, a significant number of men are presenting on testosterone replacement therapy. This can suppress spermatogenesis and should be assessed for alternative forms of medical therapy or cessation of replacement prior to reversal.

12.3.1 Obstructive Interval

The obstructive interval is defined as the length of time from the original vasectomy. Historically, an obstructive interval of greater than 10 years was thought to portend a poorer prognosis for vasectomy reversal. More recent publications, however, demonstrate that the classic dogma may not be true. The vasectomy study group examined their experience with nearly 1,500 reversals and found that the patency and pregnancy rates did decrease with time and that the pregnancy rate was proportional to the obstructive interval [11]. When grouped by obstructive interval, patency and pregnancy rates were 97% and 76%, respectively, for less than 3 years, 88% and 53% for 3–8 years, 79% and 44% for 9–14 years, and 71% and 30% for intervals greater than 15 years [11]. In contrast, in another series of 334 patients Magheli reported that obstructive interval did not influence

patency or pregnancy rates even in the group with intervals longer than 15 years [12]. Kolettis et al. retrospectively examined a group of 70 patients with extended obstructive intervals and found a patency and pregnancy rate of 74% and 40%, respectively, for obstructive intervals of 10–15 years, 87% and 36% for 16–19 years, and 75% and 27% for those with obstructive intervals longer than or equal to 20 years [13]. With good microsurgical techniques reasonable patency can be achieved after extended obstructive intervals, but the effect on pregnancy rate is less clear and likely contains many confounding factors.

12.3.2 Partner History

The age of the female partner significantly impacts post vasectomy reversal pregnancy rates as potential female fertility potential drops in women older than 40 years [13,14]. Gerrard and colleagues examined patency and pregnancy rates in a series of 249 couples in which the male underwent vasectomy reversal. Postoperative pregnancy and patency rates were 90% and 67%, respectively, for female partner age of 20–24, 89% and 52% for age 25–29, 90% and 57% for age 30–34, 86% and 54% for age 35–39, and 83% and 14% for female age 40 and older [14]. Similarly, Kolettis reviewed the records of men following vasectomy reversal with partners 35 years and older and noted a marked decrease in pregnancy rates in female partners 40 years or older [15].

By contrast the age of the male does not appear to independently influence patency or pregnancy after vasectomy reversal. In some series older male age is associated with longer obstructive intervals, which in turn may be associated with increased need to performed VE [13]. In couples where the partner's age may compromise natural pregnancy following reversal, additional evaluation and a discussion of assisted reproductive techniques should be considered.

12.3.3 Previous Reconstruction

Patients who have failed a previous vasectomy reversal should be considered for a repeat attempt at reconstruction. Paick reviewed a series of 62 repeat vasectomy reversals and demonstrated a patency and pregnancy rate of 92% and 52%, respectively [16]. Of note the authors performed a bilateral VV in all (97%) patients unless technically not feasible regardless of the quality of the intravasal fluid [16]. In a series by Hernandez and Sabanegh 41 patients underwent repeat vasectomy reversals, of which 20 required at least a unilateral VE with an overall patency and pregnancy rate of 79% and 31%, respectively [17]. Repeat surgical intervention should be considered even after failed prior VE. Pasqualottto reported a patency and pregnancy rate of 67% and 25%, respectively; in a series of 18 patients who underwent a repeat VE after a failed prior VE [18]. In patients who have failed a prior vasectomy reversal the literature supports a repeat attempt, but the surgeon should be prepared to perform a VE if required.

12.4 Post-Vasectomy Pain Syndrome

Vasectomy is considered a safe and efficacious procedure to prevent pregnancy; however, a small subset of patients are at risk for developing a chronic type of scrotal pain termed post-vasectomy pain syndrome (PVPS). The incidence of PVPS is estimated at 1 in 1,000 patients, but the true incidence has not been fully validated [19]. Initial options for treatment are conservative and include oral pain control, anti-inflammatory medications, scrotal support, and local anesthesia. Should these fail, one can consider surgical intervention including vasectomy reversal [19]. Horowitz reviewed their series of vasectomy reversals and noted 23 patients (15% of vasectomy reversals) who underwent reversal for PVPS in which pain improved in 93% of them and resolved in 50% [19]. Similarly, Nangia's series of 13 men with PVPS found 69% of had complete resolution of pain after VV [20]. Vasectomy reversal represents an established treatment with good success in patients who experience PVPS after conservative measures have failed.

12.5 Physical Exam

A physical exam should be performed on the patient seeking vasectomy reversal. Exam should focus on the scrotum and contents. The testes should be examined for normal size (>20 ml volume or 4 cm in length) and consistency. The exam may also reveal testicular abnormalities or epididymal induration. The vas deferens should be palpated with a goal to locate the vasectomy defect with annotation of the length of the defect. The presence of a sperm granuloma should be noted [21]. The epididymis should be palpated to examine for fullness and/or induration, which predicts epididymal obstruction, thus the increased possibility of VE (specificity 89%, sensitivity 33%] [22].

12.6 Epididymal Obstruction and Sperm Granuloma

Multiple techniques for division of the vas deferens exist during vasectomy, including suturing, metal clips, and electrocautery. All of the various techniques purport to achieve the same end: complete deferential obstruction. The obstruction, however, leads to increased intra vas deferential and epididymal pressures, rupture, and subsequent luminal obliteration [23]. Thus, vasectomy not only disrupts the site of vas deferens removal, but has the potential to create a more proximal blockage which would require VE to bypass.

A sperm granuloma is a collection of extravasated sperm found at the proximal end of the divided vas deferens in men who have previously undergone vasectomy. These can range in size from millimeters to centimeters. Sperm granulomas are thought to act as a "pop-off" valve. Some have suggested that they protect the epididymis from increased pressure as a result of vasectomy and thus, if found, would lead to better success rates with reversal. However, the Vasectomy Study Group found no difference in either patency or pregnancy rates based on the presence of a sperm granuloma [11]. In another series of 213 men who underwent vasectomy reversal, 28% had at least a unilateral granuloma [21]. Of those who had a unilateral granuloma, 14% required VE compared with 31% in their overall series [21]. The patency and pregnancy did not statistically differ based on the presence of a granuloma (patency

95 vs 78%, $p = 0.07$; pregnancy 83 vs 78%, $p > 0.05$) [21]. These sources contrast with a third series in which sperm granuloma was found to increase both patency and pregnancy rates [24]. If a sperm granuloma is found at the time of initial exam or at reconstruction it may increase the post-surgical patency and pregnancy; and decrease the need for VE.

12.7 Surgical Technique

Since the initial publications in 1977, microsurgical vasectomy reversal has become the gold standard, setting the benchmark in terms of patency and pregnancy rates [9,10]. Microsurgical repair is superior when compared with pregnancy and patency due to loupe magnification and unmagnified repair [25–27]. General or spinal anesthesia may be preferred to local anesthesia due to the duration of the case and need for minimal to no patient movement. The patient should be placed in the supine position, and his pubic hair clipped and adequately removed to prevent interference with suture visualization. Prophylactic antibiotics should be provided and sequential compression devices used. The vasal defects should be palpated and brought to the skin. High vertical scrotal incisions directed toward the external inguinal ring no longer than 2 cm are made over the defect. The dartos is divided until the vas deferens is identified and brought up to the field.

Healthy appearing vasa deferentia are identified proximal to and distal to the vasectomy defects. The vasa are then carefully dissected with judicious electrocautery in order to preserve maximal perfusion. Battery-powered hand-operated electrocautery instruments can be useful during dissection as these have a very limited area of collateral tissue damage. Vessel loops or fine stay sutures are placed in the vasal adventia to assist with retraction. The vascular pedicle to the vasa is then ligated with 6-0 polypropylene suture to the level of the proposed anastomosis. When additional vas length is needed to perform a tension-free anastomosis, the distal vas can be mobilized on its vascular pedicle into the inguinal canal to gain several additional centimeters of length (Figure 12.2).

After mobilization and vascular control the operative microscope is moved over the operative field. The microscope should be positioned such that the surgeon and assistant can work comfortably and thus minimize unnecessary movement. Success rates are similar between anastomosis to the straight and convoluted vasa; therefore, healthy tissue should be sought [28]. The proximal vasa is then divided perpendicular to its axis with a Beaver blade or a super-sharp ophthalmic blade. The division may be performed with free hand or against a surface such as a tongue blade or a cutting guide. Fluid from the proximal vasa is obtained with the possible aid of gentle milking of the vas or epididymis, and examined under a bench-top microscope. A touch prep of the effluent can be prepared by touching a sterile slide to the proximal vas. Alternatively, the effluent can be aspirated through a small angiocatheter attached to a sterile tuberculin syringe preloaded with a small amount of saline.

The decision to continue with VV or perform a VE depends on the findings when examining the vasal effluent. Based on the gross and microscopic findings one should proceed with a

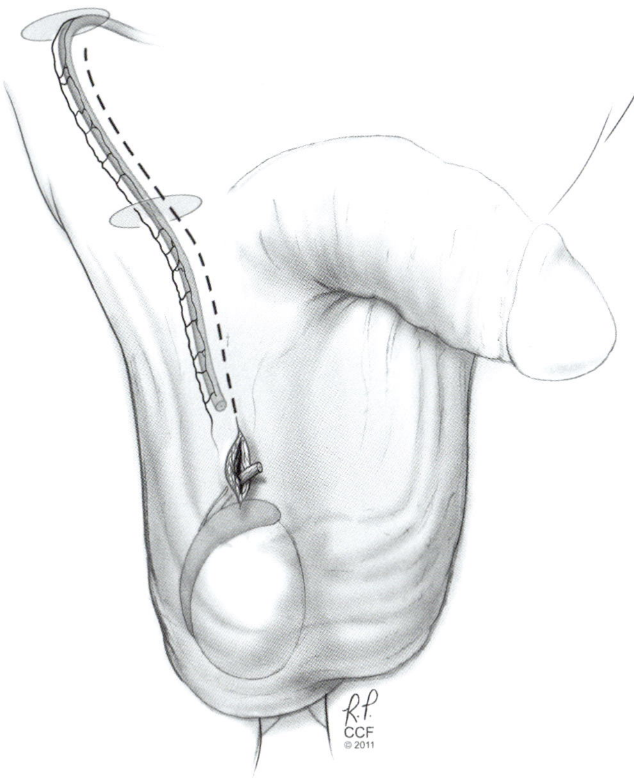

Figure 12.2 Additional vas deferens length can be obtained by extending the scrotal incision toward the external inguinal ring and mobilization of the vas. Reprinted with permission, Cleveland Clinic Center for Medical Art & Photography © 2007–2015. All Rights Reserved.

Table 12.1 Surgical Recommendation based on Gross and Microscopic Vasal Fluid Findings

Gross Vasal Fluid	Microscopic Findings	Recommendation
Creamy, cloudy, or clear	Motile sperm	VV
	Sperm, nonmotile	VV
	Sperm heads	VV
Copious clear fluid	No sperm	VV
Thick "toothpaste-like" fluid	No sperm	VE
No fluid	No sperm (after irrigation)	VE

VV or move to a VE (Table 12.1). In situations where intravasal azoospermia and an absence of fluid is encountered and VE is unable to be performed due to inadequate vasal length, a VV should be performed as a small subset will still be patent [29]. If suspicion of distal obstruction is present (childhood inguinal hernia repair, prior unsuccessful vasectomy reversal), distal vasal patency can be confirmed with a saline vasogram, radiographic vasogram, simultaneous cystoscopy and methylene blue vasal flush, or intubation with a 0-nylon suture. Often the proximal and distal ends are of discordant sizing due to the proximal vasal dilation upstream of an obstruction. Some choose to dilate the distal vasa with lacrimal duct probes or tips

of microforceps. The ends of the vasa are held in proximity with gentle traction on stay stiches or in a VV clamp. If tension is present nearby tissue can be approximated such that tension-free anastomosis can be performed. A fine-tip marker can be used to place symmetric microdots on the cut edge of the vasa to mark the planned suture exit sites to help facilitate precise suture placement [30]. VV can be performed with a two-layer anastomosis or a modified one-layer. The two techniques yield similar patency and pregnancy rates [31,32]. The two-layer anastomosis may provide better approximation for anastomosis with vasa with large discrepancies in lumen size. The two-layer anastomosis is slower than the modified one-layer, however [31].

12.7.1 Two-Layer Anastomosis

The two-layer anastomosis begins by securing the vasal adventia with two interrupted 9-0 nylon sutures on the posterior side of the anastomosis (Figure 12.3A). Next, interrupted 10-0 nylon sutures are placed in the mucosal layer starting on the posterior aspect (Figure 12.3B). The first two to three posterior sutures can be gently tied to approximate the delicate mucosal tissue. Additional interrupted 10-0 nylon sutures are placed working posterior to anterior until a total of six to eight evenly placed mucosal sutures are present (Figure 12.3C). The sutures should be placed such that the knots are outside of the vasal lumen. The second layer is completed by placing an additional four to five interrupted 9-0 nylon sutures through the advential and muscularis layer of the anterior vas (Figure 12.3D). Additional nylon sutures (up to 6-0) can be used to approximate the vasal sheath if desired.

12.7.2 Modified One-Layer Anastomosis

The approach to a modified one-layer anastomosis remains identical to that of the traditional two-layer anastomosis in terms of exposure and dissection. The technique diverges during re-anastomosis of the isolated vasal ends. Two to three full-thickness 9-0 nylon sutures are placed through the vasal mucosa, muscularis, and adventitia and secured with a knot outside of the lumen (Figure 12.4A). The surgeon can either start on the posterior aspect of the vasa and move forward, or can start anteriorly and rotate the vasa to suture posteriorly. A total of four to six evenly placed full-thickness 9-0 nylon sutures are required to create a water-tight mucosal anastomosis (Figure 12.4B). After the lumen is reconstructed a second layer of partial thickness 9-0 nylon sutures are placed in between the full-thickness sutures through the adventia and muscularis to finalize the anastomosis (Figure 12.4C).

12.7.3 Vasoepididymostomy

If an epididymal obstruction is suspected, a VE should be performed. Modern techniques for VE center upon identifying and then directly anastomosing a single-patent epididymal tubule to the much larger and sturdier lumen of the vas deferens. The early vasoepididymostomies were performed in an end-to-end fashion. The technique was gradually refined to include end-to-side anastomosis, three-suture intussusception, and two-suture intussusception [9,33–35]. End-to-end and end-to-side anastomosis allow easy examination of the

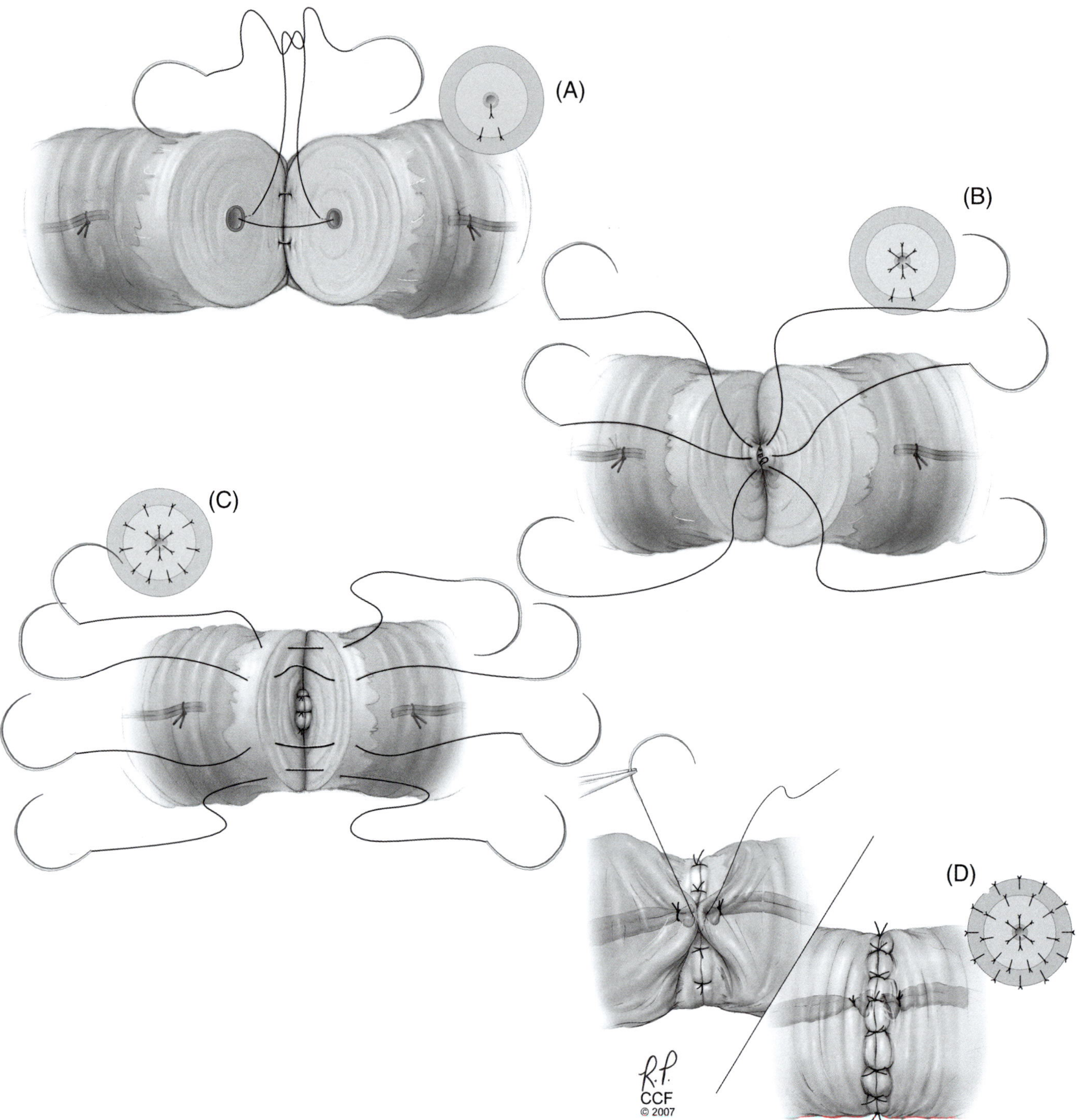

Figure 12.3 The two-layer vasovasostomy anastomosis. (A) After placement of two interrupted posterior sutures the mucosa is approximated posteriorly. (B) The anterior mucosa is then further approximated with several additional interrupted sutures. (C) After mucosal approximation the second layer is completed by four to five additional interrupted sutures through the adventitia. (D) An additional nylon suture can be used to reapproximate the vasal sheath. Reprinted with permission, Cleveland Clinic Center for Medical Art & Photography © 2007–2015. All Rights Reserved.

epididymal fluid prior to anastomosis, however, are technically more challenging. In contrast, intussusceptive techniques are easier to perform, but the surgeon cannot assess epididymal fluid prior to anastomotic setup. When the site of obstruction is clearly visible an end-to-side intussusception is the preferred technique, when unclear; however, a traditional end-to-end anastomosis will allow serial sectioning of the epididymis until effluent is visualized from a single epididymal tubule.

The vertically oriented incision described for VV can be extended inferiorly and the testis delivered into the field. The tunica vaginalis is opened and the epididymis is inspected. The site of obstruction can often be viewed as a transition point with a firm and dilated proximal epididymis. Occasionally, the location of obstruction is observed by the presence of lipofuscin, a blue-brown pigment caused by the breakdown of extravasated sperm. Less often, the level of obstruction may not be readily visualized.

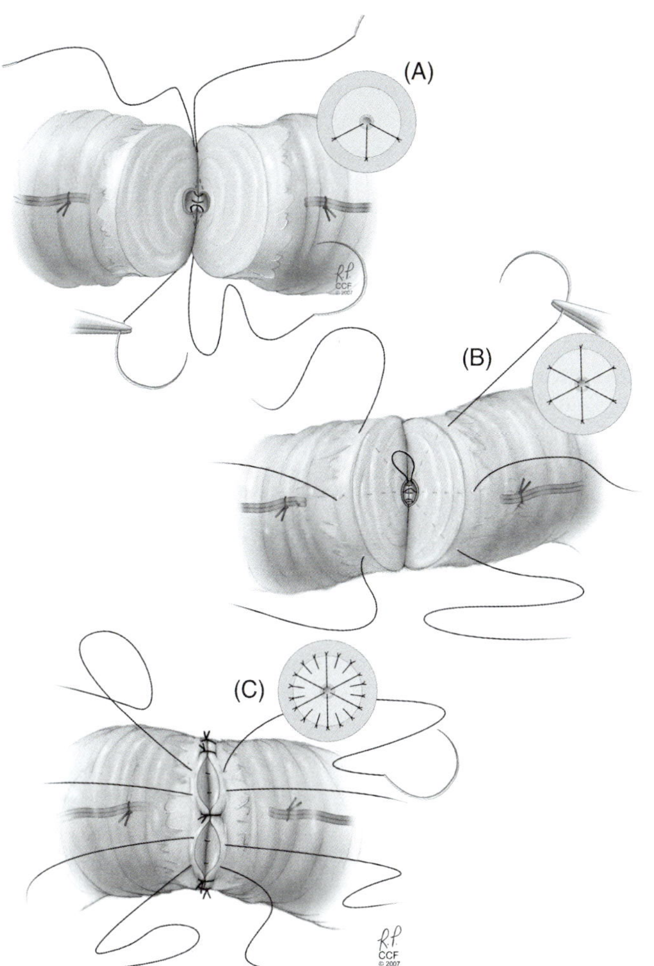

Figure 12.4 The modified one-layer anastomosis. (A) Three full-thickness sutures are placed on the posterior side of the vas deferens through all layers. (B) Three additional evenly spaced interrupted nylon sutures are placed through all layers of the vas deferens. (C) After the lumen is reconstructed one to two sutures are placed between each full-thickness suture through the adventitia and muscularis to finalize the anastomosis. Reprinted with permission, Cleveland Clinic Center for Medical Art & Photography © 2007–2015. All Rights Reserved.

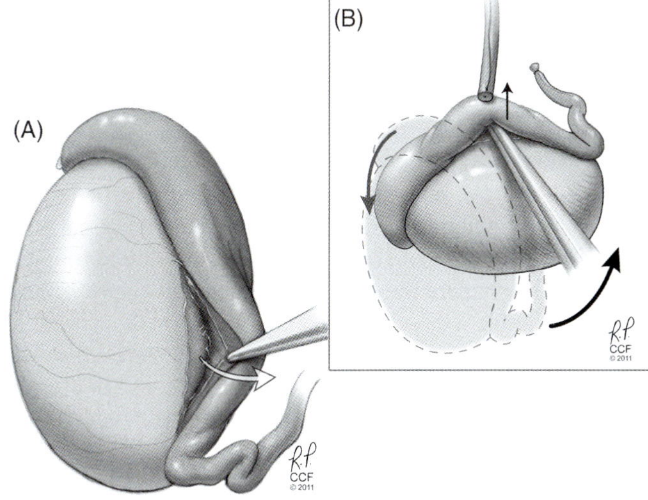

Figure 12.5 (A) The tail of the epididymis can also be mobilized by dividing the relatively avascular plane of the lateral sulcus at the junction of the epididymis and testis allowing the tail to swing superiorly. (B) If further length is needed the entire testis and epididymis can be rotated on its horizontal axis, thus inverting the testis. Reprinted with permission, Cleveland Clinic Center for Medical Art & Photography © 2007–2015. All Rights Reserved.

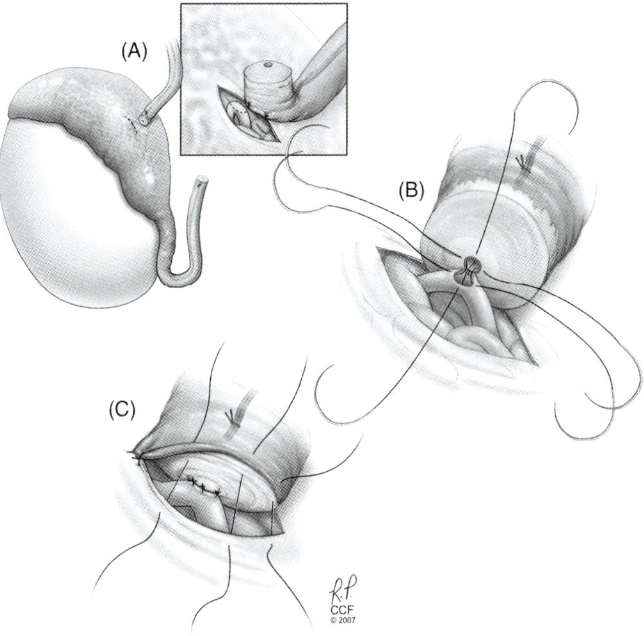

Figure 12.6 End-to-side vasoepididymostomy. (A) A 5 mm incision is made through the tunica albuginea overlying the target tubule. The adventitia of the vas is secured to the tunica albuginea with two interrupted sutures. A 1 mm incision is made longitudinally into the target epididymal tubule. (B) After incision into the tubule and assessment of the effluent three double-armed nylon sutures are placed through the epididymal wall and vasal mucosa such that the knots when tied will lay outside of the lumen. (C) After tying the anastomotic sutures the tunica albuginea is secured to the vasal adventitia. Reprinted with permission, Cleveland Clinic Center for Medical Art & Photography © 2007–2015. All Rights Reserved.

A tension-free anastomosis is of critical importance during VE and requires additional vasal mobilization compared to VV. Additional length can be obtained from inguinal vasal mobilization (Figure 12.2). Often, inguinal mobilization is performed through the scrotal incision, but when necessary, the incision can be extended superiorly to the external inguinal ring. It is important to maintain hemostasis while ensuring adequate blood supply to the vas via the pedicle. The tail of the epididymis can also be mobilized by dividing the relatively avascular plane of the lateral sulcus at the junction of the epididymis and testis allowing the tail to swing superiorly (Figure 12.5A). If further length is needed the entire testis and epididymis can be rotated on its horizontal axis, thus inverting the testis (Figure 12.5B). With careful application these maneuvers should not compromise blood supply to the testis.

Once adequate length has been dissected to obtain a tension-free anastomosis and the site of epididymal obstruction is identified a 5 mm incision is made through the tunica albuginea overlying the target tubule (Figure 12.6A). The most distal epididymal tubule without obstruction should be sought as studies suggest improved pregnancy rates, likely a reflection of the maturation function of the epididymis. Sharp dissection is continued under high magnification (25×) to mobilize the candidate tubule with extremely judicious use of bipolar cautery or handheld low-temperature cautery for hemostasis. Saline irrigation through an angiocatheter may aid in visualization. The adventitia of the vas deferens is secured to the tunica albuginea of the epididymis with a 9-0 nylon suture.

For the conventional end-to-side anastomosis a microknife or microscissors is used to make a 0.5–1 mm incision on the side of the candidate tubule. A 10-0 nylon suture is placed through the lip of the tubule to aid in identification of the mucosal edge. The effluent is assessed, and whole, preferably motile sperm, should be found. Two to three additional 10-0 nylon sutures are placed evenly around the incision to triangulate or quadrangulate the epididymal opening (Figure 12.6B). Single- or double-arm sutures may be used and all knots should lie outside of the lumen. The 10-0 sutures are passed through the corresponding sectors in the vasal mucosa and tied while supporting the vas in close proximity to the epididymal tubule. Several additional 9-0 nylon supporting sutures are placed circumferentially between the adventitia and tunica albuginea (Figure 12.6C).

An end-to-side intussusception technique can also be employed, which makes precise needle placement easier as the sutures are placed before the tubule is opened and decompressed. As with the conventional method a candidate tubule is identified and widely mobilized so it can be drawn into the vasal lumen. The adventitia of the vas is secured to the tunica albuginea of the epididymis with an interrupted 9-0 nylon suture (Figure 12.7A). The first needle of a double-armed 10-0 nylon is passed in and then out of the wall of the tubule, but the throw is not completed anchoring the body of the needle in the epididymal tubule (Figure 12.7A). An additional one to two sutures are similarly passed depending on if a two- or three-suture intussusception technique is preferred. The epididymis is then sharply incised longitudinally in between the sutures and the fluid assessed. The needles within the epididymal tubule are pulled through and then all arms are passed inside to out through the vasal mucosa (Figure 12.7B). The 10-0 nylon sutures are gently pulled and tied to invaginate the epididymis inside the lumen of the vas (Figure 12.7C). Additional 9-0 nylon sutures are placed to secure the vas deferens to the tunical albuginea of the epididymis. The tunica vaginalis, dartos, and skin are closed in accordance with standard practice with attention to hemostasis.

Postoperative care includes local dressing and ice packs for 2–3 days following surgery. Supportive underwear should be utilized for 2 weeks. Patients are advised to avoid strenuous activity and sexual intercourse for 3 weeks following VV and VE. Oral analgesics are usually sufficient for postoperative pain control. Semen analysis should be obtained every 2–3 months until sperm count returns to normal or a pregnancy is achieved.

12.8 Outcomes

Since the advent of microsurgical vasectomy reversal patency and pregnancy rates have improved significantly compared to the earlier methods. VV leads to sperm in the ejaculate in 85–99% of the cases and pregnancy in 50–60% of the reversals [11,36]. In contrast, VE leads to sperm in the ejaculate in 70–85% of the men after surgery and pregnancy in 40–55% of the cases [9,33,37]. The published rates of success after

VE represent a heterogeneous group of patients with vasal obstruction with only a subset resulting from prior vasectomy [9,33,37]. Although the majority of patients can obtain sperm in their ejaculate following reconstruction, only a subset will achieve pregnancy. An interesting study performed by Sharlip examined men who after vasectomy reversal had completely normal postoperative sperm counts ($>20 \times 10^6$/ml) and found that the rate of natural pregnancy was only 61% [38]. Rates of pregnancy depend on multiple factors including partner fertility, epididymal dysfunction, and sperm antibodies [38].

Following vasal reconstruction the mean time to observance of motile sperm are 2.1 and 5.8 months for VV and VE, respectively [39]. More than 90% of patients who have motile sperm will do so at 6 and 12 months for VV and VE, respectively [39]. Nonmotile sperm returns earlier than motile sperm [39]. Factors associated with a more rapid return of motile sperm following vasectomy reversal are an obstructive interval less than 8 years, motile sperm intraoperative, and VV (compared with VE) [40]. The late failure rate defined as the transition from patency to azoospermia is 4–12% for VV and 10–20% for VE [11,39,41]. Patients are considered a reversal failure 3–6 months after VV and 12 months after VE. If failure is encountered men may be offered a repeat attempt or may pursue assisted reproductive technology.

Complications following vasectomy reversal are uncommon. The most common complication is hematoma, which can be prevented with meticulous hemostasis. If a hematoma develops the surgeon should consider evacuation to prevent interference with the fragile vasal anastomosis. Infections are uncommon with good sterile technique and perioperative antibiotics. If an infection develops it should be treated with oral antibiotics and local wound care. Devascularization of the testis can be prevented with cautious dissection to avoid injury of the testicular artery.

12.9 Vasectomy Reversal and Assisted Reproductive Technology

In the era of advanced assisted reproductive technologies, microsurgical vasectomy reversal remains an important modality. Reversal provides an opportunity for couples to create a spontaneous pregnancy and thus avoid the expense, limitations, and risks of in vitro fertilization (IVF) or intracytoplasmic sperm injection (ICSI). IVF with ICSI is associated with a 30% risk of multiple gestations, many times higher than that of spontaneous pregnancy [42]. Further, ovarian hyperstimulation syndrome is a potentially life-threatening condition associated with IVF and is estimated to occur in a moderate and severe form in 3–6% and 0.1–2% of the patients, respectively [43]. Additionally, there exists risks for the progeny including low birth weight, prematurity, and chromosomal abnormalities [44,45]. Although the best options for some couples will be ICSI/IVF, in those without significant female factor infertility the safety of natural conception and the options for multiple sequential pregnancies remain compelling justifications for surgical vasectomy reversal.

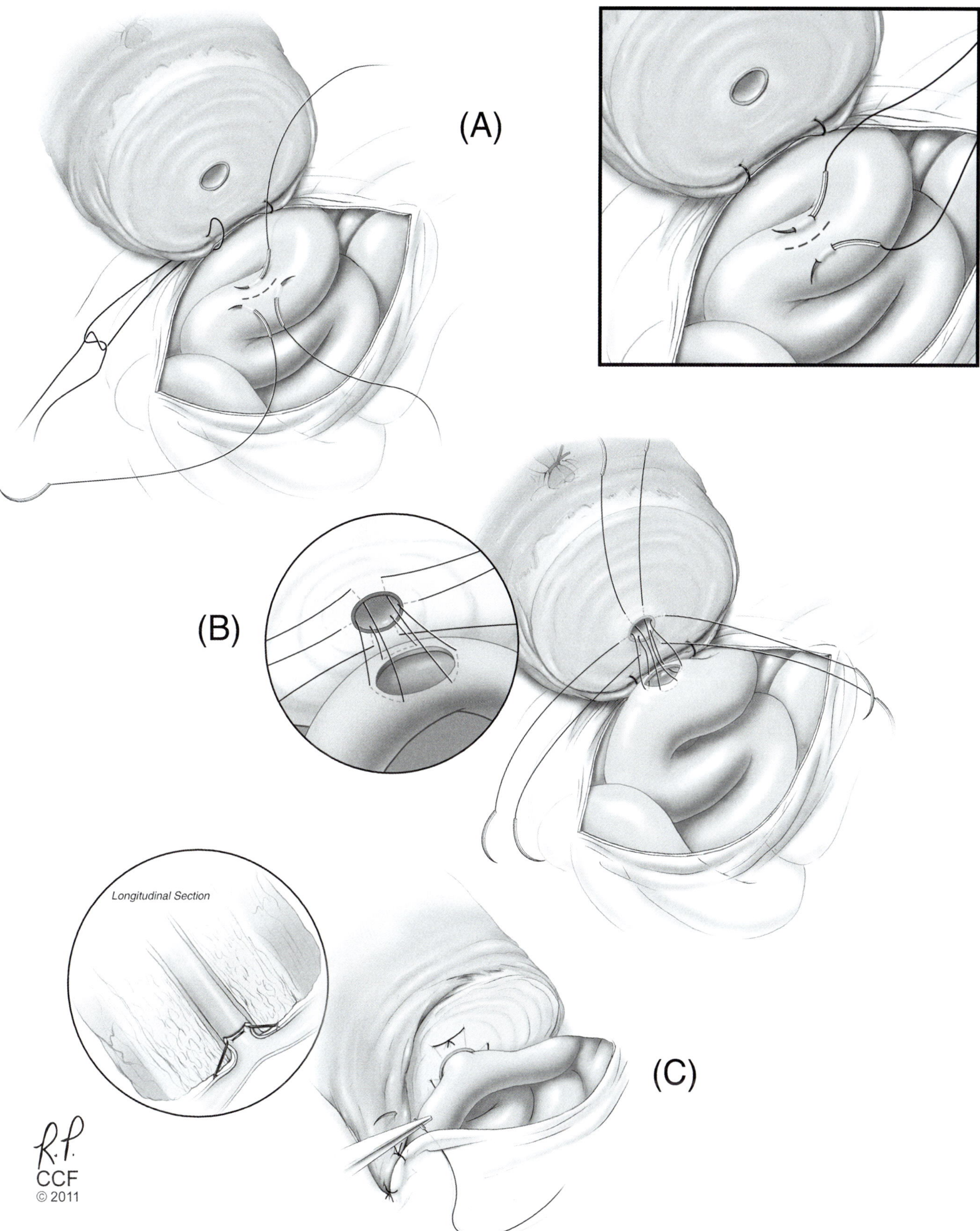

Figure 12.7 End-to-side intussusception vasoepididymostomy. (A) After opening the tunica albuginea and securing the vasal adventia to the tunica albuginea in a similar fashion to the traditional end-to-side anastomosis, three double-armed sutures are placed such that the needle remains in the tubule. Inset – alternatively two sutures can be placed. (B) The epididymis is the incision in between the sutures and the needle throws are completed and the same needles are passed inside-out in the vasal mucosa. (C) The nylon sutures are gently pulled and tied to invaginate the epididymis inside the lumen of the vas, then the tunica albuginea is secured to the adventitia of the vas. Reprinted with permission, Cleveland Clinic Center for Medical Art & Photography © 2007–2015. All Rights Reserved.

Another argument in favor of microsurgical vasectomy reversal compared with IVF/ICSI is the decreased cost. A series comparing the success rates and cost of those undergoing VV and IVF appreciated a higher rate of pregnancy (52% vs 22.5%) and a decreased cost (€29,000 vs €15,000) in the VV group [46]. Another analysis concluded that the more complex and less successful VE was still more cost effective than IVF/ICSI [47]. Decision analysis modeling suggests that in order for microsurgical vasectomy reversal to be cost effective compared with IVF a patency rate of 79% or greater is required [48]. During vasectomy reversal, especially if VE is required, sperm can be harvested in the event that future ICSI or IVF is required, which would lead to decreased expense in the event of failure [49]. Currently, there remains a fundamental role for microsurgical vasectomy reversal in patients who wish to restore their fertility.

12.10 New Advances

12.10.1 Robotic Vasectomy Reversal

The Da Vinci robotic surgical system (Intuitive Surgical, Inc., Sunnyvale, CA) has been applied to multiple surgical domains including urology. Some have hypothesized that the reduced motion and surgeon tremor dampening may allow improved outcomes compared to traditional microsurgical vasectomy reversal [50]. In humans, the procedure involves specialized microneedle drivers and a specialized video system showing the Da Vinci Si 3D camera view, 16–20× optical camera lens system, and a high magnification view from the andrology lab [51]. Although the series reports an improved robotic-assisted VV outcome compared with microsurgical VV (>1 million sperm count 96% vs 80%) the microsurgical success rate is generally lower than the majority of published series [11,51]. The report concludes that their microsurgical and robotic-assisted VE patency and pregnancy rates are similar [11,51]. Robotic-assisted vasectomy reversal is an appealing advancement, but is associated with a significant increase in cost with only equivocal outcomes, and therefore is not widely recommended at the current time.

12.10.2 Anastomotic Adjuncts

Further attempts to improve outcomes and ease of vasectomy reversal have focused on stents and glues. In one series, VV was performed with three 9-0 nylon sutures 120° apart after which the vas deferens was sealed with fibrin glue [52]. Patency rates (85%) were acceptable with a mean operative time of 80 minutes [52]. Although fibrin glue may allow a shorter duration VV there exist concerns regarding disease transmission as the glue is derived from pooled plasma [53]. Nonabsorbable vasal stents have also been investigated in animal models during vasal reconstruction and present an interesting area of future development [54].

12.11 Conclusions

Microsurgical vasectomy reversal is a viable option following vasectomy. The rates of patency and pregnancy following VV

are excellent while those for VE are reasonable. Even in the era of advanced reproductive techniques microsurgical vasectomy reversal remains the preferred method of fertility restoration. There are numerous emerging technologies that may improve outcomes of vasectomy reversal and remain to be studied.

References

1. Dassow P, Bennett JM. Vasectomy: an update. *Am Fam Physician*. 2006;74(12):2069–74.

2. Eisenberg ML, Lipshultz LI. Estimating the number of vasectomies performed annually in the United States: data from the National Survey of Family Growth. *J Urol*. 2010;184(5):2068–72.

3. Sandlow JI, Nagler HM. Vasectomy and vasectomy reversal: important issues preface. *Urol Clin N Am*. 2009;36(3):xiii–xiv.

4. Potts JM, Pasqualotto FF, Nelson D, Thomas AJ, Agarwal A. Patient characteristics associated with vasectomy reversal. *J Urol*. 1999;161(6):1835–9.

5. Horovitz D, Tjong V, Domes T, Lo K, Grober ED, Jarvi K. Vasectomy reversal provides long-term pain relief for men with the post-vasectomy pain syndrome. *J Urol*. 2012;187(2):613–17.

6. Chan PT. The evolution and refinement of vasoepididymostomy techniques. *Asian J Androl*. 2013;15(1):49–55.

7. Herrel L, Hsiao W. Microsurgical vasovasostomy. *Asian J Androl*. 2013;15(1):44–8.

8. O'Conor VJ. Anastomosis of the vas deferens after purposeful division for sterility. *J Urol*. 1948;59(2):229–33.

9. Silber SJ. Microscopic vasoepididymostomy: specific microanastomosis to the epididymal tubule. *Fertil Steril*. 1978;30(5):565–71.

10. Owen ER. Microsurgical vasovasostomy: a reliable vasectomy reversal. *Aust N Z J Surg*. 1977;47(3):305–9.

11. Belker AM, Thomas AJ, Jr., Fuchs EF, Konnak JW, Sharlip ID. Results of 1,469 microsurgical vasectomy reversals by the Vasovasostomy Study Group. *J Urol*. 1991;145(3):505–11.

12. Magheli A, Rais-Bahrami S, Kempkensteffen C, Weiske WH, Miller K, Hinz S. Impact of obstructive interval and sperm granuloma on patency and pregnancy after vasectomy reversal. *Int J Androl*. 2010;33(5):730–5.

13. Kolettis PN, Sabanegh ES, D'Amico AM, Box L, Sebesta M, Burns JR. Outcomes for vasectomy reversal performed after obstructive intervals of at least 10 years. *Urology*. 2002;60(5):885–8.

14. Gerrard ER, Jr., Sandlow JI, Oster RA, Burns JR, Box LC, Kolettis PN. Effect of female partner age on pregnancy rates after vasectomy reversal. *Fertil Steril*. 2007;87(6):1340–4.

15. Kolettis PN, Sabanegh ES, Nalesnik JG, D'Amico AM, Box LC, Burns JR. Pregnancy outcomes after vasectomy reversal for female partners 35 years old or older. *J Urol*. 2003;169(6):2250–2.

16. Paick JS, Park JY, Park DW, Park K, Son H, Kim SW. Microsurgical vasovasostomy after failed vasovasostomy. *J Urol*. 2003;169(3):1052–5.

17. Hernandez J, Sabanegh ES. Repeat vasectomy reversal after initial failure: overall results and predictors for success. *J Urology*. 1999;161(4):1153–6.

18. Pasqualotto FF, Agarwal A, Srivastava M, Nelson DR, Thomas AJ, Jr. Fertility outcome after repeat vasoepididymostomy. *J Urol.* 1999;162(5):1626–8.

19. Horovitz D, Tjong V, Domes T, Lo K, Grober ED, Jarvi K. Vasectomy reversal provides long-term pain relief for men with the post-vasectomy pain syndrome. *J Urol.* 2012;187(2):613–17.

20. Nangia AK, Myles JL, Thomas AJ. Vasectomy reversal for the post-vasectomy pain syndrome: a clinical and histological evaluation. *J Urol.* 2000;164(6):1939–42.

21. Boorjian S, Lipkin M, Goldstein M. The impact of obstructive interval and sperm granuloma on outcome of vasectomy reversal. *J Urol.* 2004;171(1):304–6.

22. Kolettis PN. Is physical examination useful in predicting epididymal obstruction? *Urology.* 2001;57(6):1138–40.

23. Silber SJ. Epididymal extravasation following vasectomy as a cause for failure of vasectomy reversal. *Fertil Steril.* 1979;31(3):309–15.

24. Bolduc S, Fischer MA, Deceuninck G, Thabet M. Factors predicting overall success: a review of 747 microsurgical vasovasostornies. *Cuaj-Can Urol Assoc.* 2007;1(4):388–94.

25. Lee L, McLoughlin MG. Vasovasostomy: a comparison of macroscopic and microscopic techniques at one institution. *Fertil Steril.* 1980;33(1):54–5.

26. Dewire DM, Lawson RK. Experience with macroscopic vasectomy reversal at the Medical College of Wisconsin. *Wis Med J.* 1994;93(3):107–9.

27. Jee SH, Hong YK. One-layer vasovasostomy: microsurgical versus loupe-assisted. *Fertil Steril.* 2010;94(6):2308–11.

28. Patel SR, Sigman M. Comparison of outcomes of vasovasostomy performed in the convoluted and straight vas deferens. *J Urol.* 2008;179(1):256–9.

29. Sheynkin YR, Chen ME, Goldstein M. Intravasal azoospermia: a surgical dilemma. *BJU Int.* 2000;85(9):1089–92.

30. Goldstein M, Li PSH, Matthews GJ. Microsurgical vasovasostomy: the microdot technique of precision suture placement. *J Urol.* 1998;159(1):188–90.

31. Fischer MA, Grantmyre JE. Comparison of modified one- and two-layer microsurgical vasovasostomy. *BJU Int.* 2000;85(9):1085–8.

32. Sharlip ID. Vasovasostomy: comparison of two microsurgical techniques. *Urology.* 1981;17(4):347–52.

33. Thomas AJ, Jr. Vasoepididymostomy. *Urol Clin North Am.* 1987;14(3):527–38.

34. Berger RE. Triangulation end-to-side vasoepididymostomy. *J Urol.* 1998;159(6):1951–3.

35. Marmar JL. Modified vasoepididymostomy with simultaneous double needle placement, tubulotomy and tubular invagination. *J Urol.* 2000;163(2):483–6.

36. Chan PT, Goldstein M. Superior outcomes of microsurgical vasectomy reversal in men with the same female partners. *Fertil Steril.* 2004;81(5):1371–4.

37. Chan PT, Brandell RA, Goldstein M. Prospective analysis of outcomes after microsurgical intussusception vasoepididymostomy. *BJU Int.* 2005;96(4):598–601.

38. Sharlip ID. What is the best pregnancy rate that may be expected from vasectomy reversal. *J Urol.* 1993;149(6):1469–71.

39. Matthews GJ, Schlegel PN, Goldstein M. Patency following microsurgical vasoepididymostomy and vasovasostomy: temporal considerations. *J Urol.* 1995;154(6):2070–3.

40. Yang G, Walsh TJ, Shefi S, Turek PJ. The kinetics of the return of motile sperm to the ejaculate after vasectomy reversal. *J Urol.* 2007;177(6):2272–6.

41. Jarow JP, Sigman M, Buch JP, Oates RD. Delayed appearance of sperm after end-to-side vasoepididymostomy. *J Urol.* 1995;153(4):1156–8.

42. Boulet SL, Mehta A, Kissin DM, Warner L, Kawwass JF, Jamieson DJ. Trends in use of and reproductive outcomes associated with intracytoplasmic sperm injection. *JAMA.* 2015;313(3):255–63.

43. Delvigne A. Symposium: update on prediction and management of OHSS. Epidemiology of OHSS. *Reprod Biomed Online.* 2009;19(1):8–13.

44. Hansen M, Kurinczuk JJ, Bower C, Webb S. The risk of major birth defects after intracytoplasmic sperm injection and in vitro fertilization. *New Engl J Med.* 2002;346(10):725–30.

45. Schieve LA, Meikle SF, Ferre C, Peterson HB, Jeng G, Wilcox LS. Low and very low birth weight in infants conceived with use of assisted reproductive technology. *New Engl J Med.* 2002;346(10):731–7.

46. Heidenreich A, Altmann P, Engelmann UH. Microsurgical vasovasostomy versus microsurgical epididymal sperm aspiration/testicular extraction of sperm combined with intracytoplasmic sperm injection. A cost-benefit analysis. *Eur Urol.* 2000;37(5):609–14.

47. Kolettis PN, Thomas AJ, Jr. Vasoepididymostomy for vasectomy reversal: a critical assessment in the era of intracytoplasmic sperm injection. *J Urol.* 1997;158(2):467–70.

48. Meng MV, Greene KL, Turek PJ. Surgery or assisted reproduction? A decision analysis of treatment costs in male infertility. *J Urol.* 2005;174(5):1926–31; discussion 31.

49. Glazier DB, Marmar JL, Mayer E, Gibbs M, Corson SL. The fate of cryopreserved sperm acquired during vasectomy reversals. *J Urol.* 1999;161(2):463–6.

50. Schiff J, Li PS, Goldstein M. Robotic microsurgical vasovasostomy and vasoepididymostomy: a prospective randomized study in a rat model. *J Urol.* 2004;171(4):1720–5.

51. Parekattil SJ, Gudeloglu A, Brahmbhatt J, Wharton J, Priola KB. Robotic assisted versus pure microsurgical vasectomy reversal: technique and prospective database control trial. *J Reconstr Microsurg.* 2012;28(7):435–44.

52. Ho KL, Witte MN, Bird ET, Hakim S. Fibrin glue assisted 3-suture vasovasostomy. *J Urol.* 2005;174(4 Pt 1):1360–3; discussion 3.

53. Kolettis PN. Restructuring reconstructive techniques – advances in reconstructive techniques. *Urol Clin North Am.* 2008;35(2):229–34, viii–ix.

54. Vrijhof EJ, de Bruine A, Zwinderman AH, Nijeholt AABL, Koole LH. The use of a newly designed nonabsorbable polymeric stent in reconstructing the vas deferens: a feasibility study in New Zealand white rabbits. *BJU Int.* 2005;95(7):1081–5.

Varicocele Repair

Christopher M. Deibert, Brooke A. Harnisch, and Jay I. Sandlow

13.1 Introduction

Varicoceles are the most common diagnosis of male subfertility (Table 13.1). In the general population, varicocele affects about 13% of men, while 35–40% of subfertile men have varicoceles. The presence of a varicocele can impair testicular function and sperm production [1].

13.2 Effect of Varicoceles

Several proposed mechanisms have been described regarding how the varicocele negatively impacts testicle function. Increased testicular temperature, reflux of renal metabolites and toxins, and reactive oxygen species (ROS) accumulation have all been the suggested mechanisms. Increased temperature has the most likely pathologic effect on sperm production, likely due to disruption of the countercurrent heat exchange system within the scrotum. It is known to cause both Leydig and Sertoli cell dysfunction, decreased protein synthesis, and germ cell damage [2]. When affected, subfertile men with varicoceles can present with any combination of seminal abnormalities. Varicoceles may also increase the DNA fragmentation in sperm [3].

13.3 Diagnosis and Grading

Physical examination remains the most valuable tool for the diagnosis of varicocele. Careful physical examination of the subfertile male may reveal varicocele. It is imperative to examine the men in both upright and supine positions with Valsalva in each position. Exam may also demonstrate testicular asymmetry in size or consistency of the testes. Varicocele grades are based exclusively on clinical examination (Box 13.1). The left side is most commonly affected, with some men presenting with bilateral varicocele. Isolated right-sided varicocele is uncommon and suggests further evaluation for intraabdominal venous obstruction affecting the right side.

Radiographic imaging, though not necessary, may include ultrasound, venography, or radionucleotide scan. Ultrasound is the most commonly used modality and again here the ultrasonographer should perform the exam similarly to the physical exam: both upright and supine with and without Valsalva. This can demonstrate vessel size, reversal of flow, and a volume measurement of each testicle.

13.4 Treatment Indications

The Male Infertility Best Practice Policy Committee of the American Urological Association (AUA) initially provided guidance on treatment indications in 2001. More recently, the American Society of Reproductive Medicine has updated this guidance [4]. Varicocele repair should be offered to men who meet the following criteria: (1) A varicocele is palpable; (2) the couple has documented infertility; (3) the female has normal fertility or potentially correctable infertility; and (4) the male partner has one or more abnormal semen parameters or sperm function test results.

Other recommendations include offering repair to adult men who have a palpable varicocele and abnormal semen analyses but are not currently attempting to conceive. Young men who have a varicocele and normal semen analyses should be followed with semen analyses every 1–2 years. Finally, adolescents who have a varicocele and objective evidence of reduced ipsilateral testicular size should be offered repair. If these adolescents have normal testicular size, they should be offered follow-up with monitoring through an annual objective measurement of testicular size and/or semen analyses [4].

13.5 Surgical Approaches

Men offered repair of the varicocele should be apprised of the current available approaches and best-practice recommendations. Best practice is a microscopic varicocele ligation, generally via a subinguinal approach. Alternatives include inguinal and retroperitoneal (Palomo) approaches with or without the use of the microscope or laparoscopic ligation [4]. An original scrotal approach with scrotal excision and clamping of the varicocele veins was described over a century ago by Hartman [5]. This has been abandoned as it posed a higher risk of testicular artery damage and recurrence.

In this next section, each technique will be described in detail. All procedures should be completed under either general or monitored sedation anesthesia with generous use of local injectable analgesia. Intravenous antibiotics are routinely utilized immediately preoperatively and postoperative analgesics include standing oral anti-inflammatories for 1 week and narcotic prescription available as needed. Scrotal support also provides additional value in the first days to week after surgery.

Use of the microscope allows ready visualization of the spermatic vessels including the veins, vas deferens, and, critically, the testicular artery and associated lymphatics. A micro Doppler probe is used throughout the procedure to identify and isolate the testicular artery(ies). Some surgeons opt to use

Table 13.1 Distribution of Final Diagnostic Categories Found in Male Fertility Clinic

Category	Number	%
Varicocele	603	42.2
Idiopathic	324	22.7
Obstruction	205	14.3
Normal/female factor	119	7.9
Cryptorchidism	49	3.4
Immunological	37	2.6
Ejaculatory dysfunction	18	1.3
Testicular failure	18	1.3
Drug/radiation	16	1.1
Endocrinopathy	16	1.1
Others (all <1.0%)	31	2.1
Total	1,430	100.0

Source: Sigman M, in Lipshultz LI, Howards SS, eds. *Infertility in the Male*, 3rd ed. St. Louis, MO: Mosby-Year Book, Inc, p. 530, 1997. Reprinted with permission.

Box 13.1 Varicocele Grading

Subclinical	Not detected on physical exam; found on radiologic imaging only
Grade I	Only palpable during Valsalva on physical exam
Grade II	Routinely palpable without Valsalva on physical exam
Grade III	Visible and palpable on physical exam

surgical loupes alone to augment their visualization. Magnified visualization reduces the recurrence and hydrocele complication rate [4,6].

13.5.1 Subinguinal

This is our preferred approach to varicocele ligation (see video). We feel that the subinguinal incision spares muscle splitting of the other surgical approaches, leading to more rapid convalescence and return to work in these relatively young men.

A 3 cm subinguinal incision is made just lateral to the penis and just superior to the scrotum (Figure 13.1). Some authors incise just below the level of the external inguinal ring. The dissection is carried down through Camper's and Scarpa's fascia. Army-Navy retractors placed parallel to the cord allow for blunt dissection of the loose connective tissues overlying the cord (Figure 13.2). Once the cord is seen, Metzenbaum scissors are used to spread both lateral and medial to the cord to allow identification of the cord itself. The cord is then grasped with an atraumatic Babcock clamp and brought into the incision (Figure 13.3). A finger is placed under the cord and using a small gauze sponge, noncord structures are swept away from the cord, and the finger is allowed to fully encircle the cord. An Army-Navy retractor is placed under the cord, raising it, and the space below the cord is inspected to ensure that all spermatic cord vessels are included above. Once placed flat against the patient's body, the retractor serves to keep the

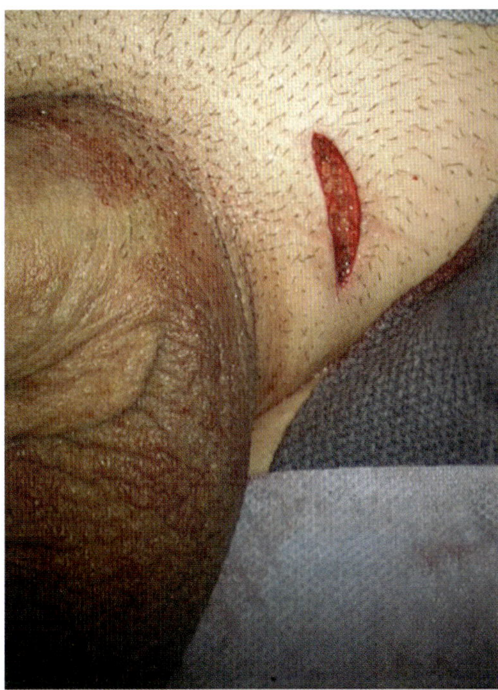

Figure 13.1 A 2–3 cm incision is typically made in a subinguinal location, just lateral to the scrotum and base of penis, a few centimeters caudal to the external ring.

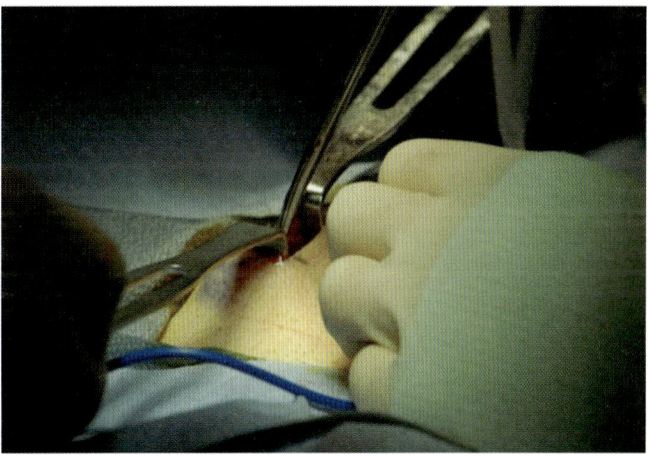

Figure 13.2 Army-Navy retractors are used to bluntly dissect tissue down to Scarpa's fascia, which is entered bluntly with the retractors or by spreading with the tips of a Metzenbaum scissors.

cord above the skin level and in the field throughout the procedure (Figure 13.4). Some surgeons choose to use one or two penrose drains snapped to the drapes to keep the cord elevated.

The operating microscope is brought onto the field and set to 10–20× magnification. The internal spermatic fascia and tissue overlying the cord is grasped with Pierce pickups, and a hemostat and electrocautery are used to incise and open the space. The cremasteric fibers are dissected and tagged medially and laterally into two separate packets and placed in vessel loops for future ligation (Figures 13.5 and 13.6). Using the fine Jacobsohn hemostat, the vas deferens and its related structures are dissected away from the remainder of the cord and placed in a separate vessel loop. The remaining spermatic cord is then dissected using a combination of sharp and blunt dissection

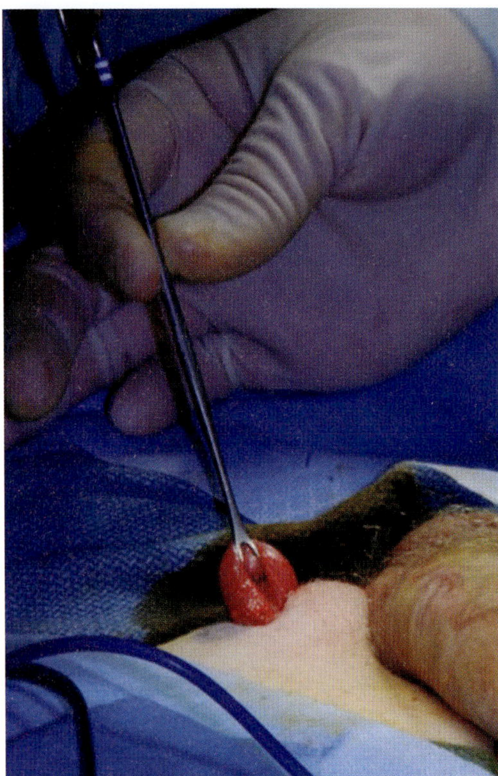

Figure 13.3 Babcock clamp is used to bring the spermatic cord up through the skin incision.

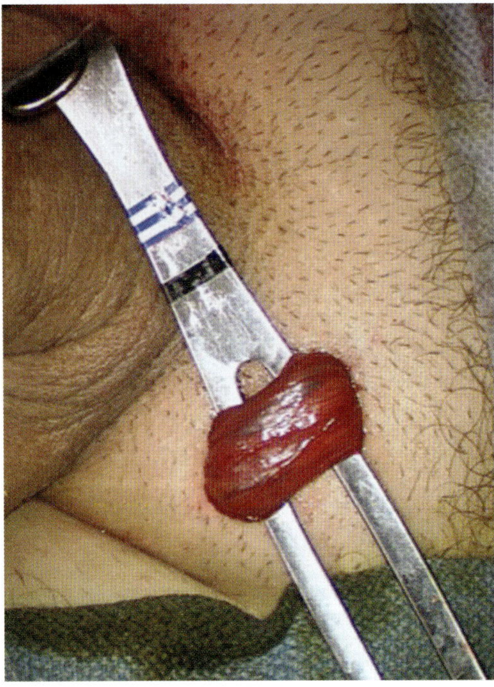

Figure 13.4 After isolating the cord, it is suspended above the skin by passing an Army-Navy under the cord.

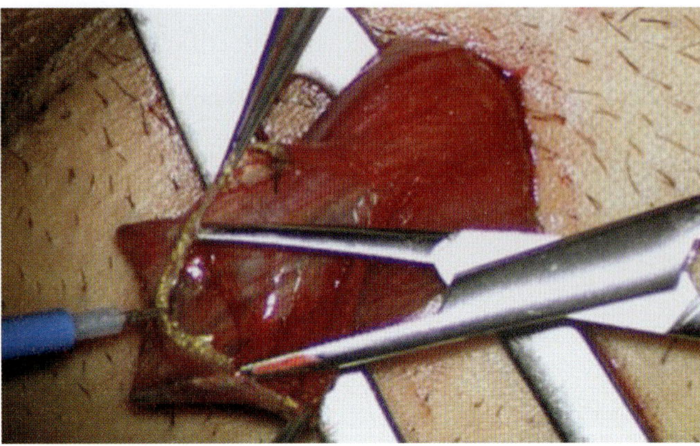

Figure 13.5 Under microscopic view, the external spermatic fascia, cremasteric muscle fibers, and internal spermatic fascia are opened along the direction of the cord with fine-point electrocautery.

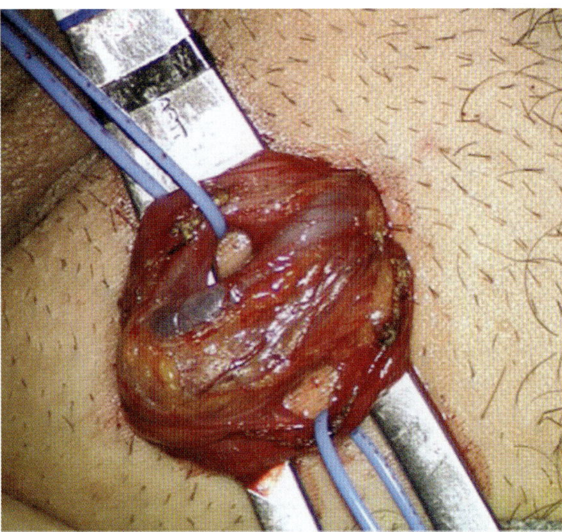

Figure 13.6 The spermatic fasciae and cremasteric muscle fibers are isolated medially and laterally and retracted from the cord with blue microvessel loops.

with the Jacobsohn hemostat. It is important to identify individual lymphatic vessels early and tag these with vessel loops for preservation. The micro Doppler is first used here to identify the section of cord that contains the artery and to determine if multiple arteries are present (Figures 13.7 and 13.8). The Doppler should be used prior to each and every venous ligation to ensure that no artery is included with that vein and that the artery has signal elsewhere in the cord bundle. The internal spermatic veins are then dissected and clip- or suture-ligated, based on surgeon preference, and divided. The spermatic artery(ies) is separated from the often adherent spermatic veins (Figure 13.9). If needed, a curved microneedle holder can be used for dissection of particularly adherent vessels. The microneedle holder is more likely to puncture a vessel wall than the Jacobsohn and must be used with care. Papaverine (30 mg/cc, 1 cc in 4 cc of sterile water) can be drip-applied to the field in small volume to increase arterial signal and combat any vasospasm caused by dissection. The spermatic artery is also isolated and preserved in a vessel loop. Once it appears that all veins have been ligated, all lymphatic vessels and arteries should be placed within a single vessel loop. With gentle retraction of this new bundle, the surgeon can determine if any tissue or vessels remain to be ligated and do so. Doppler is used again to confirm arterial waveform. Cremasteric fibers are then

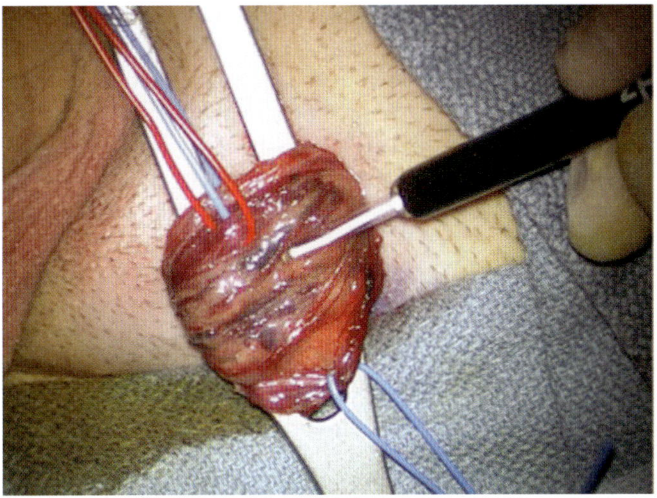

Figure 13.7 A 20 MHz microvascular Doppler (Vascular Technology, Nashua, NH) is used to identify arteries in the cord.

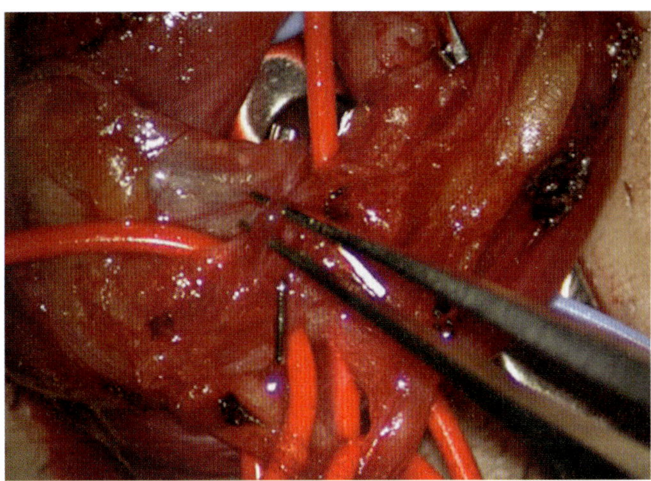

Figure 13.9 Spermatic/testicular artery is carefully dissected from adherent veins.

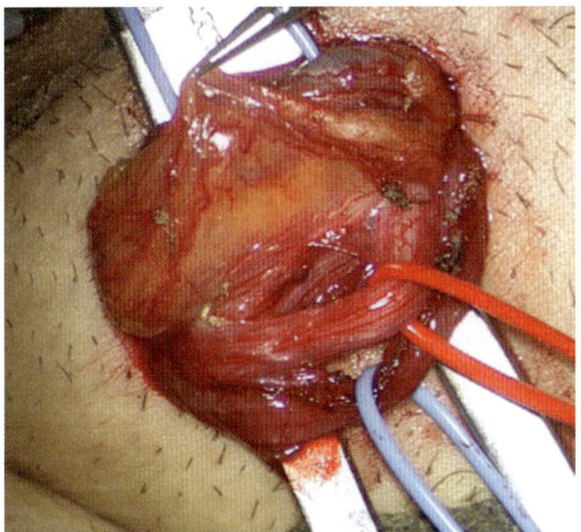

Figure 13.8 Vas and vasal vessels are isolated to avoid inadvertent injury to these vital structures.

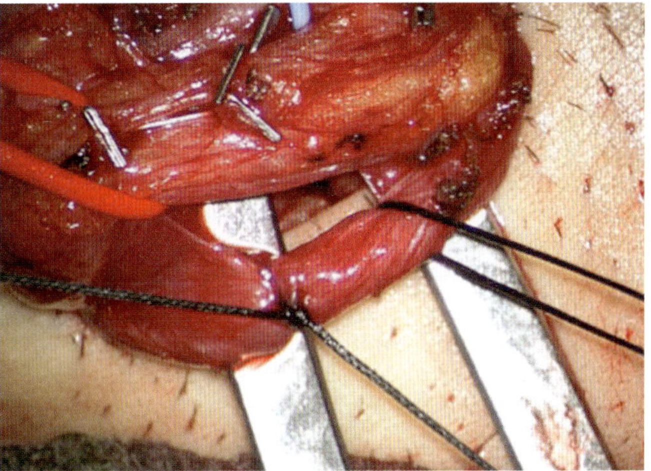

Figure 13.10 The cremasteric fibers are ligated and divided. They are ligated and sharply divided with cautery.

ligated and cauterized (Figure 13.10). If the cremaster on either side is very thick, consider separating it into two packets and ligating each separately. One cremaster packet should be ligated but not cauterized so that the cord retains some strength and the testicle does not rely on the artery and lymphatics alone for support. If there is concern for injury to the spermatic artery, then cremaster fibers, which often contain a small accessory artery, should not be ligated. Any large cremaster veins can be isolated and ligated from the remainder of the cremaster fibers to prevent recurrence. Hemostasis can be achieved with bipolar electrocautery where necessary. The preserved cord structures are then replaced into the incision and the testis is very gently drawn caudad to its natural position. Scarpa's fascia is then closed with interrupted 3-0 Vicryl suture. The skin is closed with a running subcuticular 4-0 Monocryl stitch.

13.5.2 Inguinal

The inguinal procedure is also called the Ivanissevich approach. A skin crease incision is made between the internal and external inguinal rings. An incision may be made parallel to the inguinal ligament for a standard hernia repair if this approach is more comfortable for the surgeon. The external oblique fascia is identified. It is then incised and opened in the direction of the fibers, just above the inguinal ring. It is at this point that the ilioinguinal nerve must be identified and protected. The spermatic cord is identified and brought up and into the operative field, secured at the level of the skin by either penrose drains or an Army-Navy retractor. The operating microscope, if used, is now brought over the field.

The procedure then continues similar to that described in the subinguinal approach in Section 13.5.1. Any large veins identified in the cremasters are also ligated. Once all veins are ligated, lymphatics and artery(ies) preserving the cord is returned to the canal. Some surgeons opt to close the cremaster muscle at this point, while others do not. The external oblique fascia is closed with either running or interrupted 2-0 or 3-0 absorbable sutures, recreating the anterior wall of the inguinal canal and the external inguinal ring.

The inguinal approach may be easier for surgeons more accustomed to an inguinal incision. At this level, the veins are typically larger in size and fewer in number. Though fewer veins require ligation here, the same attention to preservation of the artery and lymphatics is critical to both operative success and minimizing complications.

13.5.3 Retroperitoneal/Palomo
Open or Laparoscopic

First described in 1949, this retroperitoneal approach allows access to the cord above the vas deferens [7]. This approach may be used in any patient, although it is simpler if the man is thin. A horizontal incision is made medial and inferior to the anterior iliac crest, at a point about 2 cm superior to the internal inguinal ring. This is carried down though the subcutaneous adipose and other tissues to the external oblique fascia. Here it is opened in the direction of the fibers. The internal inguinal ring is identified. Using a blunt-tipped clamp, the internal oblique and transversalis muscles are entered and spread, revealing the retroperitoneal space. The peritoneum is medially retracted, resulting in exposure of the spermatic cord as it travels lateral to the ureter and toward the internal ring. The spermatic veins can be ligated at this point. Generally, two to three veins are present at this level. Preservation of the artery and lymphatics remains paramount. After confirming hemostasis, the transversalis muscle and internal oblique are reapproximated with 2-0 absorbable suture. Next the external oblique is closed with the same suture. The overlying subcutaneous tissues and skin are closed in a standard fashion.

A transperitoneal laparoscopic approach to varicocelectomy has also been reported. This essentially provides access to the same space as the Palomo but from the peritoneum. This approach can spare the artery and lymphatics if care is taken during the dissection [8–10].

13.5.4 Embolization

Embolization is a viable option for some men with varicoceles. This technique was first described in 1978 [11]. It can be used for men as primary treatment or for men in whom varicoceles recur or persist after surgical intervention. Importantly, a skilled interventional radiologist should perform the procedure to maximize possible patient benefit. The procedure is performed as an outpatient. Typically it allows the patient a rapid return to all activities.

Access to the veins occurs via canalization of the right femoral vein with a 7 French guiding catheter, which is directed into the left gonadal vein under fluoroscopic guidance with nonionic contrast. A 4 French catheter extends from the 7 French catheter to gain access to the distal veins closer to the scrotum. The tip of the catheter is placed level with the sacroiliac and coils are released into the vein. The catheter is then drawn slightly back and upward with additional coils released. A dextrose solution is then injected to promote thrombus development around the coils. Alternatively, sclerotherapy with a variety of sclerosing agents has been investigated and may be used by radiologist preference [12]. A final venogram demonstrates occlusion of the vessels.

The right side is often more difficult to access in the case of bilateral varicoceles. Surgery remains an option if embolization fails for both first-time treatment and recurrence of the condition. Embolization may be of benefit to men in whom surgery may be particularly difficult, such as the obese. Typically, interventional radiologists perform this procedure. It can be done under local or moderate sedation but does not require general anesthesia.

13.6 Outcomes of Repair

Surgical intervention eliminates varicoceles successfully 90–98% of the time. Regarding the improvement in semen analysis, it is more difficult to describe, mainly as there is no standard definition of "improvement." Between 65% and 75% of men can expect some improvement in semen parameters following repair [13,14]. This improvement generally takes 3–6 months, which corresponds to one to two full spermatogenic cycles.

Some men will improve to a degree where the type of artificial reproductive technology (ART) or need for ART can be altered. A large cohort of men with palpable varicocele underwent microsurgical varicocelectomy. They were followed for at least 1 year. The men were subdivided by type of ART most likely to benefit them. These groups included ICSI (0–1.5 million sperms), IVF (1.5–5 million sperms), intrauterine insemination (5–20 million sperms), and spontaneous pregnancy (20 million or higher sperm count). Overall, 50% of men had improvement in semen parameters. Thirty-one percent of men improved from an absolute indication for in vitro fertilization (IVF)/intracytoplasmic sperm injection (ICSI) to intrauterine insemination (IUI) or spontaneous pregnancy and another 42% improved from IUI to sufficient concentration and motility of sperm to enable natural conception [15].

In one randomized controlled trial, 60% of men achieved pregnancy after repair, compared to just 10% for those who did not have surgery. Thereafter, the untreated second group had surgery with a subsequent natural conception rate of 66% over the next 2 years [16]. In a more recent trial, 145 men were randomized to subinguinal microscopic varicocele repair or observation [17]. Surgical patients had spontaneous pregnancy in 32% vs 13.9% in untreated men. There does not appear to be a difference in pregnancy rates for the different surgical approaches, though the complication rates differ from one approach to another [18]. An additional randomized controlled study (RCT) of 125 couples did not show any difference in pregnancy rates at 1 year compared to observation (29 vs 25.4%) [19]. In meta-analyses, including a Cochrane review, varicocelectomy has an improved pregnancy rate compared to no intervention for men with idiopathic male infertility [20,21].

13.7 Complications

The rate of recurrence (13.9% vs. 1.9%) and postoperative hydrocele (7.3% vs.0.4%) were significantly lower for microscopic approach [13,18,22,23]. The lower recurrence and hydrocele formation rates are likely because of the increased visibility of the microscope. The scope allows identification and ligation of even the smallest veins, preventing recurrence from residual veins.

Similarly, the careful dissection and preservation of lymphatic vessels under the scope limits hydrocele formation. Postoperative hematoma formation or infection is rare with all approaches.

For patients, common surgical questions relate to time off from work and activity. Time to return to work varies from 5 to 7 days after surgery, a similar timing regardless of approach. Though one group has shown faster return by 1 day for the microsurgical or laparoscopic approach compared to open procedure, other groups did not show any difference [13,22].

Limitations and complications can also present with the interventional radiology approach to varicocele repair. In up to 8% of men, embolization and occlusion are not possible because of inability to access the gonadal vein, intimal vessel dissection/injury, or evidence of significant vessel communication with systemic venous circulation [24]. Unperformable rates as high as 30% have been reported, but most contemporary studies have put this figure around 8–10% [4,25]. Recurrence rates after a technically successful procedure are around 15% [4,25]. Percutaneous embolization results are dependent on the skill and experience of the interventional radiologist performing the procedure [4]. Coil migration has been described whereby the coil is dislocated to another vascular bed, rarely leading to pulmonary embolism [26].

13.6 Conclusion

None of the methods has been proven to be superior to the others in their ability to improve fertility. However, the microscopic approach to varicocelectomy does have the lowest rate of recurrence and complications [4]. Around 65–75% of men should expect an improvement in their semen parameters, notably in concentration or motility. They should be followed for 1 year after repair or until their partner becomes pregnant.

References

1. World Health Organization. The influence of varicocele on parameters of fertility in a large group of men presenting to infertility clinics. *Fertil Steril.* 1992;57(6):1289–93.

2. Williams DH, Karpman E, Lipshultz LI. Varicocele: surgical techniques in 2005. *Can J Urol.* 2006;13 Suppl 1:13–17.

3. Moazzam A, Sharma R, Agarwal A. Relationship of spermatozoal DNA fragmentation with semen quality in varicocele-positive men. *Andrologia.* 2015;47(8):935–44.

4. Practice Committee of the American Society for Reproductive Medicine, Society for Male Reproduction and Urology. Report on varicocele and infertility: a committee opinion. *Fertil Steril.* 2014;102(6):1556–60.

5. Noske HD, Weidner W. Varicocele – a historical perspective. *World J Urol.* 1999;17(3):151–7.

6. Goldstein M, Gilbert BR, Dicker AP, Dwosh J, Gnecco C. Microsurgical inguinal varicocelectomy with delivery of the testis: an artery and lymphatic sparing technique. *J Urol.* 1992;148(6):1808–11.

7. Palomo A. Radical cure of varicocele by a new technique; preliminary report. *J Urol.* 1949;61(3):604–7.

8. Tan SM, Ng FC, Ravintharan T, Lim PH, Chng HC. Laparoscopic varicocelectomy: technique and results. *Br J Urol.* 1995;75(4):523–8.

9. Tu D, Glassberg KI. Laparoscopic varicocelectomy. *BJU Int.* 2010;106(7):1094–104.

10. Jarow JP, Assimos DG, Pittaway DE. Effectiveness of laparoscopic varicocelectomy. *Urology.* 1993;42(5):544–7.

11. Lima SS, Castro MP, Costa OF. A new method for the treatment of varicocele. *Andrologia.* 1978;10(2):103–6.

12. Li L, Zeng XQ, Li YH. Digital subtraction angiography-guided percutaneous transcatheter foam sclerotherapy of varicocele: a novel tracking technique. *AJR Am J Roentgenol.* 2009;193(4):978–80.

13. Al-Kandari AM, Shabaan H, Ibrahim HM, Elshebiny YH, Shokeir AA. Comparison of outcomes of different varicocelectomy techniques: open inguinal, laparoscopic, and subinguinal microscopic varicocelectomy: a randomized clinical trial. *Urology.* 2007;69(3):417–20.

14. Baazeem A, Belzile E, Ciampi A, et al. Varicocele and male factor infertility treatment: a new meta-analysis and review of the role of varicocele repair. *Eur Urol.* 2011;60(4):796–808.

15. Cayan S, Erdemir F, Ozbey I, Turek PJ, Kadioglu A, Tellaloglu S. Can varicocelectomy significantly change the way couples use assisted reproductive technologies? *J Urol.* 2002;167(4):1749–52.

16. Madgar I, Weissenberg R, Lunenfeld B, Karasik A, Goldwasser B. Controlled trial of high spermatic vein ligation for varicocele in infertile men. *Fertil Steril.* 1995;63(1):120–4.

17. Abdel-Meguid TA, Al-Sayyad A, Tayib A, Farsi HM. Does varicocele repair improve male infertility? An evidence-based perspective from a randomized, controlled trial. *Eur Urol.* 2011;59(3):455–61.

18. Al-Said S, Al-Naimi A, Al-Ansari A, et al. Varicocelectomy for male infertility: a comparative study of open, laparoscopic and microsurgical approaches. *J Urol.* 2008;180(1):266–70.

19. Nieschlag E, Hertle L, Fischedick A, Abshagen K, Behre HM. Update on treatment of varicocele: counselling as effective as occlusion of the vena spermatica. *Hum Reprod.* 1998;13(8):2147–50.

20. Marmar JL, Agarwal A, Prabakaran S, et al. Reassessing the value of varicocelectomy as a treatment for male subfertility with a new meta-analysis. *Fertil Steril.* 2007;88(3):639–48.

21. Kroese AC, de Lange NM, Collins J, Evers JL. Surgery or embolization for varicoceles in subfertile men. *Cochrane Database Syst Rev.* 2012;10:CD000479.

22. Ding H, Tian J, Du W, Zhang L, Wang H, Wang Z. Open non-microsurgical, laparoscopic or open microsurgical varicocelectomy for male infertility: a meta-analysis of randomized controlled trials. *BJU Int.* 2012;110(10):1536–42.

23. Cayan S, Kadioglu TC, Tefekli A, Kadioglu A, Tellaloglu S. Comparison of results and complications of high ligation surgery and microsurgical high inguinal varicocelectomy in the treatment of varicocele. *Urology.* 2000;55(5):750–4.

24. Gazzera C, Rampado O, Savio L, Di Bisceglie C, Manieri C, Gandini G. Radiological treatment of male varicocele: technical, clinical, seminal and dosimetric aspects. *Radiol Med.* 2006;111(3):449–58.

25. Iaccarino V, Venetucci P. Interventional radiology of male varicocele: current status. *Cardiovasc Intervent Radiol.* 2012;35(6):1263–80.

26. Verhagen P, Blom JM, van Rijk PP, Lock MT. Pulmonary embolism after percutaneous embolization of left spermatic vein. *Eur J Radiol.* 1992;15(3):190–2.

Surgical Sperm Retrieval Methods

Phil V. Bach and Peter N. Schlegel

14.1 Introduction

Azoospermia, or the absence of sperm in the ejaculate, affects approximately 1% of the general male population and 10–20% of men with infertility and may be caused by obstructive or nonobstructive etiologies [1]. In the past, azoospermia has been a considerable therapeutic challenge for urologists, with donor insemination or adoption being the only therapeutic options. However, the advent of intracytoplasmic sperm injection (ICSI) has enabled the potential for very small numbers of live sperm to produce offspring in conjunction with in vitro fertilization (IVF). As a result, men with azoospermia now have the ability to successfully father their own biological children.

The goal of sperm retrieval is to obtain a maximal amount of viable sperm while minimizing the amount of damage to the reproductive tract. Different techniques are available for use in men with obstructive azoospermia (OA) and for those with nonobstructive azoospermia (NOA), with each technique presenting its own advantages and disadvantages. In this chapter, we will describe the various surgical sperm retrieval techniques from the vas deferens, epididymis, and testicle of the azoospermic male and highlight important considerations regarding clinical evaluation, postoperative care, and outcomes for each.

14.2 Clinical Evaluation

Patients presenting with azoospermia or severe oligospermia need to be thoroughly evaluated in order to ascertain the cause of infertility and to identify an appropriate treatment plan. At a minimum, physicians should obtain a complete history and physical exam, two semen analyses, and hormonal studies (including testosterone and FSH). To rule out female factors for infertility, a focused evaluation or referral of the partner to a reproductive endocrinologist should also be included in the clinical evaluation of the infertile couple.

Men with congenital bilateral absence of the vas deferens on physical exam (CBAVD) should undergo genetic testing for cystic fibrosis (cystic fibrosis transmembrane regulator [CFTR]) mutations. If any mutations are detected on genetic testing, the patient and his partner should be advised to seek genetic counseling.

Men with bilateral atrophic testes on physical exam should be evaluated for primary versus secondary testicular failure. Elevated FSH levels coupled with normal or low serum testosterone levels suggest primary testicular failure whereas low FSH

and serum testosterone levels are consistent with secondary testicular failure. Men with suspected primary testicular failure likely have NOA and should undergo genetic testing with karyotype and Y microdeletion testing. Secondary testicular failure, or hypogonadotrophic hypogonadism, is often caused by hypothalamic pathologies, such as Kallman syndrome or pituitary disorders (e.g., pituitary tumors). Further hormonal evaluation (with prolactin and LH) and pituitary imaging by computed tomography (CT) or magnetic resonance imaging (MRI) should be pursued as appropriate.

When the vasa and testes are normal on physical exam, the semen volume and FSH become critical in determining the cause of azoospermia. Patients with low semen volume (<1.0 mL) may have ejaculatory dysfunction or ejaculatory duct obstruction. Postejaculatory urinalysis for sperm may help diagnose retrograde ejaculation whereas the diagnostic tool of choice for ejaculatory duct obstruction is transrectal ultrasound (TRUS). The presence of midline cysts, dilated seminal vesicles (>1.5 cm), or dilated ejaculatory ducts are suggestive of ejaculatory duct obstruction. If dilated seminal vesicles are seen on TRUS, TRUS-guided seminal vesicle aspiration may be performed to confirm the diagnosis. Patients with unilateral absence of the vas deferens and low-volume azoospermia may have a variant of CBAVD and should undergo CFTR testing before TRUS.

In patients with normal semen volume, serum FSH can help delineate between OA and NOA. Markedly elevated serum FSH is diagnostic of impaired spermatogenesis and of NOA whereas low-normal serum FSH is more consistent with OA. Testicular biopsy can help to delineate OA from NOA, but because a biopsy only samples less than 5% of the seminiferous tubules within a testis, it has minimal utility in prognosticating whether or not sperm are present elsewhere in the testis of a man with NOA. Studies have shown that the testis is highly heterogeneous both histologically and in terms of spermatogenesis, which explains the poor correlation between diagnostic testicular biopsies and sperm retrieval rates in men with NOA [2]. As a result, we do not perform diagnostic testicular biopsies routinely in our clinical evaluation of azoospermia. Men with suspected OA (normal volume testes, intact vas deferens, normal serum FSH) may have diagnostic testicular biopsy performed at the time of reconstruction.

Men with NOA or severe oligospermia (<5 million sperm/mL) should undergo genetic testing. Genetic testing, namely karyotype and Y microdeletion testing, can help identify the cause of impaired spermatogenesis in 15–20% of men with NOA and provide important prognostic information. Men with Klinefelter syndrome (47XXY) or AZFc deletions have a 65–75% chance of sperm retrieval with microtesticular sperm extraction (microTESE) while those with complete deletions of AZFa, AZFb, or AZFb+c have a very poor prognosis (near 0% chance of sperm retrieval) [3,4].

14.3 Indications

The critical classification that will determine the type of surgical sperm retrieval method used is whether the patient has OA or NOA. Vasal and epididymal sperm retrievals can only be considered for those presenting with OA while testicular sperm retrievals (especially microdissection testicular sperm extraction) can be considered for those with OA or NOA.

14.4 Preoperative Preparation

Because men with NOA have severely impaired spermatogenesis, their limited production should be optimized prior to surgery. Men with prior scrotal surgery should wait at least 6 months before surgical sperm retrieval to allow for resolution of any hematoma or inflammation that may impair sperm production, which usually takes 3 months [5]. Those with varicocele may also benefit from varicocelectomy to optimize sperm production and potentially allow for the return of sperm to the ejaculate. However, the benefits from varicocelectomy may take 6 months or longer to be realized and while up to 39% of men may have return of motile sperm to the ejaculate, less than 10% of men have sufficient sperm in the ejaculate to avoid TESE [6,7]. While early studies suggest that performance of varicocelectomy has no effect on sperm retrieval rates at TESE, more recent studies have noted significantly higher rates of sperm retrieval at TESE following varicocelectomy [7–9]. Finally, men with NOA often have compromised serum testosterone levels and relatively increased estradiol levels that could be caused by increased testicular aromatase activity. Treatment of these men with low serum testosterone (<300 mg/dL) and decreased testosterone:estradiol ratios (<10) with an aromatase inhibitor (such as anastrozole, 1 mg P.O. daily) reliably increases circulating testosterone and decreases estradiol, thereby enhancing intratesticular testosterone levels and improving spermatogenesis [10].

Additionally, all patients scheduled for surgical sperm retrieval procedures should refrain from taking aspirin and nonsteroidal anti-inflammatory medications for 1 week preoperatively and discontinue anticoagulants perioperatively. Patients may receive a single dose of IV antibiotics 30 minutes prior to incision.

14.5 Techniques

14.5.1 Vasal Aspiration

Following administration of adequate anesthesia (either regional or general), the patient is placed in the supine position and the genitalia prepped as per the usual aseptic technique. The testicle is delivered via either a midline raphe or a high transverse incision along the scrotal skin lines. The straight vas deferens is palpated along the spermatic cord using the thumb and forefinger and stabilized using a Babcock clamp. Blunt dissection of the vasal adventitia is carried out using a curved mosquito clamp, taking care to not damage the perivasal vasculature. Bipolar cautery can be used to maintain adequate hemostasis. Once the vas is completely isolated, a Penrose drain can be used to separate the bare vas from its adventitia. A straight mosquito clamp is then placed below the bare vas to serve as a platform on which the vas can be hemitransected using a 15° ultrasharp microknife in a single motion. A 24G angiocatheter attached to a tuberculin syringe containing 0.1 mL of sperm wash medium can be used to aspirate sperm from the testicular vas lumen. A small sample should be placed on a slide for examination under a bench microscope for the presence of motile sperm while the rest is gently flushed into sperm wash medium.

Once adequate amount of motile sperm are aspirated, the vasotomy can be closed in two layers. First, three 10-0 nylon sutures are used to reapproximate the vasal mucosa before three 9-0 nylon sutures are used to close the vasal muscularis and adventitia, taking great care to not obliterate the vasal lumen. A 0.25% Marcaine solution is infused within the spermatic cord and the testicle is replaced within the scrotum. The dartos fascia and skin are both closed separately with fine absorbable suture. The incision can be infiltrated with 0.25% Marcaine solution with epinephrine to ensure adequate postprocedural anesthesia. Finally, Bacitracin ointment, fluff gauze, and a scrotal supporter are applied.

14.5.2 Percutaneous Epididymal Sperm Aspiration

Percutaneous epididymal sperm aspiration (PESA) can be performed in an office setting with local anesthesia. To perform PESA, one requires a 22–26G needle attached to a tuberculin syringe containing 0.1 mL of sperm-washing medium. There should be an air bubble maintained within the syringe to prevent contact between the rubber and the sperm-washing medium.

After the patient is placed in the supine position, the scrotum is cleaned with an antiseptic solution and rinsed with saline to remove any residual antiseptic. Local anesthesia is administered via cord block and skin infiltration using 2% lidocaine. The head of the epididymis is then palpated and isolated between the thumb and index finger. The 22–26G needle is then used to puncture the epididymis through the scrotal skin. Once within the epididymis, the plunger of the tuberculin syringe should be pulled all the way back to create a suction force. While maintaining the suction force, the needle is carefully advanced and withdrawn partially throughout the epididymis, taking care to remain within the epididymis at all times. The needle can be rotated 180° and the angle of entry can be varied slightly with each pass (while maintaining suction) to ensure that multiple areas of the epididymis are sampled. Once this position is satisfied, the suction can be partially released and the needle removed from the epididymis. One should not expect a significant amount of epididymal fluid following PESA (can be anywhere from 0.3 to 1 mL) and the epididymal aspirate may, in fact, be invisible.

The epididymal fluid should be flushed into an Eppendorf tube containing sperm-washing medium and a small sampled placed on a slide for examination under the bench microscope. If no motile sperm are detected, the procedure can be repeated at a more proximal portion of the epididymis (toward the epididymal head). Multiple passes may be required before motile sperm are found. If no motile sperm are found, PESA can be performed on the contralateral side or one can proceed to testicular sperm aspiration (TESA). If no motile sperm are found on PESA or TESA, the patient can be booked for future microsurgical epididymal sperm aspiration (MESA) or microdissection testicular sperm extraction (microTESE).

14.5.3 Microsurgical Epididymal Sperm Aspiration

Unlike PESA, MESA requires microscopic magnification and is ideally performed with general anesthesia. Following induction of anesthesia, the patient is placed in the supine position and the testis is delivered through either a scrotal midline raphe incision or a high-transverse incision along the scrotal skin lines. The tunica vaginalis is incised using electrocautery and the epididymis is inspected under the operating microscope in order to identify dilated epididymal tubules containing golden, semitranslucent fluid for aspiration. Opaque, yellow tubules typically contain sperm heads and debris and should be avoided.

The structure of the epididymis consists of numerous ducts that coalesce at the junction of the epididymal head and body into a single epididymal duct that travels through the epididymal tail into the vas deferens. In order to minimize the risk of inducing an epididymal obstruction, the safest area to perform a MESA is in the epididymal head, where damage to

a single duct will not cause obstruction to the entire outflow tract. In OA, the likelihood of finding motile sperm in the epididymal head is higher than normal [2].

Jeweler forceps are used to pick up the tunica of the epididymis, which is then incised with a small microscopic curved scissors to reveal the dilated tubule. Blunt dissection with the microscopic needle holder can be used to further expose the dilated tubule. Bipolar cautery can be used judiciously to ensure meticulous hemostasis, taking care to not damage the exposed tubule. At this point, a glass micropipette with a sharpened tip can be used to both puncture the tubule and aspirate the epididymal fluid. Alternatively, a 15° ultrasharp microknife can be used to incise the exposed tubule and a regular glass 0.5 μL micropipette (0.5 mm luminal diameter and 0.9 mm outer diameter) used to collect the epididymal fluid using capillary action (Figure 14.1).

A small sample of the epididymal fluid should be placed on a slide and examined immediately under a bench microscope to confirm the presence of motile sperm. Once motile sperm are visualized, the epididymal fluid can be flushed from the micropipettes into sperm wash media and given to the IVF lab personnel for processing and storage. If no motile sperm are visualized, a more proximal epididymal tubule can be isolated and punctured until motile sperm are found. Manual compression of the testis and/or epididymis during aspiration can maximize the amount of fluid retrieved. Aspiration is continued until no more fluid can be obtained. About 10–20 μL of epididymal fluid can usually be aspirated.

Once aspiration is complete, the incised epididymal tubule can be closed using either 10-0 nylon sutures or the bipolar cautery. The tunica vaginalis is closed with absorbable suture in a running fashion and the intratunical space is infused with 0.25% Marcaine before the testicle is returned to the scrotum. The dartos fascia is also closed with fine absorbable suture in a running fashion and the subdermal layer is infused with 0.25% Marcaine with epinephrine prior to skin closure with a 5-0 Monocryl suture. Finally, Bacitracin ointment, fluff gauze, and a scrotal supporter are applied.

14.5.4 Testicular Sperm Aspiration

One can perform TESA in an office setting using two different methods requiring different pieces of equipment – either a biopsy gun or a 19G butterfly needle attached to a 20 cm³ syringe and Cameco piston syringe handle. Both techniques will be described in the following section.

Once the patient is placed in the supine position, the scrotum is cleaned with an antiseptic solution and rinsed with saline to remove any residual antiseptic. Local anesthesia is administered via cord block and skin infiltration using 2% lidocaine at the planned aspiration sites. In order to minimize potential damage to the epididymis, we recommend using the inferior pole of the testicle as the entry site for aspiration. The testis is then grasped up near the scrotal skin and stabilized with the nondominant hand. If using a biopsy gun, the biopsy gun is fired with the entry point of the needle at the inferior pole of the testis (Figure 14.2). Once removed, pressure is held at the site of the biopsy while the testicular tissue is placed in

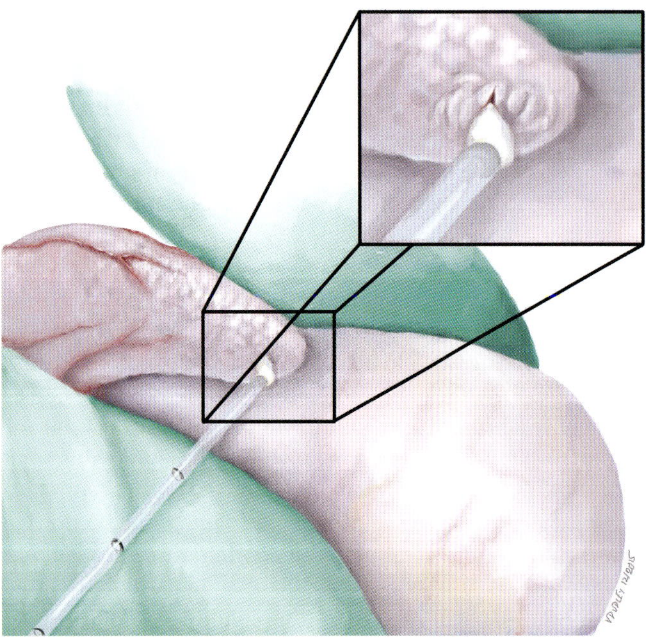

Figure 14.1 After incision of the dilated epididymal tubule, a glass micropipette is used to aspirate the epididymal fluid using simple capillary action.

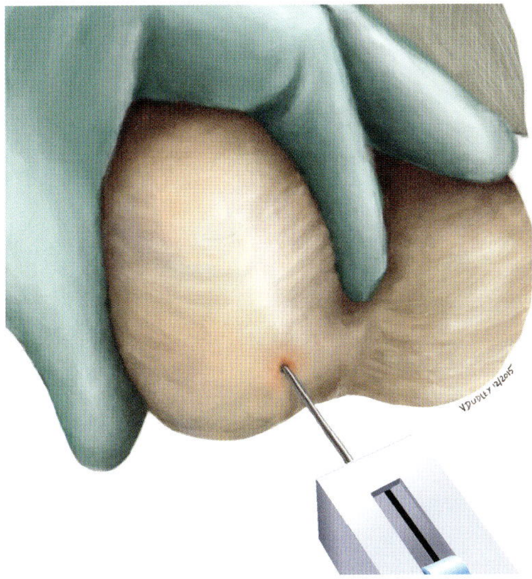

Figure 14.2 With the testicle stabilized using the nondominant hand, a biopsy gun is fired into the inferior pole.

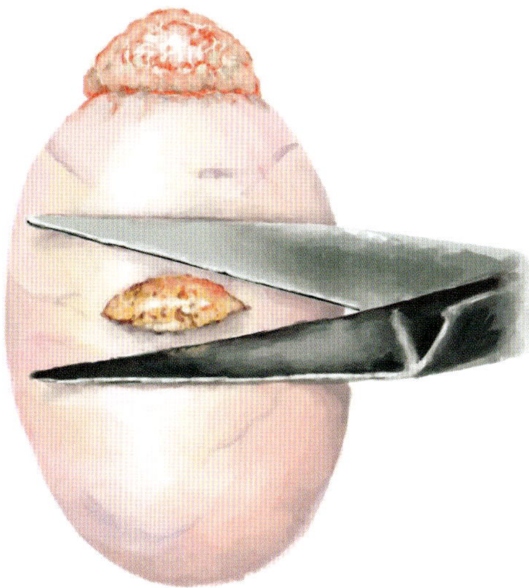

Figure 14.3 In TESE, manual compression of the testicle causes extrusion of the testicular tissue, which is then excised sharply using a curved iris scissor.

sperm-wash medium. If the 19G butterfly needle attached to the 20 cm³ syringe is used, then the needle is used to puncture the testicle at the inferior pole through the scrotal skin. The Cameco piston syringe is used to produce and maintain a suction force as multiple passes are made through the same puncture site. The aspirated tissue and fluid are then gently flushed into sperm-wash medium.

The testicular tissue aspirated should then be passed through a 24G angiocatheter to promote suspension of sperm from the testicular tissue into the sperm-wash medium. A sample can then be placed on a slide and examined immediately under a bench microscope for the presence of mature, viable sperm. Multiple aspirations may be taken to ensure enough tissue and sperm are obtained for at least three fresh IVF cycles. If no mature, viable sperm are detected, TESA may be performed on the contralateral testicle.

Once satisfied, continuous pressure should be applied to the biopsy sites to promote adequate hemostasis. A sterile dressing and fluff gauze are applied and held in place by a scrotal supporter.

14.5.5 Testicular Sperm Extraction

TESE, also known as an open testicular biopsy, can be done under local, regional, or general anesthesia and with or without the assistance of a microscope. A microdissection TESE (or microTESE) will be discussed later on.

Once appropriate anesthesia is administered, the patient is placed in a supine position and the genitalia are prepped with an antiseptic solution. Using either a midline raphe incision or a high-transverse incision along the scrotal skin lines, the testis is delivered. The tunica vaginalis is incised using electrocautery and the testis is inspected. Use of an operating microscope during this stage greatly enhances visibility of the testicular blood supply and allows for the subsequent transverse incision of the tunica albuginea to occur between blood vessels. A 1 cm transverse incision is then made along the anterior surface of

the testicle between the blood vessels using a 15° ultrasharp microknife. Bipolar cautery is used to ensure adequate hemostasis, especially of subtunical blood vessels. Testicular tubules are extruded from the testicle using manual compression and are excised sharply from the base using curved iris scissors (Figure 14.3). The specimen is then placed in an Eppendorf tube containing tubal fluid media. The testicular tissue can be minced sharply and then passed sequentially via a 24G angiocatheter to release the sperm from the seminiferous tubules into the tubal fluid media. Processing of the testicular tissue in this manner increases sperm yield by up to 470% [11]. A small sample is placed on a slide for microscopic examination of mature, viable sperm.

Multiple testicular tissue samples can be collected from the same incision or from various tunical incisions. Once satisfied, bipolar cautery is again used to achieve adequate hemostasis and the tunica albuginea is closed with 5-0 absorbable sutures in an interrupted fashion. The tunica vaginalis is also closed with a fine absorbable suture before the testicle is replaced within the scrotum. Finally, the dartos fascia and skin layers are closed with absorbable suture in a running fashion. The incision is infiltrated with 0.25% Marcaine with epinephrine to ensure adequate postprocedural anesthesia. The same procedure can also be repeated on the contralateral testicle if inadequate amounts of mature, viable sperm were found. Bacitracin ointment and fluff gauze are applied to the incision before a scrotal supporter is placed.

14.5.6 Microdissection Testicular Sperm Extraction

A critical understanding that has led to the development of microTESE was the documentation of the heterogeneity of sperm production within the testicle by Jow et al., who found sperm within the testes of one-third of men with NOA [2]. Goldstein described a technique of identification of the subtunical blood vessels that decreased the risk of damage to the testicular blood supply and which introduced the concept

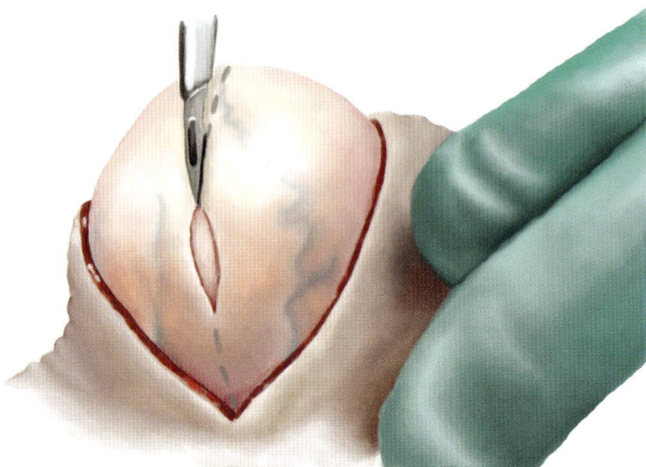

Figure 14.4 In microTESE, a 15° ultrasharp microknife is used to make a wide equatorial incision around the midportion of the testicle.

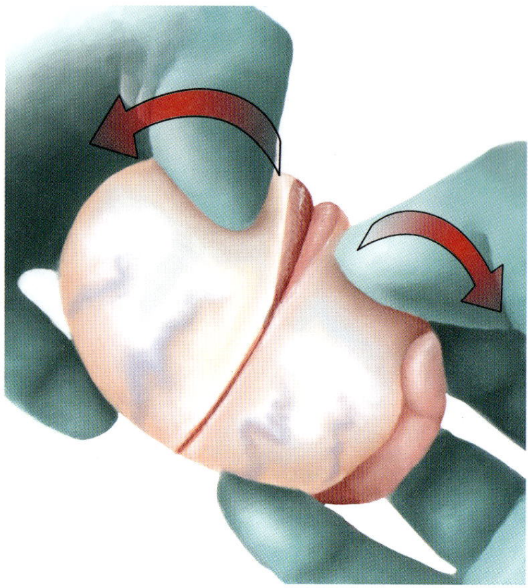

Figure 14.5 The testicle is opened up along the equatorial incision to provide maximal exposure of the seminiferous tubules.

of using an operating microscope for testicular procedures [12]. With the magnification provided by an operating microscope, the identification of sites within the testis that have sperm production is possible.

After the patient is induced under general anesthesia, he is placed in the supine position and the genitalia are prepped as per the usual aseptic technique. A median raphe incision is made and the dartos fascia dissected with electrocautery. The testicle is delivered via the median raphe incision and the tunica vaginalis is incised using electrocautery. A 15° ultrasharp microknife is used to open the testicle widely in an equatorial plane along the midportion of the testis (Figures 14.4 and 14.5). Bipolar cautery is used to control any subtunical blood vessels. With this incision, the seminiferous tubules are visualized in a physiologic approach that mimics the blood supply of the testis and maintains intratesticular blood flow.

By using the operating microscope at 15–20× magnification, seminiferous tubules likely to harbor spermatogenesis can be identified. In theory, seminiferous tubules with normal sperm production contain more cells and are therefore larger and more opaque than those without sperm (Figure 14.6). Selection and careful extraction of these specific seminiferous tubules improves the yield of sperm retrieval while minimizing the amount of testicular tissue removed.

In order to examine the entire testis, careful microdissection of the seminiferous tubules must be done while respecting the testicular architecture. Seminiferous tubules are divided by very fine septae with centrifugal blood vessels running in parallel to the tubules and the septae. Dissection must occur between the tubules to access deeper sections of tubules right down to the level of the tunica albuginea. Digital pressure under the tunical albuginea can help to evert the testicular tissue and facilitate dissection of tissues deep within the testicular parenchyma. Continuous gentle pressure across the tubules is also critical to allow for blunt separation of the tissue and for identification of tissue planes between the tubules. Dissection between tubules minimizes damage to the blood supply along the tubules and prevents separation of the tubules from the tunica albuginea,

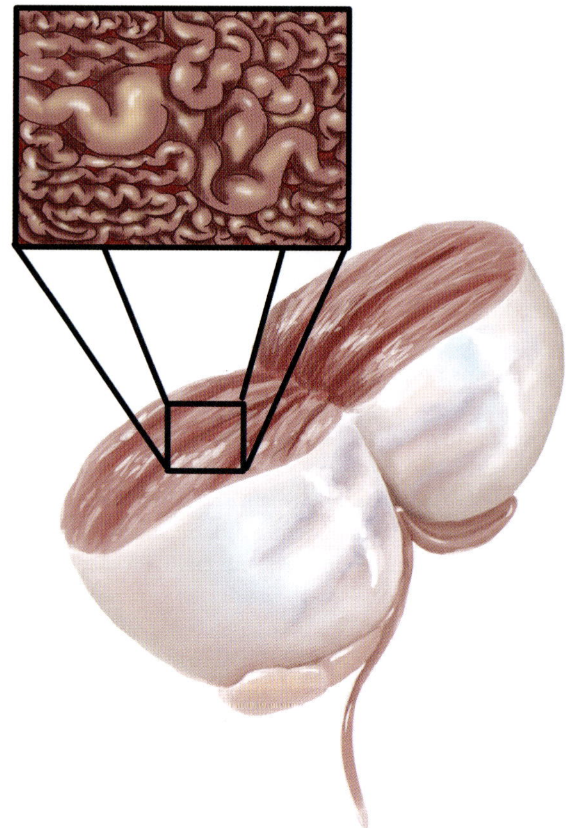

Figure 14.6 Seminiferous tubules that harbor intact spermatogenesis contain more cells and are therefore larger and more opaque than those without spermatogenesis.

where there is an extensive array of subtunical blood vessels that are prone to excessive bleeding. Bipolar cautery should be used throughout the dissection to maintain meticulous hemostasis that will minimize scarring and postoperative testicular hypofunction.

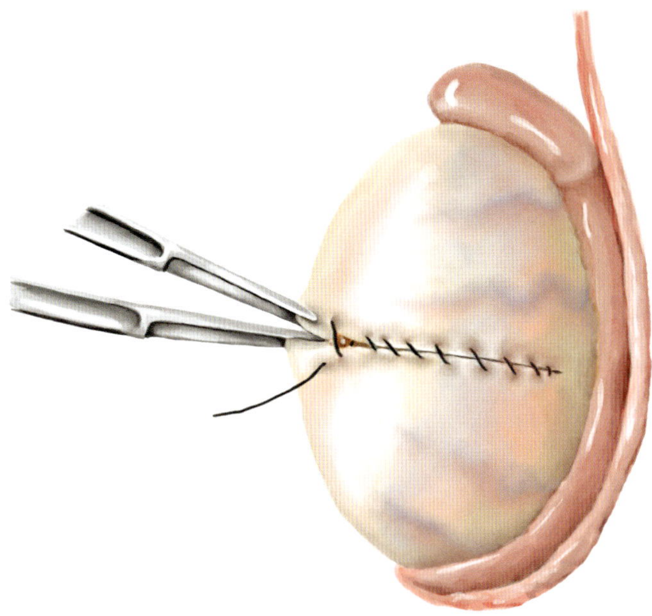

Figure 14.7 Once complete, the tunica albuginea is closed with 5-0 Prolene in a running fashion.

As seminiferous tubules are selected and removed from the testicle, they are placed in a dish containing sperm-wash fluid. The tubules are minced sharply with iris scissors until the tissue can be passed sequentially through a 24G angiocatheter. It is important to sequentially process and examine seminiferous tubule specimens for the presence of sperm in the operating room since the procedure can be terminated once a sufficient number of sperm are found.

Once satisfied, bipolar cautery is used to ensure meticulous hemostasis. The testicular parenchyma is reapproximated and the tunica albuginea closed with 5-0 Prolene in a running fashion (Figure 14.7). The tunica vaginalis is also closed with a fine absorbable suture and the intratunical space infused with 0.25% Marcaine. After using 0.25% Marcaine to provide a spermatic cord block, the testicle is replaced into the scrotum. If inadequate sperm were found, then a microTESE of the contralateral testicle can be performed at this time. Once complete, the dartos fascia is closed with a fine absorbable suture. The skin is also closed with 5-0 Monocryl in a running fashion and the incision infiltrated with 0.25% Marcaine with epinephrine to ensure adequate postprocedural anesthesia. Bacitracin ointment, fluff gauze, and a scrotal supporter are applied.

14.6 Postoperative Care

All surgical sperm retrieval procedures are typically performed on an outpatient basis, either in a hospital, ambulatory surgical center, or office. At our institution, patients are instructed to wear the scrotal supporter and to apply ice to the incisions for 48 hours to minimize scrotal swelling and edema. Patients can shower after 48 hours and may return to desk work and light activity after 2–3 days. No sexual intercourse is allowed for 1 week postoperatively and the patient should refrain from heavy work, strenuous activity, or sports for 2 weeks postoperatively.

All patients are discharged with oral opioid analgesics to be taken on an as needed basis as well as a scheduled anti-inflammatory medication (unless otherwise contraindicated), which has been shown to significantly decrease postoperative pain and opioid use in a randomized, double-blind, placebo-controlled trial [13].

14.7 Outcomes

14.7.1 Obstructive Azoospermia

Success rates for surgical sperm retrieval in patients with OA range from 90% to 100% (see Table 14.1). Each method is associated with its own anesthetic requirements, safety profiles, surgical skill requirements, and sperm retrieval yields. A 2008 Cochrane meta-analysis of various sperm retrieval techniques on pregnancy and fertilization rates in ICSI noted that "there was insufficient evidence to recommend any specific sperm retrieval technique" [17]. Similarly, an earlier meta-analysis examining ICSI outcomes using testicular or epididymal sperm from men with OA did not find any differences in fertilization, implantation, or pregnancy rates.[18]. Ultimately, in men with OA, the decision on which technique to choose depends heavily on both patient preferences and on surgeon experience.

Complications from surgical sperm retrieval techniques can include pain, bleeding/hematoma, hydrocele, and infection, with incidences ranging from 0% to 70% [19]. Percutaneous procedures tend to result in higher rates of hematoma, likely because of the inability to ensure adequate hemostasis [19]. More severe complications from vasal and epididymal sperm retrieval techniques include vasal and epididymal obstruction that can complicate or preclude future reconstruction.

14.7.2 Nonobstructive Azoospermia

Unlike in men with OA, there is considerable variation in the sperm retrieval rates (SRR) among the various testicular sperm extraction techniques. Further complicating a direct comparison between the techniques is the variable sperm retrieval rates associated with different pathologies.

While there are no RCTs comparing all three techniques of testicular sperm extraction, controlled observational studies have shown TESA, while simple and cheap, to have a lower SRR when compared to TESE with multiple biopsies, especially in those with Sertoli cell-only or maturation arrest on histology [20]. In the original description of microTESE by Schlegel, the historical SRR for TESE of 45% increased to 63% with microTESE [21]. These original results have been corroborated by other studies also showing higher SRR with microTESE compared to TESE, with the differences most pronounced in patients with a predominantly Sertoli cell-only pattern (that accentuates the difference in seminiferous tubule size). A systematic review examining surgical sperm retrieval for men with NOA identified microTESE as the most effective approach for surgical sperm retrieval, especially in those with a predominant Sertoli cell-only pattern [20]. A recent review presented an update of the microTESE experience at

Table 14.1 Clinical Characteristics of Sperm Retrieval Techniques for Men with OA [14–16]

Procedure	Anesthesia	Sperm Retrieval Rate	Advantages	Disadvantages
Vasal aspiration	General/regional or local	100%	Source of most mature sperm	Requires delicate microsurgical reconstruction of vasotomy
PESA	Local	80–100%	Office procedure Minimal recovery period	Hematoma May not retrieve adequate sperm Higher likelihood of inducing epididymal obstruction
MESA	General/regional or local	95–100%	High likelihood of obtaining adequate sperm May perform simultaneous reconstruction	Requires operating room and microsurgical skills
TESA	Local	52–100%	Office procedure Minimal recovery period	Hematoma May not retrieve adequate sperm
TESE	General/regional or local	100%	Fast procedure No microsurgical skills required	Risk of testicular atrophy and hypofunction Requires operating room More invasive and longer recovery period

Table 14.2 MicroTESE Sperm Retrieval and Pregnancy Rates for Azoospermia Patient Subsets at Weill Cornell Medical Center [22]

Patient Condition	Sperm Retrieval Rate	Pregnancy Rate (%)
Klinefelter syndrome	65% (100/155)	40
AZFc deletion	72% (39/54)	46
Cryptorchidism	64% (116/181)	50
Post-chemotherapy	48% (55/114)	40
All patients	56% (794/1414)	48

Weill Cornell Medicine and demonstrated continued respectable SRRs for a variety of patient subsets with NOA, such as Klinefelter syndrome, post-chemotherapy, AZFc deletion, and cryptorchidism (Table 14.2).

Another advantage of microTESE when compared to other testicular sperm extraction techniques is its low rate of complications. The aforementioned systematic review reported that microTESE had the lowest complication rate, ahead of TESA and TESE [20]. While TESA may appear to be a minimally invasive technique, the inability to ensure meticulous hemostasis means the adverse consequences within the testicle and on testicular function may be more significant than expected. In fact, TESA has been associated with testicular hemorrhage [23]. Complications from TESE range from transient inflammatory changes or hematomas detected on ultrasound lasting for up to 6 months postoperatively in up to 80% of patients to complete devascularisation of the testicle [24]. Other groups performing TESE have reported hypogonadism requiring hormone replacement therapy in 2.5% of patients, testicular atrophy in 25% of patients, and chronic testicular changes seen on ultrasound in 23% of patients [25]. On the other hand, patients undergoing microTESE have fewer acute and chronic changes as detected on scrotal ultrasound and appear to have less disruption in serum testosterone levels than those undergoing TESE [26,27].

14.8 Summary

Men with azoospermia due to OA or NOA can be managed with surgical sperm retrieval and advanced reproductive technologies. Those with OA can be managed with sperm retrieval from the vas deferens, epididymis, or testicle while those with NOA are limited to testicular sperm extraction. While the SRRs are similar among sperm retrieval techniques for men with OA, microTESE is the preferred surgical sperm retrieval technique for men with NOA due to its higher SRR and lower complication rate.

References

1. Jarow JP, Espeland MA, Lipshultz LI. Evaluation of the azoospermic patient. *J Urol.* 1989;142(1):62–5.

2. Jow WW, Steckel J, Schlegel PN, Magid MS, Goldstein M. Motile sperm in human testis biopsy specimens. *J Androl.* 1993;14(3):194–8.

3. Ramasamy R, Ricci JA, Palermo GD, Gosden LV, Rosenwaks Z, Schlegel PN. Successful fertility treatment for Klinefelter's syndrome. *J Urol.* 2009 Sep;182(3):1108–13.

4. Hopps CV, Mielnik A, Goldstein M, Palermo GD, Rosenwaks Z, Schlegel PN. Detection of sperm in men with Y chromosome microdeletions of the AZFa, AZFb and AZFc regions. *Hum Reprod.* 2003;18(8):1660–5.

5. Schlegel PN, Su LM. Physiological consequences of testicular sperm extraction. *Hum Reprod.* 1997;12(8):1688–92.

6. Weedin JW, Khera M, Lipshultz LI. Varicocele repair in patients with nonobstructive azoospermia: a meta-analysis. *J Urol.* 2010;183(6):2309–15.

7. Schlegel PN, Kaufmann J. Role of varicocelectomy in men with nonobstructive azoospermia. *Fertil Steril.* 2004;81(6):1585–8.

8. Inci K, Hascicek M, Kara O, Dikmen AV, Gürgan T, Ergen A. Sperm retrieval and intracytoplasmic sperm injection in men with nonobstructive azoospermia, and treated and untreated varicocele. *J Urol.* 2009;182(4):1500–5.

9. Haydardedeoglu B, Turunc T, Kilicdag EB, Gul U, Bagis T. The effect of prior varicocelectomy in patients with nonobstructive azoospermia on intracytoplasmic sperm injection outcomes: a retrospective pilot study. *Urology.* 2010;75(1):83–6.

10. Raman JD, Schlegel PN. Aromatase inhibitors for male infertility. *J Urol.* 2002;167(2, Part 1):624–9.

11. Ostad M, Liotta D, Ye Z, Schlegel PN. Testicular sperm extraction for nonobstructive azoospermia: results of a multibiopsy approach with optimized tissue dispersion. *Urology.* 1998;52(4):692–6.

12. Dardashti K, Williams RH, Goldstein M. Microsurgical testis biopsy: a novel technique for retrieval of testicular tissue. *J Urol.* 2000;163(4):1206–7.

13. Mehta A, Hsiao W, King P, Schlegel PN. Perioperative celecoxib decreases opioid use in patients undergoing testicular surgery: a randomized, double-blind, placebo controlled trial. *J Urol.* 2013;190(5):1834–8.

14. Levine LA, Fakouri BJ. Experience with vasal sperm aspiration. *J Urol.* 1998;159(5):1551–3.

15. Qiu Y, Wang S, Yang D, Wang L. Percutaneous vasal sperm aspiration and intrauterine insemination for infertile males with anejaculation. *Fertil Steril.* 2003;79(3):618–20.

16. Bernie AM, Ramasamy R, Stember DS, Stahl PJ. Microsurgical epididymal sperm aspiration: indications, techniques and outcomes. *Asian J Androl.* 2013;15(1):40–3.

17. Van Peperstraten A, Proctor ML, Johnson NP, Philipson G. Techniques for surgical retrieval of sperm prior to intra-cytoplasmic sperm injection (ICSI) for azoospermia. *Cochrane Database Syst Rev.* 2008;(2):CD002807. doi(2):CD002807.

18. Nicopoullos JDM, Gilling-Smith C, Almeida PA, Norman-Taylor J, Grace I, Ramsay JWA. Use of surgical sperm retrieval in azoospermic men: a meta-analysis. *Fertil Steril.* 2004 Sep;82(3):691–701.

19. Esteves SC, Miyaoka R, Orosz JE, Agarwal A. An update on sperm retrieval techniques for azoospermic males. *Clinics (Sao Paulo).* 2013;68 Suppl 1:99–110.

20. Donoso P, Tournaye H, Devroey P. Which is the best sperm retrieval technique for non-obstructive azoospermia? A systematic review. *Hum Reprod Update.* 2007;13(6):539–49.

21. Schlegel PN. Testicular sperm extraction: microdissection improves sperm yield with minimal tissue excision. *Hum Reprod.* 1999;14(1):131–5.

22. Dabaja AA, Schlegel PN. Microdissection testicular sperm extraction: an update. *Asian J Androl.* 2013;15(1):35–9.

23. Friedler S, Raziel A, Strassburger D, Soffer Y, Komarovsky D, Ron-El R. Testicular sperm retrieval by percutaneous fine needle sperm aspiration compared with testicular sperm extraction by open biopsy in men with non-obstructive azoospermia. *Hum Reprod.* 1997;12(7):1488–93.

24. Schlegel PN, Su LM. Physiological consequences of testicular sperm extraction. *Hum Reprod.* 1997;12(8):1688–92.

25. Okada H, Dobashi M, Yamazaki T, et al. Conventional versus microdissection testicular sperm extraction for nonobstructive azoospermia. *J Urol.* 2002;168(3):1063–7.

26. Ramasamy R, Yagan N, Schlegel PN. Structural and functional changes to the testis after conventional versus microdissection testicular sperm extraction. *Urology.* 2005;65(6):1190–4.

27. Deruyver Y, Vanderschueren D, Van der Aa F. Outcome of microdissection TESE compared with conventional TESE in non-obstructive azoospermia: a systematic review. *Andrology.* 2014;2(1):20–4.

15.1 Introduction

Obstruction of the ejaculatory ducts can negatively impair semen quantity and quality to the extent of azoospermia, compromising fertility. Further, it may lead to symptoms including ejaculatory disorders (e.g., painful ejaculation, nonprojectile ejaculation, diminished sense of orgasm, or hematospermia), dysuria, and variable extents of pelvic and genital pain [1,2]. Anatomically, the left and right ejaculatory ducts enter the prostatic urethra at the level of the utricle of the prostate. Bilateral complete obstruction of ejaculatory ducts typically leads to low-volume azoospermia with acidic pH in semen that is negative for fructose. Some patients who have acquired this condition may present with painful ejaculation or general pelvic pain. Unilateral or incomplete ejaculatory duct obstruction (EDO), on the other hand, may lead to variable deterioration of semen parameters. In the context of male infertility, ejaculatory duct obstruction may be managed surgically by transurethral resection of the ejaculatory duct (TURED) to remove the obstructed segment of the excurrent ductal system within the prostate. The approach to TURED will be the focus of this chapter. Other surgeries of the seminal vesicles for other pathologies such as cyst or neoplasia will not be discussed in this chapter.

Normally, the ejaculatory ducts contain a valve-like mechanism that prevents reflux of urine into the excurrent ductal system. Though TURED can relieve the obstruction, reflux of urine up the excurrent ductal system may develop in a significant portion of men after successful TURED [3], causing chemical and/or bacterial epididymitis. Not infrequently, additional significant complications (see Section 15.7, "Complications") may develop postoperatively. Thus, TURED should not be considered a benign procedure and should only be done by experienced surgeons after careful evaluation and counseling with patients. Alternative options for management of symptoms of ejaculatory obstruction (e.g., for pelvic pain or pain with ejaculation) and infertility (e.g., with sperm retrieval in conjunction with assisted reproduction) must be discussed prior to undertaking TURED.

15.2 Preoperative Evaluations

A detailed history should focus on any history of infertility, symptoms of pelvic/genital pain, sexual, ejaculatory, and voiding dysfunction. Drugs that are known to impair ejaculation, such as α-adrenergic antagonists, selective serotonin reuptake inhibitors, thiazides, or certain antipsychotic and antihypertensive agents, should be discontinued. A thorough physical examination focusing on the prostate and genital examination (such as scrotal and spermatic cord anomalies, testicular size and texture, epididymal fullness and anomalies, presence of vas deferens, prostate volume, and anomalies) must be carefully documented. Postejaculation urinalysis should confirm the absence of retrograde ejaculation. Urine culture and urinalysis should be performed prior to surgery to confirm the absence of urinary tract infection. Hormonal profile including morning serum total or bioavailable testosterone, estradiol, luteinizing hormone, and follicle-stimulating hormone should be performed.

In men with ejaculatory duct obstruction, semen analyses, performed according to the standards of the WHO [4], generally reveal low-volume azoospermia with acidic pH. However, patients with incomplete obstruction (e.g., unilateral or partial) may have variable semen parameters. Surgical correction of ejaculatory duct obstruction is not contraindicated in non-azoospermic symptomatic men (e.g., those with pelvic or ejaculatory pain, low volume of semen or infertility) or men with coexisting spermatogenic dysfunction (as indicated by elevated serum FSH level, hypogonadism, hypotrophic testis). However, patients with this presentation should be clearly informed that even after successful surgical correction of ejaculatory duct obstruction, there may not be any or adequate amount of sperm returning to the ejaculate for fertility purpose.

Transrectal ultrasound (TRUS) to evaluate the prostate to document any intraprostatic cysts, dilatation (e.g., seminal vesicle transverse diameter > 1.5 cm, vasal ampulla transverse diameter > 6 mm, ejaculatory diameter > 2 mm) [5] or anomalies (e.g., cysts, stones, or calcifications) of the ejaculatory ducts or seminal vesicles can provide additional information important for the planning of TURED. Generally, a single large midline prostatic cyst (Mullerian duct cyst) viewed on TRUS may represent an obliterated cavity where the outflow of the ejaculatory duct empties (Figure 15.1). Resection to unroof such a cavity may unobstruct the ejaculatory ducts. In the absence of such a cavity, transurethral resection will be a challenge as the surgeon must carefully make consecutive shallow resections until confirmation of patency of the ejaculatory ducts. It should be noted that occasionally intraprostatic cysts, particularly when they are multiple, small in size, or off the midline, do not necessarily represent a cavity obstructing the outflow of the ejaculatory ducts. In this setting, the surgeon

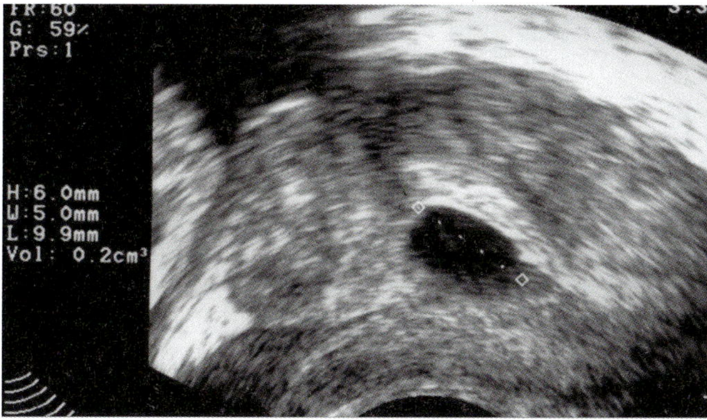

Figure 15.1 Sagital view of TRUS revealing a midline cystic cavity within the center of the prostate.

must also carefully make shallow resection until patency of the ejaculatory ducts is confirmed.

Genetic evaluation for mutations of the cystic fibrosis transmembrane regulator (CFTR) should be performed in men with congenital anomalies of the male excurrent ductal system such as the unilateral or bilateral absence of the vasa deferentia, obstruction, and partial agenesis of the epididymides. In these men the cause of infertility is often solely due to obstruction at the levels of vasa deferentia and epididymides. CFTR gene mutation evaluation may also be considered in men with congenital ejaculatory duct obstruction in spite of the vasa deferentia being palpable. Even for men with palpable vasa and intact epididymides presenting with isolated anomalies of the seminal vesicles (IASV) or bilateral EDO, mutations of the CFTR genes have been reported in 13% of IASV and as high as 86% of bilateral EDO patients [6]. As these men will have a reasonably good chance for procreation, particularly with assisted reproduction, appropriate genetic counseling for men with documented CFTR mutations should be offered. Additional workup, such as pelvic imaging with computed tomography (CT) or magnetic resonance imaging (MRI) [7], testicular biopsy, and cystoscopy may be performed as indicated based on the clinical presentation and findings of the patients. Seminal vesicle aspiration [8], for examination of sperm, can be an alternative to testicular biopsy to confirm spermatogenic activities. Less commonly performed investigations such as seminal vesicle manometry [9], vesiculoscopy, vesiculography, chromotubation [10,11], and scintigraphy [12] have been described as alternative means to confirm the diagnosis of ejaculatory duct obstruction.

15.3 Preoperative Counseling

When obtaining informed consent, patients should be counseled on the potential complications of TURED, which include, in addition to anesthesia-related complications and general surgical complications (such as wound infection, vascular injury, and pain) – from highest to the lowest rates of occurrence – urine reflux to the excurrent ductal system, vasal obstruction, persistent ejaculatory duct obstruction, retrograde ejaculation, ejaculation of urine, incontinence, rectal injury, and urethral stricture. Thus, TURED should not be considered a benign procedure and should only be done by experienced surgeon after

careful evaluation and counseling with patients. Alternative options for management of symptoms of ejaculatory obstruction (e.g., for pelvic pain or pain with ejaculation) and infertility (e.g., with sperm retrieval in conjunction with assisted reproduction) must be discussed prior to undertaking TURED.

Men with unilateral or incomplete bilateral ejaculatory duct obstruction may present with nonazoospermic infertility (i.e., semen parameters ranging from a combination of oligo-asthenoteratospermia to normal semen parameters) or ejaculatory or pelvic/genital pain symptoms. Unfortunately, these men will usually not be investigated specifically for incomplete ejaculatory duct obstruction. Instead, their presentations are often considered idiopathic and managed with assisted reproduction for infertility and analgesic/antibiotics for pain, both with variable success. With the increase in the access of various imaging modalities including TRUS and MRI, some of these men, particularly those who are refractory to other forms of therapies for their symptoms, may be correctly diagnosed to have incomplete ejaculatory duct obstruction that require surgical management. However, it is important to emphasize that these men must be properly counseled on the potential risks and benefits prior to undergoing TURED. Alternative options for symptomatic management and fertility management such as with assisted reproduction must be discussed and, as mentioned earlier, sperm cryopreservation prior to surgery and intraoperatively must be offered. Though invasive and uncommonly performed, seminal vesicle manometry [9] may be considered to establish the presence of a significant obstruction prior to considering surgical management.

15.4 Surgical Approach to TURED

15.4.1 Vasography

When performing TURED, particularly when there is a sizable single prostatic midline cyst, many fertility specialists proceed with TURED without performing a vasography in the same setting. As vasography carries risks of vasal obstruction (see Section 15.7.2), this consideration is especially important when TURED is performed by surgeons who do not routinely perform vasal surgeries that require microscopic surgical skills and special equipment. However, a concomitant vasography provides the following benefits in managing men with EDO: (1) it allows for evaluation if there is epididymal obstruction that would suggest not to proceed with TURED (see later); (2) it allows for retrieval of sperm for cryopreservation for assisted reproduction should reconstruction fail; (3) it allows for intraoperative confirmation of patency of the excurrent ductal system after TURED is performed (see Section 15.4.5). Generally, vasography should be performed in the same setting with surgical correction of ejaculatory duct obstruction [13]. The surgical procedure described in the following begins with a high scrotal incision for vasography. It should be noted that alternative approaches such as percutaneous delivery of the vas deferens for vasography (e.g., using techniques similar to no-scalpal vasectomy), transrectal vasography, or seminal vesiculography [14] may also be used. In the latter two approaches, the same bowel prep and antibiotic coverage used for transrectal prostate biopsy should be employed.

15.4.2 Anesthesia

General anesthesia or spinal anesthesia is generally required.

15.4.3 Perioperative Antibiotics

Urinary tract infection should be treated before surgery. While most experts agree that perioperative prophylactic antibiotics should be used for transurethral resection of prostate (TURP), there is a lack of literature evaluating their values for TURED, which is generally less extensive a surgery compared to TURP.

15.4.4 Position

The patient should be in supine position for the vasography and then placed in lithotomy position for the transurethral part of the surgery.

15.4.5 Procedure

After prepping and draping the scrotal, inguinal, and perineal area with antiseptic solution while the patient is in a supine position, bilateral high scrotal incision is made to expose the vas deferens at the junction of the straight and convoluted portions. Under an operating microscope at 10-power magnification, the vasal sheath is longitudinally incised to minimize damage to the vasal vessels. A clean segment of bare vas is delivered and, under 25-power magnification, a 15° microknife is used to transversely hemitransect the vas until the lumen is revealed (Figure 15.2). Any fluid exuding from the lumen is examined microscopically for sperm. Cryopreservation of the vasal fluid for sperm prior to TURED should be considered, particularly if motile sperm are found. This can be achieved with repeated aspiration of the vasal fluid with a 24 G angiocatheter attached to a 1 ml tuberculin syringe.

If the vasal fluid is devoid of sperm despite repeated sampling after milking the epididymis and convoluted vas, epididymal obstruction is likely present (in the absence of any clinical suspicion of ipsilateral testicular dysfunction). In the presence of epididymal obstruction, if the ipsilateral distal vas deferens or ejaculatory duct are obstructed, it is best to abandon attempts at reconstruction and simply perform microsurgical epididymal sperm aspiration or testicular sperm retrieval and cryopreservation for future IVF/ ICSI. This is because the overall success of simultaneous vasoepididymostomy and TURED, two technically challenging procedures, are generally low [15].

To evaluate if the distal vas deferens and ejaculatory duct are patent, the lumen of the vas toward the ejaculatory duct is then cannulated with a 24-G angiocatheter sheath and injected with 1 mL of lactated Ringer solution with 1 mL tuberculin syringe to confirm its patency (Figure 15.3). If the Ringer solution passes easily, formal vasography and ejaculatory duct resection are not necessary. If further proof of obstruction of the excurrent ductal system is desired, 1 mL of 1:20 diluted indigo carmine or methylene blue may be injected intravasally toward the ejaculatory duct and the bladder catheterized. The absence of blue/green dye in the urine confirms obstruction of the ipsilateral vas and ejaculatory duct.

Once obstruction is confirmed toward the ejaculatory duct, a 2-0 Proline suture can be passed intravasally toward

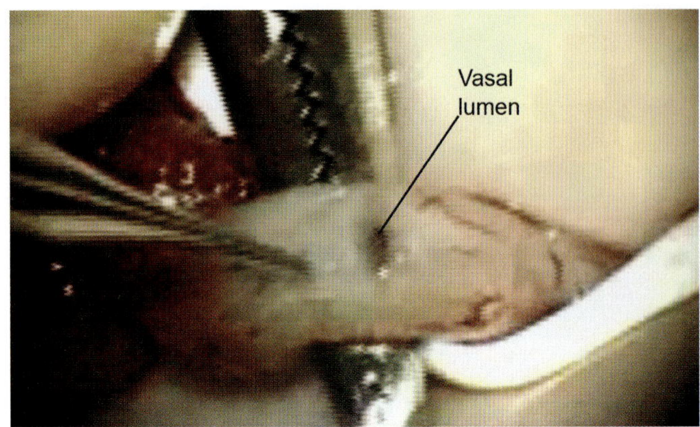

Figure 15.2 A clean segment of bare vas is delivered and, transversely hemitransected with a #11 blade to reveal the vas lumen. Any fluid exuding from the lumen is examined microscopically for sperm.

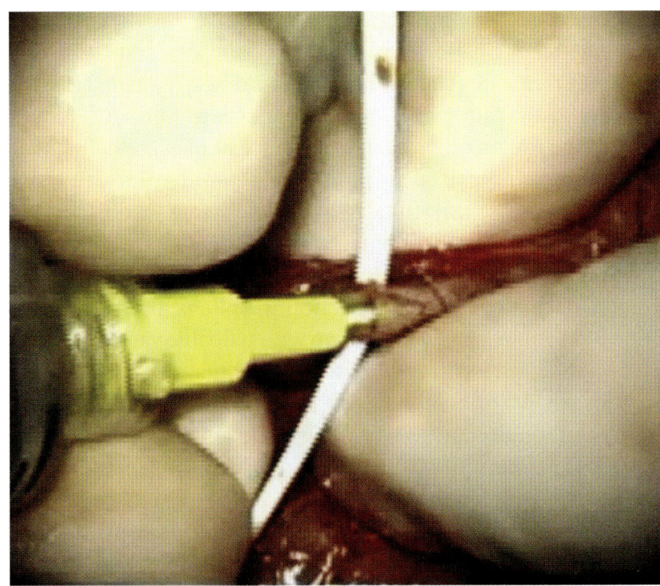

Figure 15.3 The vas is cannulated with a 24-gauge angiocatheter with fluid injected towards the abdominal end.

the ejaculatory duct and a clamp placed on the suture when it passes no farther. This is particularly useful in patients who had undergone ipsilateral inguinal surgery, such as a hernia repair, to allow confirmation that the vasal obstruction is not at the inguinal area but farther at the ejaculatory duct. Formal vasography may be performed by passing a 3 French whistle-tip ureteral catheter toward the seminal vesicle end of the vas. A 16 French Foley catheter is placed in the bladder, and the balloon is filled with 5 mL of air. Placing the balloon on gentle traction before vasography prevents reflux of contrast into the bladder, which can obscure detail. The air-filled balloon also identifies the location of the bladder neck relative to any obstruction. Vasogram is performed with the injection of 0.5 mL of water-soluble contrast media. Only if the vasogram confirms obstruction is at the level of the ejaculatory duct, instead of at the vas deferens, should one proceed to perform a transurethral resection of the ejaculatory duct. The ureteral catheter should be left in place inside the vas for later during the transurethral resection of the ejaculatory duct.

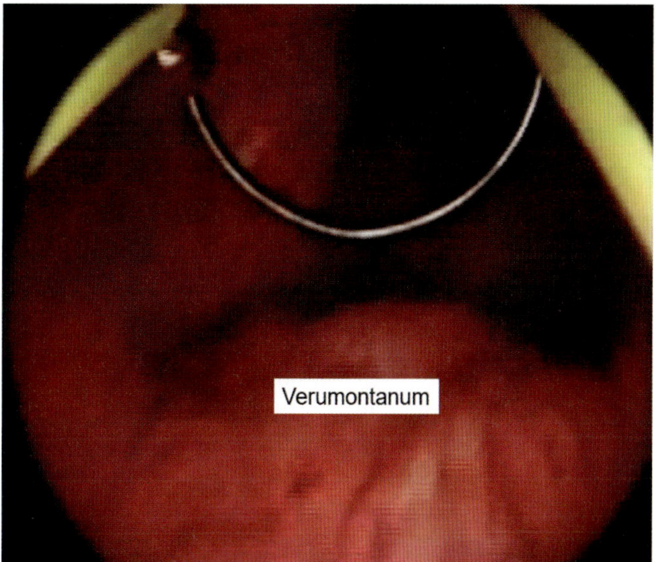

Figure 15.4 TURED is performed by resecting the verumontanum.

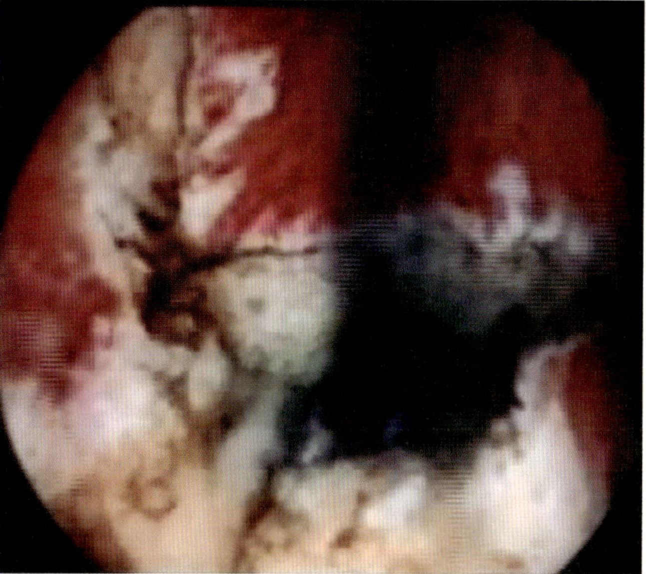

Figure 15.5 Efflux of indigo carmine from the dilated prostatic cystic cavity confirms adequate resection.

A similar procedure should be performed on the contralateral side. The dilution for indigo carmine or methylene blue for the second side should be more concentrated at 1:5 to allow visual distinction of the two sides during intravasal injection. The patient is then carefully placed in lithotomy position and prepped and draped for transurethral procedure.

The setup is identical to TURP. Although the use of holmium laser for TURED has been described [16,17], fertility specialists who do not perform prostate resection with laser routinely may choose to use conventional TURP setup as described here. Cold knife incision alone almost always leads to reobstruction and is not a treatment of choice for TURED. It is advisable to use an O'Connor-type drape in which a rectal hole is provided to allow prostate digital palpation during the resection. Keep in mind that patients undergoing TURED are generally younger with thinner prostates than men undergoing TURP for benign prostate hyperplasia/lower urinary tract symptoms (BPH/LUTS). The tactile sensation when palpating the prostate during TURED can help to minimize the risk of too deep a resection that can potentially lead to rectal damage. The resectoscope, with the 24 French cutting loop, is engaged with a finger placed in the rectum providing anterior displacement of the posterior lobe of the prostate (Figure 15.4). The ejaculatory ducts course between the bladder neck and the verumontanum and exit at the level of and along the lateral aspect of the verumontanum. Resection of the verumontanum will often reveal the dilated ejaculatory duct orifice or cyst cavity where blue dye injected through the vasa comes out (Figure 15.5). Resection should be carried out in this region with great care in order to preserve the bladder neck proximally, the striated sphincter distally, and the rectal mucosa posteriorly. In case of unilateral TURED, a Collins knife may be used and aim at an angle to resect only one side of the verumontanum (Figures 15.6 and 15.7). Efflux of indigo carmine from dilated orifices confirms adequate resection. Avoid excessive coagulation that can lead to scarring and reobstruction of the ejaculatory ducts (Figure 15.8).

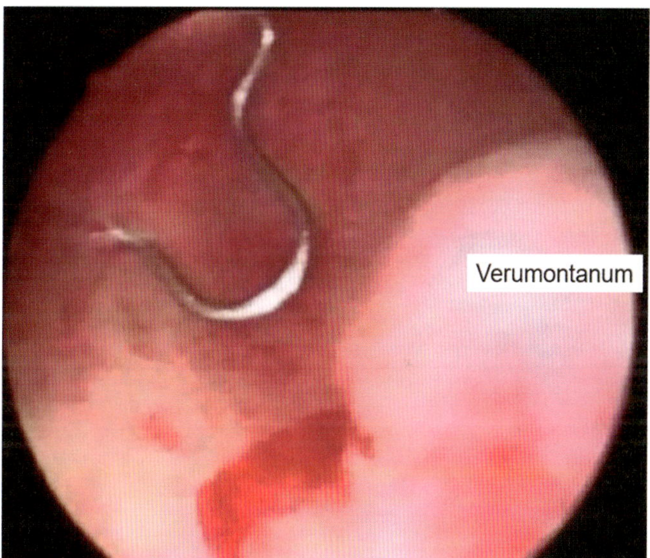

Figure 15.6 Unilateral ejaculatory duct obstruction can be resolved by resection at only the orifice involved.

If the ejaculatory duct orifices are visualized but no dye efflux is seen, there may be obstruction in the distal vas proximal to the point of resection. This may be a bilateral or unilateral phenomenon. The resectoscope may be withdrawn and replaced with a 6 or 7 French flexible ureteroscope. A small balloon dilation catheter or ureteral serial dilators over a fine (0.032 inch) guidewire may be inserted into the ejaculatory duct toward its medial aspect into the vas through the ureteroscope. Retrograde contrast injection under fluoroscopic guidance may establish the location of obstruction in the vas. Gentle balloon dilatation may be performed to correct the obstruction using similar principles as the management of ureteral stricture. Prior to completely withdrawing the fine balloon catheter from the ejaculatory duct, radio-opaque contrast should also be injected toward the ipsilateral seminal vesicle to confirm its

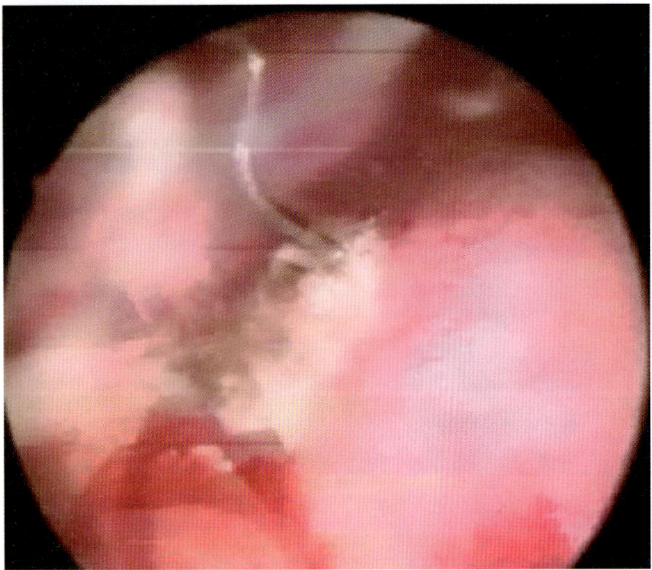

Figure 15.7 Unilateral TURED for obstruction of the right ejaculatory duct.

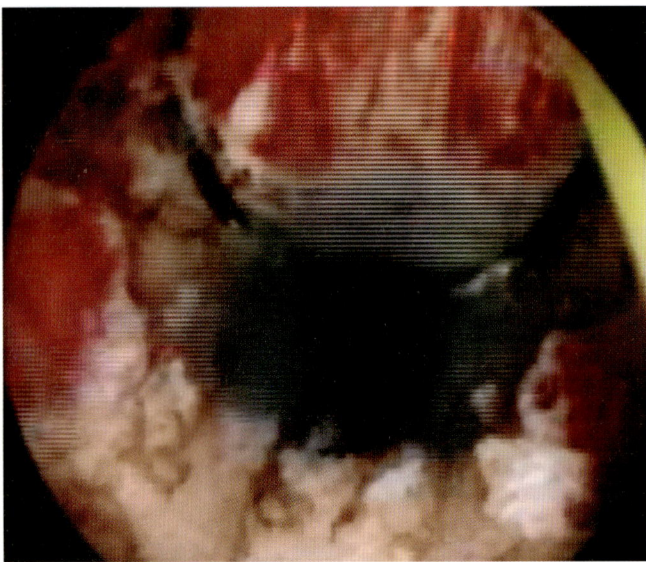

Figure 15.8 Avoid excessive coagulation that may lead to scarring and reobstruction of the ejaculatory ducts.

patency. Successful dilatation of the vas should be confirmed by establishing efflux of dye through the vasal antegrade injection with minimal resistance after withdrawal of the ureteral catheter from the ejaculatory duct. In addition to stricture, occasionally the obstruction is caused by stones in the vas or seminal vesicle. Similar techniques can be used to extract the stones using a 4 French basket and dilate the stricture in the seminal vesicle. The hemivasostomy sites are carefully closed employing microsurgical technique with 8-0 to 10-0 sutures.

Surgeons who perform these procedures in seminal vesicle, distal vas, and ampulla should be experienced in endoscopic techniques with appropriate tools and equipment. Excessive manipulations may cause further damage. If one fails to achieve patency despite various manipulations, the procedure should be abandoned before causing any further damage to the excurrent ductal system. The patient should then be counseled for alternative management postoperatively such as sperm retrieval for assisted reproduction.

15.5 Postoperative Care

Immediately post-op, a 16–20 French Foley catheter is left overnight for straight drainage. If extensive resection has been performed and there is significant hematuria, continuous bladder irrigation with a three-way Foley catheter may be needed. Oral hydration is encouraged to minimize accumulation of clots if hematuria persists. The patient is advised to abstain from ejaculation for at least 2 weeks. Self-limiting hematospermia is common immediately post-op. Semen analysis may be performed 1–2 months after surgery to evaluate any changes in semen parameters postoperatively. Surgeons should inform the laboratory to accurately remeasure semen volume, pH, and fructose levels in addition to other parameters for comparison. If semen parameters improve and no complications are observed, a repeated TRUS or cystoscopy postoperatively is generally not required.

15.6 Outcomes

TURED results in improvement in semen parameters in 50–70% of patients. Natural pregnancy rates are based on case reports and small series and are estimated to be 20–40% at 1 year postoperatively [11,18–22]. If viable sperms appear in the ejaculate but the quantity and quality are poor, assisted reproduction with intrauterine insemination (IUI), in vitro fertilization (IVF), or intracytoplasmic sperm injection (ICSI) should be recommended based on, among other factors, postoperatively semen parameters and the female partner's reproductive status. Significant relief of symptoms such as postcoital and perineal pain after TURED can be expected in 60% of patients [10,23].

15.7 Postoperative Complications

15.7.1 Urinary Reflux to the Excurrent Ductal System

Normally, the ejaculatory ducts contain a valve-like mechanism that prevents reflux of urine into the excurrent ductal system. Though TURED can relieve the obstruction, reflux of urine up the excurrent ductal system may develop in a significant portion of men after successful TURED [3], causing chemically induced inflammation and/or bacterial infection. The true incidence of this complication is probably underestimated and under-reported. Reflux of urine can lead to inflammation to any part of the excurrent ductal system and commonly presents as scrotal/pelvic pain or epididymitis. Epididymitis can be either acute or chronic and bacterial or chemical. With regards to fertility, post-TURED recurrent epididymitis often results in suboptimal improvement in semen parameters or eventual epididymal obstruction. Voiding cystourethrogram can document some cases of urinary reflux to the excurrent ductal system post-TURED.

Chronic low-dose antibacterial suppression similar to that employed for vesicoureteral reflux may be helpful in men with recurrent epididymal infection until pregnancy is achieved. If epididymitis is chronic and recurrent, vasectomy or even epididymectomy may be necessary. However, if symptoms are due to vesiculitis secondary to urinary reflux, vasectomy may not ameliorate the symptoms.

15.7.2 Vasal Obstruction

This complication occurs during surgical access to the scrotal vas for TURED. Vasal ischemia, mucosal damage, and leaky closure of a vasography site leading to the development of a sperm granuloma can result in stricture or obstruction of the vas. Microsurgical techniques for a water-tight closure of the vasography sites are the key to avoid this complication.

15.7.3 Persistent Ejaculatory Duct Obstruction

Ejaculatory duct obstruction may persist despite TURED. Typically this occurs when a long segment of the ejaculatory duct or distal vas deferens are obliterated such that despite repeated resections of the verumontanum and prostate or with balloon dilatation, obstruction remains. Even when patency of the ejaculatory duct is confirmed at the end of TURED, inflammation and fibrosis may reobstruct the excurrent ductal system. For men with incomplete obstruction (e.g., unilateral obstruction) who still have variable amounts of sperm found in the ejaculate, sperm cryopreservation should be offered pre- and intraoperatively as these patients may have complete obstruction leading to azoospermia postoperatively [24].

15.7.4 Retrograde Ejaculation

This bothersome complication occurs when the bladder neck is resected or undermined. However, even when care has been taken to spare the bladder neck, retrograde ejaculation is common after TURED. Pseudoephedrine 120 mg orally, 90 minutes before ejaculation, or Ornade Spansules (chlorpheniramine and phenylpropanolamine) twice a day [15] for a week may help in some cases. If this is not successful, sperm can be retrieved from alkalinized urine and used for either IUI or IVF with ICSI.

15.7.5 Ejaculation of Urine at Orgasm

Sometimes referred to as "climacturia," this complication is seen in approximately 20% of patients. It is a very disturbing postoperative complication characterized by a high volume (> 5 cc) of watery ejaculation. Evaluation of creatinine levels of ejaculate confirms the presence of urine. The mechanisms of this complication may include (1) urine collection in the cystic cavity post-TURED that is forced out during ejaculation; (2) urine reflux into the excurrent ductal system (particularly the seminal vesicles and/or vasal ampullae) that is forced out during ejaculation; (3) transient hyperactive bladder trigone with weakened bladder neck closure during orgasm leading to urine expulsion. The exact cause of this complication in an individual patient is often difficult to delineate. Though

conservative managements such as complete voiding prior to sexual activities and a trial of medical management using agents similar those used for overactive bladder, lower urinary tract symptoms, retrograde ejaculation may be considered, little can be offered for those who are refractory to these conservative managements.

15.7.6 Incontinence

This complication occurs due to damage to the bladder neck or external sphincter. Careful evaluation of the various anatomical landmarks during TURED should minimize or prevent this complication.

15.7.7 Rectal Injury

One of the most devastating complications of TURED is rectal injury. As these patients are generally young with small prostates, the importance of performing the surgery with prostate rectal palpation through an O'Connor-type drape (see Section 15.4.5) cannot be overemphasized.

15.7.8 Urethral Stricture

Urethral stricture is rarer in TURED compared to transurethral resection of prostate (TURP) as the former procedure is generally shorter in duration and is therefore associated with a lower risk of ischemic damage to the urethra.

15.8 Long-Term Management

Up to 50% of TURED cases may have no significant improvement postoperatively. If the ejaculate volume remains low with no significant improvement in sperm concentration and motility or if he remains azoospermic, he may have (1) incomplete unroofing of the cystic cavity where the ejaculatory ducts empty into; (2) incomplete resection of the obstructed portion of the ejaculatory duct; (3) contracture of the resection leading to reobstruction of the ejaculatory duct; (4) the obstructed ejaculatory ducts or seminal vesicles do not empty into the cystic cavity resected. Cystoscopic examination can be performed postoperatively to evaluate for contracture of the resected areas and, if necessary, cannulation of the ejaculatory duct and seminal vesicles for fluoroscopic examination should be performed to confirm their patency (Figures 15.9 and 15.10). Retrograde cannulation of the vas deferens (medially) or seminal vesicle duct (laterally) may be attempted under anesthesia through the ejaculatory duct opening (Figure 15.11) for balloon dilatation.

Postoperatively, if the patient's semen volume normalizes but without improvement in sperm concentration and motility or remains azoospermic, the patient may have persistent or recurrent obstruction of the vasa ampullae despite patency in the seminal vesicle ducts (assuming that a proper intraoperative vasography was performed to confirm the absence of epididymal obstruction). Cystoscopy in this scenario may reveal a properly opened prostatic cyst or patent seminal vesicle ducts. Seminal vesiculoscopy will reveal patent seminal vesicles. Antegrade (through scrotal vasal exploration) or retrograde (if the opening of the ejaculatory duct is clearly visualized in

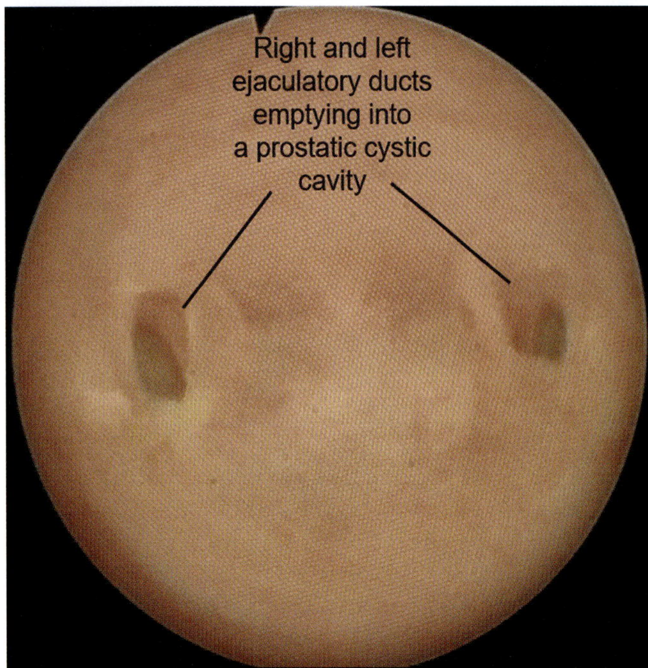

Figure 15.9 Cystoscopic inspection of the unroofed cystic cavity revealed that the ejaculatory ducts are opened bilaterally. Fluoroscopic evaluation using radio-contrast injected via retrograde cannulation of the ejaculated ducts may be required to confirm patency.

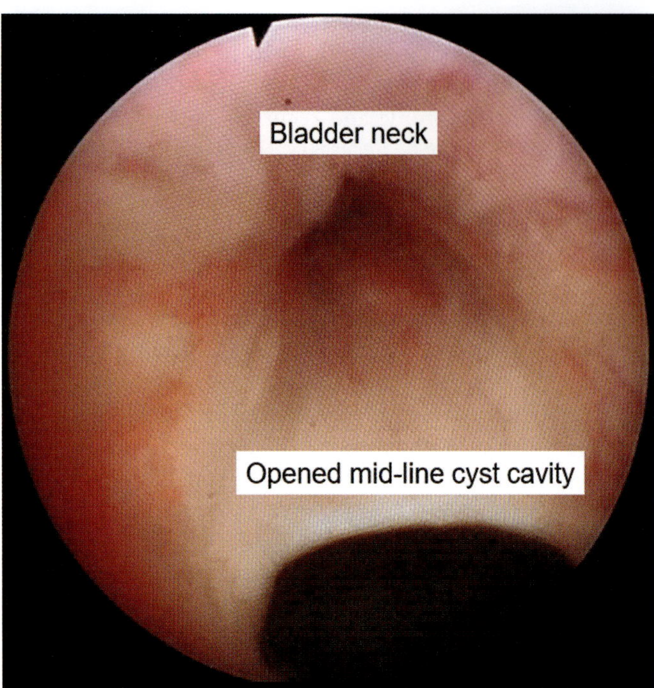

Figure 15.11 Cystoscopic evaluation post-TURED. Note the unroofed mid-line cyst cavity remains opened postoperatively.

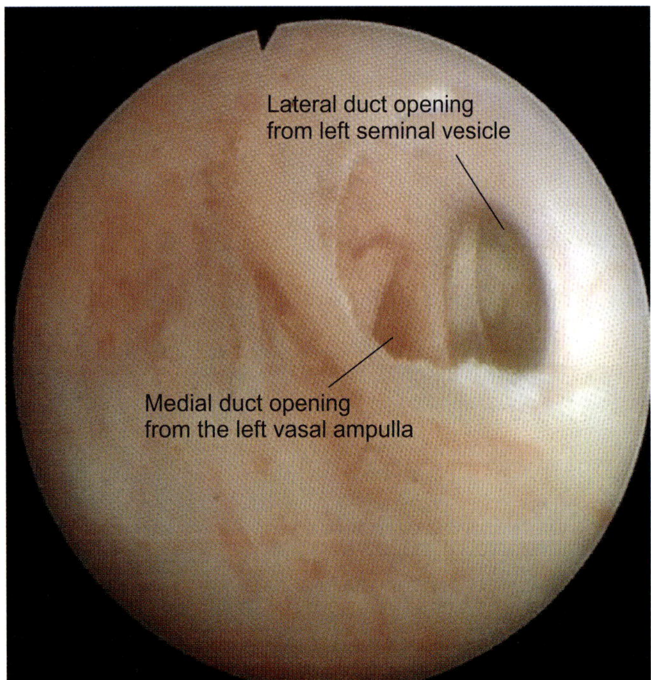

Figure 15.10 Inspection of the left ejaculatory duct revealing the medial duct opening from the vasal ampulla and lateral duct opening from the seminal vesicle.

cystoscopy) cannulation of the vas deferens for balloon dilatation may be attempted to correct the obstruction.

As discussed earlier, the best way to minimize the occurrence of these scenarios is to properly perform intraoperative vasography, which, in addition to confirming the absence of epididymal obstruction and allowing for cryopreservation of sperm, can permit confirmation of patency of ejaculatory ducts and vasa post resection.

References

1. Pryor JP, Hendry WF. Ejaculatory duct obstruction in subfertile males: analysis of 87 patients. *Fertil Steril.* 1991;56(4):725–30.

2. Johnson CW, Bingham JB, Goluboff ET, et al. Transurethral resection of the ejaculatory ducts for treating ejaculatory symptoms. *BJU Int.* 2005;95(1):117–19.

3. Vazquez-Levin MH, Dressler KP, Nagler HM. Urine contamination of seminal fluid after transurethral resection of the ejaculatory ducts. *J Urol.* 1994;152(6 Pt 1): 2049–52.

4. World Health Organization (WHO). *WHO Laboratory Manual for the Examination and Processing of Human Semen.* 5th ed. Cambridge, UK: Cambridge University Press; 2010.

5. Engin G, Kadioğlu A, Orhan I, Akdöl S, Rozanes I. Transrectal US and endorectal MR imaging in partial and complete obstruction of the seminal duct system. A comparative study. *Acta Radiol.* 2000;41:288–95.

6. Meschede D, Dworniczak B, Behre HM, et al. CFTR gene mutations in men with bilateral ejaculatory-duct obstruction and anomalies of the seminal vesicles. *Am J Hum Genet.* 1997;61(5):1200–2.

7. Xu Chen, Hua Wang, Rong Mincho Pei Wu, et al. The performance of transrectal ultrasound in the diagnosis of seminal vesicle defects: a comparison with magnetic resonance imaging. *Asian J Androl.* 2014;16:907–11.

8. Engin G, Celtik M, Sanli O, Aytac O, Muradov Z, Kadioglu A. Comparison of transrectal ultrasonography and transrectal

ultrasonography-guided seminal vesicle aspiration in the diagnosis of the ejaculatory duct obstruction. *Fertil Steril.* 2009;92(3):964–70.

9. Eisenberg ML, Walsh TJ, Garcia MM, Shinohara K, Turek PJ. Ejaculatory duct manometry in normal men and in patients with ejaculatory duct obstruction. *J Urol.* 2008;180(1):255–60.

10. Purohit RS, Wu DS, Shinohara K, Turek PJ. A prospective comparison of 3 diagnostic methods to evaluate ejaculatory duct obstruction. *J Urol.* 2004;171(1):232–5.

11. Smith JF, Walsh TJ, Turek PJ. Ejaculatory duct obstruction. *Urol Clin North Am.* 2008;35(2):221–7.

12. Orhan I, Duksal I, Onur R, B, TA, Poyraz K, Firdolas F, Kadioglu A. Technetium Tc 99m sulphur colloid seminal vesicle scintigraphy: a novel approach for the diagnosis of the ejaculatory duct obstruction. *Urology.* 2008;71:672–6.

13. Goldstein M. Surgical management of male infertility. In: Wein AJ, Kavoussi LR, Partin AW, Peters CA (eds), *Campbell's Urology*, 11th ed. Amsterdam: Elsevier; 2016, Chapter 25.

14. Jarow JP. Seminal vesicle aspiration in the management of patients with ejaculatory duct obstruction. *J Urol.* 1994;152:899–901.

15. Goldstein M. Surgical management of male infertility. In: Wein AJ, Kavoussi LR, Novick AC, Partin AW, Peters CA (eds), *Campbell's Urology*, 10th ed. Amsterdam: Elsevier; 2011, Chapter 22.

16. Lee JY, Diaz RR, Choi Y, Kang SC. Hybrid method of transurethral resection of ejaculatory ducts using holmium:yttriumaluminium garnet laser on complete ejaculatory duct obstruction. *Med J.* 2013;54(4):1062–5.

17. Oh TH, Seo IY. Endoscopic treatment for persistent hematospermia: a novel technique using a holmium laser. *Scand J Surg.* 2016;105(3):174–7.

18. Goldwasser BZ, Weinerth JL, Carson CC 3rd. Ejaculatory duct obstruction: the case for aggressive diagnosis and treatment. *J Urol.* 1985;134(5):964–6.

19. Paick J, Kim SH, Kim SW. Ejaculatory duct obstruction in infertile men. *BJU Int.* 2000 Apr;85(6):720–4.

20. Ozgök Y, Tan MO, Kilciler M, Tahmaz L, Kibar Y. Diagnosis and treatment of ejaculatory duct obstruction in male infertility. *Eur Urol.* 2001;39(1):24–9.

21. Fuse H, Mizuno I, Iwasaki M, Akashi T. Transurethral treatment of ejaculatory duct obstruction in infertile men. *Arch Androl.* 2003;49(6):429–31.

22. Yurdakul T, Gokce G, Kilic O, Piskin MM. Transurethral resection of ejaculatory ducts in the treatment of complete ejaculatory duct obstruction. *Int Urol Nephrol.* 2008;40(2):369–72.

23. Farley S, Barnes R. Stenosis of ejaculatory ducts treated by endoscopic resection. *J Urol.* 1973;109(4):664–6.

24. Turek PJ, Magana JO, Lipshultz LI. Semen parameters before and after transurethral surgery for ejaculatory duct obstruction. *J Urol.* 1996;155(4):1291–3.

Fertility Considerations in Scrotal Surgery

Katherine Rotker and Mark Sigman

16.1 Introduction

Scrotal surgeries comprise a small but significant part of a general urologic practice and can include hydrocele repair, spermatocele excision, orchidopexy, orchiectomy, sperm retrieval (epididymal or testicular), and vasectomy. The indications for scrotal surgery can include malignancy, fertility preservation, pain, and a desire for contraception. With the exceptions of vasectomy, which intentionally results in infertility, and sperm retrieval, which is specifically performed for fertility preservation or infertility treatment, the remaining procedures may inadvertently affect fertility. This chapter will review fertility concerns that arise from common scrotal surgical procedures.

16.2 Hydrocelectomy

A hydrocele is an accumulation of fluid between the parietal and visceral tunica vaginalis of the testis. Hydroceles can be congenital or acquired. Congenital hydroceles are generally found in children and are secondary to a patent processus vaginalis, allowing peritoneal fluid to collect within the scrotum. Acquired hydroceles are most commonly idiopathic but can be secondary to trauma, infection, or malignancy [1]. Underlying malignancy can be evaluated with scrotal ultrasound in those cases in which it is suspected. As hydroceles are generally painless and asymptomatic, most do not require intervention but they can grow in size and lead to discomfort or cosmetic concerns. Hydroceles can be treated with surgical excision or aspiration and sclerotherapy. A 2014 Cochrane review found that postoperative complications such as infection and fever were less when aspiration and sclerotherapy was performed. However, the recurrence rate was approximately 50% by 3–6 months with aspiration/sclerotherapy and less than 5% with surgery. Because of the recurrence rates, surgical excision is considered the standard of care with aspiration/sclerotherapy usually reserved for poor surgical candidates [2,3].

Congenital hydroceles often have a patent process vaginalis in the spermatic cord while adult hydroceles generally do not. Because of this difference, when correcting a congenital hydrocele, an inguinal approach is generally taken where the cord is separated from the patent processus vaginalis or hydrocele sac, which is subsequently transected. When performing an adult hydrocele excision, a scrotal approach is generally taken. Once the hydrocele sac is delivered via a scrotal incision, multiple methods for repair can be applied including sac excision and oversewing of the edges, a bottleneck technique (Jaboulay) where edges of the sac are inverted and sewn on the posterior aspect of the cord, or a plication technique (Lord) where the edges of the sac are sewn with radially placed stitches.

In all the methods, the complications associated with hydrocele excision include hematoma formation, infection, persistent swelling, recurrence of hydrocele, injury to the spermatic vessels, and chronic pain. Additionally, a theoretical risk of injury to the epididymis or vas deferens exists with hydrocele excision, which can occur during dissection or resection of the hydrocele sac, suturing of the hydrocele sac, or from electrocautery injury. Anatomically, the epididymis and vas deferens commonly are splayed out over the distended hydrocele sac, especially at the tail of the epididymis. Unless specifically identified, both structures may not be noticed during excision and portions may be inadvertently excised, resulting in obstruction on that side. A 2004 study looked at 378 patients who underwent hydrocelectomy and found that 5.62% had epididymal tissue or a portion of vas deferens in the pathology specimen. The authors also noted that this complication rate likely underestimated the true risk as it didn't include injuries to the epididymis from electrocautery or ill-placed sutures [4]. Patients with normal testes and ductal systems bilaterally may not demonstrate infertility following injury; however, those patients with preexisting contralateral defects on one side may be rendered azoospermic during hydrocele repair. In addition, unilateral obstruction may result in the development of antisperm antibodies, which may affect fertility.

Aspiration and sclerotherapy is an alternative treatment option for hydrocele that may be appropriate for patients who cannot tolerate anesthesia or refuse surgical treatment. This technique involves aspirating the hydrocele fluid and instilling a sclerosing agent such as tetracycline, alcohol, or phenol. Sclerotherapy avoids a general anesthetic, involving only a needle puncture into the scrotum and therefore rates of hematoma formation and fever are lower than with surgical excision [2]. However, sclerotherapy complications can include recurrence, scrotal pain, and even chemical epididymoorchitis [5]. To our knowledge, no large, randomized studies have looked at the effect of sclerotherapy on fertility, while studies with short follow-up have suggested that sperm counts may decrease following treatment [6]. An uncontrolled study of 69 men looked at postsclerotherapy semen analysis and found reductions in sperm concentration, motility, and morphology but that patients returned to normal parameters by 12 months post-procedure

[7]. A randomized trial comparing hydrocelectomy to phenol sclerotherapy reported slight decreased in sperm concentration at 6 and 12 months in both treatment groups but there were no statistical differences between the groups [8]. It should be noted that, in these studies, patients with unilateral and bilateral procedures were included but the effect of bilateral procedures was not controlled for.

Risk to fertility can occur with elective hydrocele surgery and possibly with aspiration and sclerotherapy. Careful counseling prior to elective surgery regarding this risk should be undertaken with any patient still desiring children, bilateral procedures should be avoided in this population and careful counseling should occur with those patients who elect to proceed regarding the risk to fertility. Finally, when proceeding with surgery, surgeons should be meticulous in identifying the scrotal structures prior to excision of the tunica vaginalis.

16.3 Spermatocele Excision

A spermatocele is a cystic dilation of an epididymal tubule. Spermatoceles are benign and common, occurring incidentally in up to 30% of men on high-resolution ultrasound [9]. They are usually asymptomatic and rarely require intervention but can grow in size and occasionally lead to discomfort requiring surgical correction. While aspiration with sclerotherapy has been reported, it is not standard of care and there is no data on the effect of isolated spermatocele sclerosis on semen parameters [10–12]. Spermatocele excision remains the current standard for symptomatic spermatoceles. The procedure involves a scrotal incision, entrance into the tunica vaginalis, delivery of the testicle, and identification of the spermatocele. The spermatocele should be dissected away from surrounding structures with the wall intact until the neck of the spermatocele is identified. The neck may then be ligated and the spermatocele excised. This dissection is aided with the use of optical magnification with either loupes or the operating microscope.

Postoperative complications associated with spermatocele excision include hemorrhage, infection, recurrence, pain, obstruction, and infertility. The epididymis is a tubular structure. The caput consists of multiple separate efferent ductules that coalesce by the corpus (body) of the epididymis into a single epididymal tubule. Given this anatomy, puncture or entrance into the epididymis can result in complete epididymal obstruction. Since most spermatoceles arise in the caput prior to the joining of all efferent ductules, injury in the caput to the epididymis should not completely obstruct the entire epididymis, while injury distal to the caput may completely obstruct the epididymis. Therefore, during spermatocele excision, care must be taken to avoid excising a portion of the epididymis with the spermatocele sac or injuring the epididymis during dissection of the sac. A 2004 study of 96 men sought to determine the actual risk of epididymal injury during spermatocele surgery. The authors found that on careful pathologic review, epididymal tissue was present in the specimen in 17.12% of the patients undergoing spermatocele excision. The authors concluded that the risk of damage to the epididymis

during spermatocelectomy was at least 17% and likely greater given the possible additional number who sustained injury to the epididymis during dissection [4].

Given the risk to fertility, elective spermatocele excision should be deferred in any patient interested in future fertility and any patient electing to undergo epididymal surgery should be counseled that the surgery may impair his fertility.

16.4 Orchiectomy/Orchidopexy

Indications for orchiectomy include malignancy, trauma, torsion, and chronic testicular pain. Orchidopexy is most commonly performed in children for cryptorchidism and in adolescents or adults for testicular torsion. When performed for malignancy, orchiectomy should occur via an inguinal approach. Orchidopexy performed in children for cryptorchidism is also commonly performed via an inguinal approach. When performed for trauma, testicular torsion, or chronic testicular pain, a scrotal approach to orchiectomy or orchidopexy can be utilized.

After orchiectomy for malignancy, the remaining testicle has traditionally been considered sufficient to maintain normal fertility and hormonal functions. However, evidence has shown semen abnormalities in patients with testicular cancer even before orchiectomy [13,14]. At the time of diagnosis, >50% of patients have evidence of impaired spermatogenesis, with 10–35% experiencing some degree of infertility [15]. Additionally, loss of one testicle could have psychosocial implications. Finally, adjunct treatments for testicular malignancy also have effects on fertility. Cisplatin-based chemotherapy results in azoospermia immediately following treatment in most patients. This is reversible in at least 50% of patients receiving standard-dose chemotherapy up to four cycles [16]. Radiation therapy, used in seminoma treatment, can also negatively affect fertility with impairments in spermatogenesis [17]. High doses of radiation therapy (20 Gy) can result in permanent sterility from eradication of the germ cell epithelium [18]. Lastly, retroperitoneal lymph-node dissection (RPLND), required in some testicular cancer patients, can lead to disruption of the sympathetic nervous system and may lead to impaired ejaculatory function and fertility [19]. Counseling regarding fertility preservation should be provided and sperm banking should be offered to all patients undergoing orchiectomy for malignancy prior to chemotherapy or radiation therapy. In patients with unilateral tumors and normal contralateral testes, sperm cryopreservation may be deferred until after the orchiectomy but prior to additional therapy. In patients with an absent or nonfunctioning contralateral testis, sperm cryopreservation from an ejaculated semen sample should be attempted prior to orchiectomy. Testicular sperm extraction from the normal tissue surrounding the tumor with sperm cryopreservation may be considered at the time of radical orchiectomy in those who have nonobstructive azoospermia and absent contralateral testes.

Although radical orchiectomy is considered the standard of care for testicular malignancy, partial orchiectomy can be considered for select patients including those with a small testicular mass in the setting of a solitary testicle or bilateral concurrent malignancies [20]. In fact, the current European Association of Urology guidelines support the practice of partial orchiectomy in patients with bilateral germ cell tumors [21]. Of note, the incidence of bilateral testis cancer, occurring synchronously or metachronously, is only 1–5% of testis cancer patients highlighting the fact that this applies to a small population [22]. Although no randomized controlled trials have compared partial orchiectomy with radical orchiectomy, studies have shown partial orchiectomy to be safe and feasible in patients with tumor size less than 2 cm [23,24]. Partial orchiectomy requires meticulous dissection to maintain testicular blood supply, and intraoperative biopsy of adjacent testicular parenchyma to ensure negative margins and evaluate for the presence of intratubular germ cell neoplasia (ITGCN). Local recurrence is approximately 30% following surgery alone [25]. Therefore radiation to the testis is often recommended following surgery, particularly if ITGCN is identified, which will further reduce fertility [20]. For this reason, if fertility preservation is desired after partial orchiectomy, warm ischemia time should be minimized and adjuvant radiation should be postponed until after reproduction with close follow-up [26]. Given the surgical risk to the testicle and the need for subsequent radiation, or increased risk of recurrence without it, sperm banking should be encouraged in all patients prior to partial orchiectomy.

The effect of orchiectomy or orchidopexy on fertility when performed for trauma or torsion is not fully understood. Much research exists regarding orchidopexy for cryptorchidism in the pediatric population. While current guidelines recommend earlier orchidopexy in the hope that it leads to improved fertility potential, more data is needed to validate this approach [27–29]. Of note, the cryptorchid testis is possibly abnormal at baseline and fertility in this population may not be applicable to a postpubertal testis requiring orchiopexy or one removed secondary to trauma or torsion. A study of 24 patients evaluated after testicular torsion found that both those patients who underwent orchidopexy and those who required orchiectomy had no differences in mean sperm count and average sperm motility when compared to age-matched controls. Interestingly, those who underwent orchiectomy had significantly better sperm motility than those who underwent orchidopexy. No differences in endocrine profiles were noted [30]. When placing sutures into the tunica albuginea, it is prudent to avoid subtunical vessels if possible since they are end vessels. However, there have been no studies examining whether this approach actually improves subsequent semen parameters or fertility.

The use of orchiectomy for chronic testicular pain is poorly studied and should be reserved for patients who have failed all conservative therapies and have been carefully counseled on the risks and benefits including the risk of failure and risk to fertility potential [31].

Any patient undergoing orchiectomy or orchidopexy should have a discussion regarding future fertility. In those patients with a normal contralateral testis, undergoing orchiectomy or orchidopexy for testicular torsion, trauma, or chronic pain, the risk to fertility is likely low. However, in those patients undergoing orchiectomy for malignancy, consideration should be given to fertility preservation prior to treatment and all patients should be offered sperm banking prior to chemotherapy or radiation.

16.5 Conclusion

When considering scrotal surgery it is incumbent upon the surgeon to consider the patient's fertility potential and goals. As a general rule, surgeons should consider delaying elective scrotal procedures, especially spermatocele excisions, until after the patient no longer desires fertility. When performing scrotal surgery, care should be taken to preserve the integrity of the epididymis and to avoid damage to either the testicle or cord structures. Careful counseling of men prior to scrotal surgery should include discussion of any risks to fertility potential.

References

1. Rubenstein RA, Dogra VS, Seftel AD, Resnick MI. Benign intrascrotal lesions. *J Urol.* 2004;171(5):1765–72.

2. Shakiba B, Heidari K, Jamali A, Afshar K. Aspiration and sclerotherapy versus hydrocoelectomy for treating hydrocoeles. *Cochrane Database Syst Rev.* 2014;11:CD009735.

3. Epstein A, a.N.D.E. Management of hydroceles. *AUA Update Series VII.* 1988;Lesson 19:145–9.

4. Zahalsky MP, Berman AJ, Nagler HM. Evaluating the risk of epididymal injury during hydrocelectomy and spermatocelectomy. *J Urol.* 2004;171(6 Pt 1):2291–2.

5. Lopez Laur JD, Parisi J. Sclerotherapy of hydroceles and spermatoceles with oxytetracyclines. *Actas Urol Esp.* 1989;13(6):439–40.

6. Osegbe DN. Fertility after sclerotherapy for hydrocele. *Lancet.* 1991;337(8734):172.

7. Shan CJ, et al. Sclerotherapy of hydroceles and spermatoceles with alcohol: results and effects on the semen analysis. *Int Braz J Urol.* 2011;37(3):307–12; discussion 312–33.

8. Shan CJ, Lucon AM, Arap S. Comparative study of sclerotherapy with phenol and surgical treatment for hydrocele. *J Urol.* 2003;169(3):1056–9.

9. Kavoussi PKa.C., R. A., Surgery of the scrotum and seminal vesicles. In: AJ Wein, Kavoussi LR, Novick AC, Partin AW, Peters CA (Eds), *Campbell-Walsh Urology*, 2012, Philadelphia, PA: Saunders.

10. Bullock N, Thurston AV. Tetracycline sclerotherapy for hydroceles and epididymal cysts. *Br J Urol.* 1987;59(4):340–2.

11. Daehlin L, Tonder B, Kapstad L. Comparison of polidocanol and tetracycline in the sclerotherapy of testicular hydrocele and epididymal cyst. *Br J Urol.* 1997;80(3):468–71.

12. Beiko DT, Morales A. Percutaneous aspiration and sclerotherapy for treatment of spermatoceles. *J Urol.* 2001;166(1):137–9.

13. Dieckmann KP, et al. Spermatogenesis in the contralateral testis of patients with testicular germ cell cancer: histological evaluation of testicular biopsies and a comparison with healthy males. *BJU Int.* 2007;99(5):1079–85.

14. Djaladat H, et al. The association between testis cancer and semen abnormalities before orchiectomy: a systematic review. *J Adolesc Young Adult Oncol*. 2014;3(4):153–9.

15. Spermon JR, et al. Fertility in men with testicular germ cell tumors. *Fertil Steril*. 2003;79 Suppl 3:1543–9.

16. Gospodarowicz M. Testicular cancer patients: considerations in long-term follow-up. *Hematol Oncol Clin North Am*. 2008;22(2):245–55, vi.

17. Pliarchopoulou K, Pectasides D. Late complications of chemotherapy in testicular cancer. *Cancer Treat Rev*. 2010; 36(3):262–7.

18. Bang AK, et al. Testosterone production is better preserved after 16 than 20 Gray irradiation treatment against testicular carcinoma in situ cells. *Int J Radiat Oncol Biol Phys*. 2009;75(3):672–6.

19. Donohue JP, Rowland RG. Complications of retroperitoneal lymph node dissection. *J Urol*. 1981;125(3):338–40.

20. Bazzi WM, et al. Partial orchiectomy and testis intratubular germ cell neoplasia: world literature review. *Urol Ann*. 2011;3(3):115–18.

21. Albers P, et al. EAU guidelines on testicular cancer: 2011 update. European Association of Urology. *Actas Urol Esp*. 2012;36(3):127–45.

22. Che M, et al. Bilateral testicular germ cell tumors: twenty-year experience at M. D. Anderson Cancer Center. *Cancer*. 2002;95(6):1228–33.

23. Borghesi M, et al. Role of testis sparing surgery in the conservative management of small testicular masses: oncological and functional perspectives. *Actas Urol Esp*. 2015;39(1):57–62.

24. Lawrentschuk N, et al. Partial orchiectomy for presumed malignancy in patients with a solitary testis due to a prior germ cell tumor: a large North American experience. *J Urol*. 2011;185(2):508–13.

25. Bojanic N, et al. Testis sparing surgery in the treatment of bilateral testicular germ cell tumors and solitary testicle tumors: A single institution experience. *J Surg Oncol*. 2015;111(2):226–30.

26. Heidenreich A, et al. Organ sparing surgery for malignant germ cell tumor of the testis. *J Urol*. 2001;166(6):2161–5.

27. Kollin C, et al, Surgical treatment of unilaterally undescended testes: testicular growth after randomization to orchiopexy at age 9 months or 3 years. *J Urol*. 2007;178(4 Pt 2):1589–93; discussion 1593.

28. Park KH, et al.Histological evidences suggest recommending orchiopexy within the first year of life for children with unilateral inguinal cryptorchid testis. *Int J Urol*. 2007;14(7):616–21.

29. Kolon TF, et al. Evaluation and treatment of cryptorchidism: AUA guideline. *J Urol*. 2014;192(2):337–45.

30. Arap MA, et al. Late hormonal levels, semen parameters, and presence of antisperm antibodies in patients treated for testicular torsion. *J Androl*. 2007;28(4):528–32.

31. Davis BE, et al. Analysis and management of chronic testicular pain. *J Urol*. 1990;143(5):936–9.

Index